This book is dedicated to Paul R. McHugh
and Marshal F. Folstein, who continue to teach
us about the interface of psychiatry and neurology,
and to our patients, who continue to teach
us about their illnesses and how to care for them.

Foreword

I am delighted to see the advent of this book. As a clinical practicum of real-world psychiatric problems seen by neurologists, internists, and primary practitioners, it fills a need. As a neurologist I would contend that as a group, neurologists are palpably uncomfortable and relatively ineffective in dealing with the psychiatric aspects of their patients. This contention does not of course apply to all of us, and some may not recognize their deficiencies. But the most insightful and honest among us are likely, on reflection, to acknowledge this statement. The fact that neurologists—trained students of the brain—are often insecure in dealing with prevalent behavioral disorders and practical psychiatric treatments reflects a great irony of medical science as it was in the twentieth century.

Those of us practicing now bear the legacy of our training. Neurology training for a portion of the last few decades could be completed with no psychiatry exposure at all. At best, neurology and psychiatry departments were academically separate, and most ingrained in their trainees quite different intellectual "reflexes" and approaches. Throughout the latter half of the twentieth century, training of neurologists centered on the clinical syndromes and physical signs that reflected specific lesions or diseases, and the specialists understandably came to consider behavior in a syndromic fashion. This same training often led to underemphasis on the importance of obtaining a detailed personal history, of understanding the individual's life situation, and of exploring the family dynamics. As a group, neurologists emerged from their training as relatively primitive psychopharmacologists. This may be on the whole a good thing; we tend to know a few agents well and are less likely to get into difficulty with less frequently used medications, but our patients could often benefit from wider expertise.

The irony of this separation is compounded by the fact that a high proportion of neurologists' patients have important and often treatable "psychiatric" disease. Recent data have underlined the prevalence of depression as a treatable aspect of right hemisphere stroke. Behavioral and mood symptoms are major sources of morbidity in Alzheimer's disease, and patients with Parkinson's disease benefit from "psychiatric" intervention. The "psychiatric" component of a neurologist's practice aspects can remain underrecognized and undertreated.

That neurology and psychiatry were—and still are— regarded as separate specialties reflects divergent evolution from common ancestors. In the mid-nineteenth century neurology and psychiatry began together, linked by a fascination with behavior in its broadest meaning and the belief that behavior derived from the brain. Charcot's clinic in Paris included neuroses, psychoses, and hysteria within its purview. The first great American neurologist, S. Weir Mitchell of Philadelphia, best known for his studies of peripheral nerve injuries caused by the Civil War, devoted much of his practice to treatment of neurasthenia and neuroses. He worked at the art of understanding patients' life stories, and he often solicited written descriptions of their domestic settings and their mental life from them. Still, this approach ran the risk of appearing as "soft" science. Mitchell himself flayed psychiatrists in an address to the American Medico-Psychological Association in 1894, asking: "Where are your careful scientific reports? ...You live ...out[side] of the healthy conflicts and honest rivalries that keep us [neurologists and other investigative physicians] up to the mark of the fullest possible competence." (This came from a man whose own "rest cure" for neurasthenia was based on ideas of gender differences, exercise, and nutrition that were both unfounded and untested.)

Arguably neuropathologic discoveries in diseases such as tabes, amyotrophic lateral sclerosis, and Alzheimer's disease, made by identifying disease-specific or disease-related structural changes, were partly responsible for driving a wedge between disorders with and without an obvious structural basis. And the search for a "scientific" understanding of brain diseases was of course not limited to pathology. William James was fascinated with "phosphate" theories of brain and behavior, an ironically prescient interest given the current focus on nucleic acids in molecular genetics and phosphoproteins, kinases, and phosphatases in protein biology. But even some of Charcot's students, exemplified by Freud, became discouraged with the search for pathologic or biochemical explanations for complex behaviors and developed sophisticated interview techniques to look clues to the behaviors. By the turn of the twentieth century, psychiatry was developing different diagnostic approaches and treatment methods, and psychiatric asylums were largely divorced from hospitals and medical centers.

Yet some investigators always maintained a view of the integrity of the disciplines. Adolph Meyer at Johns Hopkins University practiced a unitary approach that encompassed behavioral assessment, physical findings, and neuropathology. In an institution in which the Department of Psychiatry was highly influential, he argued forcefully for developing neurology to the same level as his department. (Despite several attempts, his vision for a department of neurology was only fulfilled after 50 years.)

Happily, the forces for divergence in the last century now conspire for a new convergent evolution of neurology and psychiatry, driven by the brain sciences. Anatomic and functional imaging, protein and gene arrays and other biomarkers, and genetics all represent shared approaches, and they are producing a single common science. That the separation of departments will decrease and that shared training components will increase can confidently be foreseen. This predicted coming-together need not entail the loss of the distinctive family histories and the rich cultural inheritances of neurology and psychiatry. Rather, these trappings will within a few decades represent "nostalgia without memory." Like third- or fourth-generation Swedish emigrants in the New World, whose celebrations of holidays are "more Swedish than the Swedes," tomorrow's brain scientists and practitioners will see the divisions of the past as quaint and perhaps endearing, but irrelevant to their work. But that is the future. At the moment, neurologists especially need and will appreciate this book.

John W. Griffin, MD
Professor of Neurology, Neuroscience, and Pathology
Former Chair of Neurology
Johns Hopkins University School of Medicine

Preface

Many neurologic diseases of the brain are associated with abnormal moods, thoughts, or behaviors. In some cases these abnormalities are—like paralysis or blindness—a direct expression of neuropathologic changes. Thus, for example, mania can be seen in Huntington's disease and major depression following left frontal strokes. In other cases, affective, cognitive, or behavioral abnormalities can be caused by treatments given for neurologic diseases. In this way, delirium can be precipitated by corticosteroids and pathologic gambling by dopaminergic agents. And in still other cases, abnormal moods, thoughts, and behaviors can arise as understandable reactions to disability, pain, and other distressing phenomena produced by the neurologic disease. Examples of such reactions can be found in the demoralization of someone with intractable epilepsy and the frustration of someone with a nonfluent aphasia.

Many neurologists would like to treat the psychiatric manifestations of neurologic diseases. In this book, our aim is to make such treatment easier by helping the reader recognize and distinguish among various psychiatric syndromes; by describing which psychiatric syndromes might be expected to occur in common or representative neurologic diseases; and by discussing the characteristics of, and indications for, psychiatric treatments.

We have not covered every psychiatric disorder and every neurologic disease, but we have focused on everyday clinical problems that might be seen primarily in adult patients and in children with Tourette's syndrome.

The chapter authors have emphasized practical approaches to these problems, and their suggestions are derived both from evidence-based medicine and considerable clinical experience. All of us have enjoyed working with, and learning from, neurologists and neuropsychologists, and we hope that this book furthers such collaborations.

We would like to thank the following members of the Johns Hopkins Department of Neurology for their help in defining the scope and structure of this book: Marilyn Albert, Eric Aldrich, Argye Hillis-Trupe, Douglas Kerr, and Richard O'Brien. We owe many thanks to Lynn Hutt for her meticulous editing of the manuscript. Finally, we would also like to thank William Lamsback of Oxford University Press for his benevolent understanding of what it takes to herd cats.

C.G.L.
P.V.R.
J.R.L.
P.R.S.

Contents

Part III. Psychiatric Treatments

Contributors

DAVID M. BLASS, MD
Adjunct Assistant Professor and
Founding Director, Fronto-
temporal Dementia Clinic,
Division of Geriatric Psychiatry
and Neuropsychiatry, Depart-
ment of Psychiatry and
Behavioral Sciences, Johns
Hopkins University School
of Medicine

KATHERINE A. L. CARROLL, MA
Sixth-Year Medical Student,
Imperial College School
of Medicine

MICHAEL R. CLARK, MD, MPH
Associate Professor and Director,
Chronic Pain Treatment Program,
Department of Psychiatry and
Behavioral Sciences, Johns
Hopkins University School of
Medicine

DEIRDRE JOHNSTON, MB, BCH
Assistant Professor and Clinical
Director, Division of Geriatric
Psychiatry and Neuropsychiatry,
Department of Psychiatry and
Behavioral Sciences, Johns
Hopkins University School of
Medicine

ADAM I. KAPLIN, MD, PHD
Assistant Professor, Division
of Geriatric Psychiatry and
Neuropsychiatry, Department
of Psychiatry and Behavioral
Sciences, Johns Hopkins
University School of Medicine;
Consultant, Multiple Sclerosis
and Transverse Myelitis Centers,
Department of Neurology, Johns
Hopkins University School of
Medicine

HOCHANG BENJAMIN LEE, MD
Assistant Professor, Division of
Geriatric Psychiatry and
Neuropsychiatry, Department of
Psychiatry and Behavioral Sci-
ences, Johns Hopkins University
School of Medicine; Attending
Psychiatrist, Neuropsychiatry and
Memory Unit, The Johns Hopkins
Hospital

SUSAN W. LEHMANN, MD
Assistant Professor, Division of
Geriatric Psychiatry and Neu-
ropsychiatry, Department of Psy-
chiatry and Behavioral Sciences,
Johns Hopkins University School
of Medicine; Director, Geriatric
Psychiatry Day Hospital, The
Johns Hopkins Hospital

JOHN R. LIPSEY, MD
Associate Professor, Department
of Psychiatry and Behavioral Sci-
ences, Johns Hopkins University
School of Medicine; Attending
Psychiatrist, Geriatric Psychiatry
Inpatient Service, The Johns
Hopkins Hospital

CONSTANTINE G. LYKETSOS, MD, MHS
The Elizabeth Plan Althouse
Professor, Division of Geriatric
Psychiatry and Neuropsychiatry,
Department of Psychiatry and
Behavioral Sciences, Johns
Hopkins University School of
Medicine; Chair of Psychiatry,
Johns Hopkins Bayview Medical
Center; founder and former
Director, Neuropsychiatry
Service, The Johns Hopkins
Hospital

RUSSELL L. MARGOLIS, MD
Professor and Director, Laboratory of Genetic Neurobiology,
Department of Psychiatry and
Behavioral Sciences, Johns Hopkins University School of Medicine; Professor, Department
of Neurology, Johns Hopkins
University School of Medicine

LAURA MARSH, MD
Associate Professor, Department
of Psychiatry and Behavioral Sci-
ences, Johns Hopkins University
School of Medicine; Associate
Professor, Department of Neurol-
ogy, Johns Hopkins University
School of Medicine; Director,
Clinical Research Program, Johns
Hopkins/Morris K. Udall Parkin-
son's Disease Research Center

CHIADI U. ONYIKE, MBBS, MHS
Assistant Professor and Director,
Frontotemporal Dementia Clinic,
Division of Geriatric Psychiatry
and Neuropsychiatry, Department of Psychiatry and Behavioral Sciences, Johns Hopkins
University School of Medicine

PETER V. RABINS, MD, MPH
Professor and Director, Division
of Geriatric Psychiatry and
Neuropsychiatry, Department of
Psychiatry and Behavioral Sciences, Johns Hopkins University
School of Medicine

VANI RAO, MD
Assistant Professor, Division of
Geriatric Psychiatry and Neuropsychiatry, Department of Psychiatry and Behavioral Sciences,
Johns Hopkins University School
of Medicine; Director, Brain Injury Clinic, Johns Hopkins Bayview Medical Center

ADAM ROSENBLATT, MD
Associate Professor and Director,
Baltimore Huntington's Disease
Center; Director for Neuropsychiatry, Division of Geriatric
Psychiatry and Neuropsychiatry,
Department of Psychiatry and
Behavioral Sciences, Johns
Hopkins University School of
Medicine

BENJAMIN N. SCHNEIDER, BS
Third-Year Medical Student,
Johns Hopkins University School
of Medicine

PHILLIP R. SLAVNEY, MD
Eugene Meyer III Professor of
Psychiatry and Medicine, Johns
Hopkins University School of
Medicine; Director, General
Hospital Psychiatry Service,
Department of Psychiatry and
Behavioral Sciences, Johns
Hopkins University School of
Medicine

MARTIN STEINBERG, MD
Assistant Professor, Division of
Geriatric Psychiatry and Neuropsychiatry, Department of Psychiatry and Behavioral Sciences,
Johns Hopkins University School
of Medicine; Attending Psychiatrist, Neuropsychiatry and
Memory Unit, The Johns Hopkins
Hospital

JOHN T. WALKUP, MD
Associate Professor and Director,
Tic, Obsessive-Compulsive,
and Anxiety Disorders Clinic,
Division of Child and Adolescent
Psychiatry, Department of Psychiatry and Behavioral Sciences,
Johns Hopkins University School
of Medicine

PART I

PSYCHIATRIC
ASSESSMENTS
AND SYNDROMES

1

The Psychiatric Examination
of the Neurologic Patient

CONSTANTINE G. LYKETSOS

A well-conducted psychiatric evaluation is central to the care of neurologic patients with psychiatric disorders. The evaluation is aimed at defining the psychiatric condition in the context of the patient's past psychiatric history and current neurologic disease. The information derived from the evaluation is used to develop a formulation, establish a diagnosis, and form a basis for treatment planning. This chapter discusses the psychiatric evaluation of the neurologic patient in detail. It includes examination techniques and questions as well as practical approaches to conducting an assessment of the patient's cognitive state. Along the way, common psychiatric symptoms encountered in neurologic patients are defined and differentiated from related symptoms. The chapter concludes by illustrating how to generate a formulation and differential diagnosis.

Taking a History

The psychiatric evaluation consists of three parts: the history; the mental status examination (MSE); and the formulation, including the differential diagnosis. The history, which is essential to defining the problem, is taken from the patient and from one or more informants. The importance of taking a history from an informant is underscored in the context of neurologic disease because patients may be forgetful, lack insight, or have language and other cognitive problems that may limit their ability to provide a good history.

History-taking begins with defining the psychiatric chief complaint and then obtaining the family and personal history. Starting in this way, rather than with the chief complaint followed by the history of present illness (HPI), makes it easier to see that the psychiatric symptoms may have been caused by, or influenced by, factors other than the neurologic disease—factors that can include psychiatric disorders as such, aspects of patients'

4

personalities, and responses patients have to the circumstances of their lives.

Table 1–1 provides an outline of important elements of the psychiatric history for neurologic patients and can be used as a checklist in clinical practice. Defining the *psychiatric chief complaint* is the physician's first task. "Psychiatric chief complaint" in this context refers to the occurrence of cognitive, affective, behavioral, or perceptual phenomena that are brought to the physician's attention by the patient, a family member or other informant, or by the physician's own observation. Most of the time the chief complaint comes from the patient in the form of a distressing mental symptom, such as feeling depressed, hearing

Table 1.1. Outline of a Psychiatric History in Patients with Neurologic Diseases

1. Identifying Data: age, marital status, race, sex, referral source
2. Chief Complaint: nature and duration
3. Family History: health status of parents, grandparents, siblings, and children; if deceased, age at death and cause; any members with psychiatric or neurologic illness
4. Personal and Social History: birth, education, work history, marital status, leisure practices, religious affiliation
5. Current Situation: living environment at present, care providers, financial state, legal problems, use of community resources, recent daily activities
6. Substance Use: lifetime and recent use of cigarettes, alcohol, and illicit drugs; history of abuse or dependency on any of the above, including prescription and over-the-counter medications
7. Medical History: past and current problems and their severity, review of systems, current medications (including over-the-counter), physicians and other health care providers
8. Personality Prior to the Neurologic Disease: traits, mood, activity, and review of prior response to stress or illness
9. Psychiatric History Prior to the Neurologic Disease: psychiatric symptoms or disorders, psychiatric assessments or treatments
10. History of Present Illness: beginning with first psychiatric symptoms after the onset of the neurologic disease; onset date, course, features, response to treatments given thus far

voices, or forgetting things. In many instances, however, the neurologist or other physician first notices the presence of a psychiatric symptom during a visit related to the neurologic disease. Once the presence of a complaint is established, the physician must define it in detail. Certain patients cannot describe the phenomenon in question, and in these cases the information has to be obtained from the informant. This may be because the patient is forgetful, lacks insight, or cannot communicate. For example, a patient with Alzheimer's disease might be oblivious to his memory loss and report that everything is well. Or a patient who has suffered a stroke might have aphasia and report feeling bad, but not use the word "sad" or "depressed" to describe her emotional state. Once the elements of the chief complaint have been defined, the physician should establish their time course in terms of their onset and duration.

After the chief complaint has been described, the physician takes a *psychiatric family history.* One way to make the transition to this part of the evaluation is to say: "Now that I see what the problem is, I'd like to get some background information that will help me understand it better." At minimum, history about grandparents, parents, siblings, and children is obtained. This is best recorded as a pedigree on a genogram, which reminds the physician to ask questions about each relative, thus increasing accuracy. This family history later assists in formulating a differential diagnosis, in assessing the current state of the family, and in identifying human resources available for the patient's care.

The family history is followed by the patient's *personal history.* Specifically, information should be obtained about any childhood cognitive and behavioral difficulties, educational achievement, work history, marital history, quality of relationships among family members, and religious background. In addition to allowing an estimation of premorbid functioning, the personal history illustrates the patient's life in a way that allows a clearer understanding of this individual and his or her response to illness. It also identifies interests and wishes that in turn will guide treatment planning.

Following the personal history, the examiner should inquire about the patient's *current psychosocial environment*. The focus here is on defining his or her living situation, ongoing family and social resources, and typical daily activities. As appropriate, this aspect of the history should inquire about caregivers involved in the patient's day-to-day life, including their availability, emotional state, health, and expertise in caring for the patient.

A *substance use* history follows. This is important because the use or abuse of certain medications or illicit drugs can produce a variety of psychiatric symptoms in addition to those of abuse or dependence themselves. Patients with neurologic diseases are especially vulnerable to the effects of alcohol, medications, or illicit substances, and certain patient populations, such as those with traumatic brain injury or chronic pain, not infrequently develop abuse or dependency on benzodiazepines or opioids. The history should estimate the use of caffeine, alcohol, tobacco/nicotine, analgesics, sedatives, hypnotics, and illicit drugs (eg, marijuana, heroin, cocaine). The specifics of use should be quantified for each substance used, including recent patterns of use, evidence of heavy use (ie, well above cultural norms for age and gender), abuse (ie, continued use despite harm or use beyond the amount prescribed), or dependence (ie, evidence of tolerance, withdrawal, or a preoccupation with obtaining and using the substance in question). Special care should be taken to explore potential abuse or dependence involving prescribed medications such as benzodiazepines, barbiturates, or opioids; if such medications are simply stopped in dependent patients, withdrawal phenomena will occur.

During the evaluation, a *medical history and review of systems* is essential. The status and treatment of all known active general medical conditions should be updated, with special attention to ones that might affect the patient's mental state. Careful attention should be given to determining current medications, including over-the-counter drugs, for anticholinergics medications (eg, antihistamines marketed as sleeping pills) can cause delirium. A review and update to the history of the primary neurologic disease is also included here.

History-taking regarding the patient's *premorbid personality* is often omitted, yet it is a critical aspect of the psychiatric evaluation. "Personality" is described in terms of traits—the enduring characteristics of individuals. The adjectives that might be used to describe personality traits include terms such as *intelligent, suspicious, cheerful, perfectionistic, gregarious, close-minded, and energetic.* The patient's personality before the apparent onset of the neurologic symptoms is important to clarifying the current psychiatric presentation. Premorbid personality shapes the patient's reaction to illness, especially chronic illness. Thus, for example, a neat or perfectionistic person might find urinary incontinence especially distressing, and a stoic person might not complain of pain.

The assessment of a patient's premorbid personality should start with questions such as: "How would you describe yourself before you became ill? What sort of a person were you? What was your personality like?" The patient's description should be augmented by someone who knew the patient before the onset of the neurologic disease. Follow-up questions are often needed about the patient's usual level of mood and mood stability (eg, "What was his usual mood?," "Did his mood change easily or quickly?"); activity; social engagements (eg, "Did she like spending time with people?, What was she like in social settings?"); habits (eg, "Did she have any set routines for things?"); reward focus (eg, "Did she respond more to encouragement or to threats?"); and future outlook (eg, "Did she tend to worry about the future or did she mostly live in the moment?").

The patient's past psychiatric history is assessed next. It is important to review all psychiatric symptoms before the onset of the neurologic disease, whether or not they were treated. Topics of inquiry should include common symptoms such as sadness and anxiety as well as signs and symptoms of dangerousness, such as a wish to die, suicidal thoughts, self-injurious behavior, suicide attempts, threats to others, and homicidal thoughts. Here, too, it should be established whether the patient has been evaluated or treated by a psychiatrist, psychologist, or social worker; whether the patient has been prescribed "psychiatric" medications by other physicians; and whether or not he or she has had psychotherapy.

The *history of present illness*, or HPI, is one of the most critical aspects of the psychiatric evaluation. The input of an informant other than the patient is crucial and should be obtained in every case, if possible, unless the patient refuses to give permission. In the context of neurologic disease, the HPI is best anchored on one of two time points: the onset of the neurologic symptoms, or the onset of the current psychiatric illness, whichever started earlier. In searching for an anchor, it is useful to ask the patient and the informant, using clues from the chief complaint, about when the patient was last well from the psychiatric point of view. As will be noted later in this book, psychiatric signs or symptoms, in particular affective changes or personality changes, are at times the first symptoms of a brain disease, occurring before the onset of neurologic symptoms. Such phenomena are often overlooked and can persist after treatment of the neurologic disorder. If psychiatric signs or symptoms clearly began after the onset of the neurologic disease, it should be established whether the psychiatric phenomena appeared following the initiation of a particular treatment (eg, forgetfulness after beginning diazepam, anxiety after corticosteroids).

Table 1.2. Psychiatric Review of Symptoms in Seven Domains

COGNITION

Forgetfulness
Language problems
Writing difficulties
Reading difficulties
Calculation difficulties
Problems recognizing people
Disorientation
Visuospatial problems
Attention and concentration
  problems
Difficulty planning and organizing

FUNCTIONING

Problems with the following:
  Working
  Cooking
  Finances
  Housekeeping
  Driving
  Shopping
  Dressing
  Bathing
  Grooming
  Mobility
  Eating
  Continence

AFFECTIVE

Depression
Crying spells
Diurnal variation in mood
Anxiety
Euphoria
Irritability
Anhedonia (loss of enjoyment)

Self-deprecating thoughts
Death wishes
Suicidal thoughts

PHYSICAL SYMPTOMS

Easy tiring
Unexplained physical complaints
Low energy level
Sleeps disturbance
Appetite disturbance
Self injury

**PERCEPTUAL/THOUGHT
CONTENT**

Suspiciousness
Delusions
Illusions
Hallucinations

PROBLEM BEHAVIORS

Disinhibition
Social inappropriateness
Explosiveness
Apathy
Loss of interest in usual activities
Social withdrawal
Verbal abusiveness
Uncooperativeness
Screaming or calling out
Physical aggression
Wandering
Hoarding
Rummaging
Intrusiveness
Self-injury

Once the temporal relationship between the psychiatric signs or symptoms and the neurologic disease has been established, the examiner should identify the earliest psychiatric phenomena and provide a chronological history of their evolution up to the present time. The examiner should begin with open-ended questions, helping the patient or informant describe the emergence and course of symptoms in his or her own words. Thus, for example, the examiner might ask, "Describe for me what it was like when these problems started?" or "Tell me how you were doing after you first started feeling depressed?" Subsequently, the examiner should follow-up with a *psychiatric review of symptoms* evaluating the occurrence of these symptoms as part of the HPI. Table 1–2 outlines such a review. In addition to helping with the differential diagnosis, a psychiatric review of symptoms aids in the identification of target problems requiring treatment. The examiner should be careful to define the recent time course of the psychiatric complaints, in particular of cognitive symptoms, so as to identify any acute changes or exacerbations that might be suggestive of delirium.

Examining the Patient

A thorough MSE is a central part of the psychiatric evaluation. The purpose of the MSE is to investigate the patient's mental state with an eye to describing his or her mental experiences and any abnormal mental phenomena. Conducting a MSE requires patience and skill so as to elicit without suggesting, while making sure the patient is comfortable with the assessment. Given a format and some practice, conducting a MSE is well within the abilities of any physician and can readily lead to an understanding of the phenomena of interest. Much of the awkwardness the physician might feel in asking MSE questions can be dispelled by approaching the examination in the same way as the physical examination is approached, with introduction to the activity. For example, the physician might say, "I would now like to ask you some questions about your thoughts, feelings, and emotions. These will help me understand better what the problem is and what it has been like for you. These questions are routine, and I ask them of anyone who presents with problems similar to yours."

Open-ended questions are preferred, but it is also necessary to use focused follow-up questions so as to better define any mental experiences uncovered. For example, the examiner might ask, "How are you feeling today?," "Could you tell me a bit about how you have been doing emotionally?," or "I don't mean you should have thought this, but have you been wishing you were dead?"

Some clinicians fear that the MSE is intrusive, whereas others are concerned that it is unreliable. Despite its reliance on the patient's subjective report, a careful MSE—one that is systematic, focused and informed by widely accepted definitions of mental experiences—is highly reliable and provides essential information for the differential diagnosis. This section provides a systematic outline for the MSE, a discussion of its elements, and definitions of common mental phenomena.

The seven major headings MSE are outlined in Table 1–3. For experienced examiners, it is not necessary to survey these areas in this sequence or to assess all aspects of individual areas at the same time. However, beginners may find reassurance by sticking to this outline and keeping it at hand, along with the definitions of mental phenomena outlined in the glossary. Some aspects of the MSE (eg, mood) can be assessed while taking the history, but general impressions must be validated by specific questions (eg, "How is your mood today?"). The following sections discuss the seven areas of the MSE in detail.

Table 1.3.   Parts of the Mental Status Examination

1. Appearance/Behavior	5. Content of Thought
2. Speech	• Delusions
• Volume	• Obsessions
• Rate	• Compulsions
• Rhythm	• Phobias
• Fluidity	6. Insight and Judgment
• Spontaneity	7. Cognition
• Latency	• Level of consciousness
• Thought disorder	• Orientation
3. Mood and Affect	• Memory
• Observed and reported, stability, reactivity, appropriateness	• Praxis
	• Language
• Vital sense	• Abstraction
• Self attitude	• Fund of knowledge
• Thoughts of death, suicide, homicide	• Attention
	• Calculation
4. Abnormal Perceptions	• Executive function
• Illusions	
• Hallucinations	

Appearance and Behavior

One thing to note at the start of the examination is whether the patient acts in a manner consonant with the context of the assessment. For example, does the patient recognize the examiner as a physician? In general, a patient's approach to the examination reflects how he or she reacts in situations that are unusual or stressful. The predominant demeanor of the patient during the assessment should be noted. How cooperative is the patient with the evaluation? Does the examiner have to work hard to put the patient at ease? Is the patient calm, tense, or distressed? What sort of body posture does the patient display? How much eye contact does the patient make? Is the patient restless or fidgety? Is there evidence of psychomotor agitation—

motor agitation driven by emotional agitation—such as pacing or rocking, or are there signs of retardation? Does the patient display frequent, easily induced changes in mood or behavior? How does he or she react to stressful questions? Observing the patient's behavior might detect hallucinations, for example, if the patient turns his or her head as if listening to sounds the examiner cannot hear, or if the patient talks to people the examiner cannot see.

Observing how the patient is dressed is also important. Are the patient's clothes neat or do they seem disheveled, mismatched, misbuttoned, or dirty? Are they appropriate for the weather? Patients who are described as always having been neat and appear dressed in messy or stained clothes may be apraxic, have dysmetria, or be so depressed that they have neglected their appearance.

Speech

Several aspects of the patient's speech should be assessed throughout the evaluation and also probed with secondary questions as needed. It is good to encourage and allow the patient to speak on his or her own for a while about a neutral topic (eg, "Tell me more about when you went on vacation last summer ..."). This permits an assessment of whether the talk is spontaneous (ie, is appropriately initiated by the patient) and focused on the topic at hand. Speech should be fluent and should demonstrate appropriate rate, rhythm, and prosody (smoothness). The pragmatics of talk (ie, appropriate use of facial expression, gestures, and other aspects of nonverbal communication in conversation) should be assessed.

Talk should be assessed for thought disorder, defined as a disturbance in the sequencing of thought as reflected in the patient's speech or writing. It is a disorder in the *form* of thought, not in the *content* of thought, as well of *how* the patient is thinking, not *what* the patient is thinking about. Thought disorder is not pathognomonic of schizophrenia, because it also occurs in delirium and dementia (conditions in which neurologists tend to see it) as well as in mania. The most common form of thought disorder is *loosening of associations* (also called *derailment*), where the sequence of the talk is not logical or linear and the patient's talk does not follow a coherent path. For example, a patient might start by talking about how he got to the hospital, then move on to talk about the death of her aunt a year ago, then ask the examiner why he is wearing a red tie. *Tangentiality* is evident when the patient repeatedly gives answers that are not directly in response to the examiner's questions. For example, if the examiner asks, "What time do you usually go to bed?" and the patient answers, "My mother always put me to bed when I was little," this is a tangential response. *Flight of ideas* refers to talk characterized by the very rapid succession of loosely related ideas, often with a "push" to get the ideas out not allowing interruptions; it is typically associated with mania.

Talk should also be assessed for language disorder. Language disorder differs from thought disorder in that the former is a disorder in the comprehension or use of language (ie, grammar, syntax, words), whereas the latter is a disorder of the flow of language in which individual segments of thought make correct use of language. Hesitant talk, in which word-finding difficulty is prominent, or speech that is telegraphic or without usual connecting words, suggests a nonfluent aphasia. Talking a great deal but saying little that makes sense may indicate a fluent aphasia. Substituting one word for another, saying words that are combinations of other words, or saying words that are not in the lexicon—phenomena called *paraphrasic errors*—also indicate a language disorder.

The patient should be able to comprehend questions and follow instructions. An inability to do so in response to a normal spoken voice might be due to a hearing deficit or may indicate receptive aphasia. Hearing problems should be suspected if the patient asks that questions and instructions be repeated or if he or she seems to understand simple and straightforward questions but to have difficulty with more complicated ones, even if the examiner maintains the same loudness of voice.

The ability to control the speed of speech can be impaired. Hesitancy or delay before answering questions and speaking very slowly can indicate depression. Rapid speech that dominates the conversation and prevents the examiner from interrupting (*"push of speech"*) suggests mania.

Mood and Affect

In this part of the MSE, the examiner first attempts to define the patient's current and recent mood states, followed by assessment of the patient's vital sense and self-attitude. The examiner must avoid the temptation to guess the patient's current mood state in the context of neurologic disease (eg, "If I had Parkinson's disease, I would be depressed, so why bother asking?"). In reality, most patients with neurologic disease are not sad or depressed and adapt quite well emotionally to their illness. This area of the MSE is critical to identifying those patients who have not adapted well or who have developed mood disorders. Many such patients are embarrassed by their abnormal moods and do not report them spontaneously.

It is best to note both how patient describes his or her mood (ie, subjective mood) and how the examiner perceives the patient's mood (ie, observed mood). The observed mood and the reported mood are usually congruent, and the patient's affect is usually appropriate for his or her mood. Questions such as "How are your spirits?" or "How is your mood today?" are appropriate. If the patient does not know what "mood" means, the examiner might ask, "Are you happy, sad, or in between?" or "Are you feeling depressed, blue, or like crying?" When there is evidence of anxiety, the examiner might ask, "Are you feeling anxious today?" or "Are you feeling worried or tense?" When euphoria is suspected, then the clinician might ask, "How good is your mood today?" or "Is this the best you have ever felt?" It is helpful to use quotations specifying the patient's exact words used in the responses they provide to the questions (eg, "The patient described his mood as 'good' and it appeared to be neutral").

The examiner should also follow up with questions that clarify whether the current mood state is reflective of the patient's usual mood state or whether a recent or sustained change has occurred. Also, the context of any changes in mood state is important. The examiner should define the relationship between any changes in mood state and life events (eg, anxiety over the threat of a job loss, distress or anger with the diagnosis of Parkinson's disease). Most affective disorders (eg, major depression, mania) involve sustained mood changes with little relationship to life events.

Another important aspect of the patient's mood state is his or her ability to feel enjoyment or pleasure. Questions such as, "How well have you been enjoying things lately?," "What sorts of things gave you pleasure in the past week?," and "What about things that you usually enjoy such as (cite examples from the personal history)?" are appropriate. If there is any evidence of a diminished capacity to enjoy things (*anhedonia*), it is important to clarify whether this represents a change and whether it has been sustained. In general, anhedonia is a worrisome symptom and is typically evidence of major depression.

Variations in mood during the course of the examination should be described if they occur. The examiner should note if patients cry or laugh easily or if they are emotionally labile in some other way (eg, displaying flashes of anger or irritability). Any sudden crying or laugher following a minor stimulus or no apparent stimulus—a phenomenon referred to as *emotional incontinence*—should be differentiated from more sustained mood changes that are appropriate to the content of the conversation. For example, patients with emotional incontinence often state that the laughing or crying is not accompanied by the moods that are typically associated with these behaviors (eg, sadness or happiness), or that the crying and laughing is beyond their control and that any associated emotions are transient. A lack of reactivity and evidence of monotony in mood should also be noted.

Irritability, anxiety, sadness, or anger when confronted with a cognitive task beyond the patient's capacity to perform—a phenomenon called a *catastrophic reaction*—may disrupt the examination. Such reactions can be seen in demented, delirious, or mentally retarded patients, as well as in those with focal cognitive deficits (eg, following a left hemisphere stroke or traumatic brain injury). These reactions should be distinguished from the reactions of paranoid patients who think the examiner is trying to embarrass them by asking certain questions that are beyond the their ability to answer.

Vital sense refers to the patient's assessment of his energy level or sense of well-being. This involves several elements, including the background or resting energy level, a sense of how the body feels, the level of interest in activities, the ability to initiate activities, and the ability to sustain activities. Patients should be asked how they feel at baseline when they are not doing much (eg, "Do you have much energy?," "How does your body feel?," "Do you feel sick or well?" "Do you have any aches or pains, abdominal fullness, headaches, or feelings of tiredness and listlessness?"). If the answers to such questions are affirmative, the examiner should assess whether the complaints are appropriate to the patient's medical condition or whether they might be physical or somatic manifestations of depression or anxiety. Other questions should clarify how interested the patient is in activities and how difficult it is to get started with activities (eg, "Is it hard to begin doing things?") or to sustain them (eg, "Do you get tired easily, more than you would expect based on what you are doing?," "Once you get started, can you keep going for a while like you used to?"). Patients who have a lack of interest in doing things but have normal mood and vital sense are apathetic as opposed to depressed.

Self-attitude refers to the patient's sense of his moral worth and capacities. Self-attitude can be elevated, with increased self-confidence and self-esteem, or lower than usual, with guilt, remorse, self-deprecation, self-blame, and feelings of incompetence and failure. Low self-attitude may be accompanied by sadness and hopelessness, whereas elevated self-attitude may coexist with an elated mood and overconfident optimism. Fluctuations in self-attitude, especially those not linked to environmental events, may be indicative of a mood disorder. Even when a cognitive disorder such as dementia is present, the identification of a change in self-attitude is a particularly important indicator of the presence of a concomitant mood disorder. To assess self-attitude, the examiner asks questions such as, "How do you feel about yourself today?," "What is your level of confidence?," "How about your self-esteem?," "Do you feel pretty good about yourself or do you feel self-critical?," "Are you having any guilty feelings?," "Do you think there is any hope for you in your condition?," "How does the future look?," or "Do you see ways in which things might get better for you?"

A critical aspect of assessment relates to investigating for thoughts of death, suicide, or homicide. Once again, these questions are routine in the MSE and can be asked without concern of "putting ideas in the patient's head." The most natural way to ask them is after inquiring about the patient's mood, "I am sorry to hear your spirits are low. Are they so low that you wished you were dead or thought of taking your life?" or "I am glad to hear your spirits are good. Sometimes, though, when people's moods are bad, they wish they were dead or think of suicide. I do not mean that you should have had such thoughts, but have you?" Other approaches might be, "Not that you should, but are there times when you think a lot about death or dying? Do you ever wish death upon yourself? If so, why? Do you think you might be better off dead?" or "Have you ever considered hurting yourself? How about taking your own life?" If patients are thinking of harming themselves, follow-up questions are important, "Do you have a plan or sense of how you would kill yourself?," "What do you think you would gain?," or "How likely are you to do this?"

Next the examiner turns to asking questions about plans to harm others, also properly prefaced as the questions about suicidal ideas. To assess for violent ideas toward others, the examiner can ask questions such as, "Are you angry with someone else?," "Are you thinking of hurting someone?," "What is the reason for this?," "What has prevented you from doing it thus far?," "How would you do it?," "Do you have a plan as to what you would do?" The examiner must remember that evidence of patients' dangerousness toward themselves or others creates a duty on the part of the examiner to take action to protect those at risk. Thus, the examiner must be prepared to explain this to the dangerous patient and also to propose an appropriate plan to handle the situation, such as involving a psychiatrist, immediate hospitalization, or warning others of the threat.

Abnormal Perceptions

In this section, the physician determines whether the patient has experienced hallucinations or illusions. Hallucinations are sensory perceptions without stimuli, whereas illusions are misperceptions or misinterpretations of stimuli. Hallucinations and illusions can occur in all sensory modalities (ie, hearing, sight, smell, taste, and proprioception), but auditory hallucinations and visual illusions are the most common. Examples of hallucinations include hearing voices talking about the patient, seeing small people come into the room, or feeling bugs crawling on the skin. Examples of illusions include seeing a face in the folds of the curtains or looking at an intravenous line and seeing a snake.

To prepare the ground for MSE questions in this area, the examiner might start by asking patients whether, while falling asleep or waking up, they have dreamlike experiences that might seem real. Such experiences are common, and can help introduce the topic in a matter-of-fact way. Phenomena that occur while falling asleep (the "hypnagogic" state) or waking up (the "hypnopompic" state) include hallucinations, which are usually visual or auditory. The examiner should then explore whether any such phenomena are in fact hallucinations and then go on to ask about the occurrence of such phenomena when the patient is fully awake. To this end, the examiner might ask, "Other than when you are falling asleep or waking up, have you had the experience of hearing sounds or voices, or seeing things that others do not hear or see?," "Are there any odors that you smell but you cannot explain or that others cannot smell?," or "Have tastes come to your mouth that you cannot explain, or sensations anywhere on your body that have been hard to explain or upsetting?" If the answer is "yes," follow-up questions are be needed to clarify the experience, such as "Did the voices sound real to you—like they were coming through your ears, or, did you hear them in your head?"

It is important to help patients distinguish between perceptions and thoughts. Sometimes patients describe their own thoughts as if they were perceptions (eg, "I hear the voice of my conscience" or "I can just see my mother standing there"). To distinguish hallucinations from illusions, the patient might be asked whether there were in fact stimuli provoking the perception (eg, "Do you think you really saw a face, or could it have been the shades of the curtains making it look like a face?"), and other informants should be questioned as to whether the patient was misperceiving a stimulus or having a perception without stimulus.

Content of Thought

In this part of the MSE, questions are asked about beliefs and other thoughts. It is here that the examiner inquires about delusions. Delusions are false, fixed (ie, unshakable), and idiosyncratic (ie, unique to that person) ideas that often lead patients to take some action. Thus, for example, patients who believe that others are trying to kill them (a *persecutory* or *paranoid delusion*) will hide, call the police, or attack the feared person. Patients who believe that they have unlimited wealth (*grandiose delusion*) may bankrupt themselves. Patients who believe that they have done terrible things (*delusion of guilt*) may commit suicide. The commonest type of delusion is persecutory and includes beliefs that others are trying to harm the patient, are spying on the patient, or are stealing from the patient.

It is important to distinguish between delusions and ideas based on culture and background. One helpful way is to ask the patient's relatives or friends whether they also believe what the patient believes. For example, the patient might have a religious belief with which the examiner is not familiar. If relatives have the same belief, then it is unlikely to be a delusion.

One way to begin a series of questions about delusions is to start with the patient's illness, "Sometimes when people are ill they think they deserve to suffer. I don't mean you should be thinking that, but I was wondering whether you have?" A transition can then be made to other types of delusions, "As well, sometimes when people are ill they might think that others are causing that illness or want to see them suffer. Have you had thoughts along these lines?" Often, it is useful to probe on how fixed any ideas might be, "Do you think this is really going on?

Can you think why? Is it possible your mind is playing tricks on you?"

Many times, the history provides clues about possible delusions (or hallucinations), and questions during the MSE can be tailored to the situation. For example, a patient with Alzheimer's disease believed that a former tenant was living in her house and stealing from her. Before the examiner had a chance to talk to another informant, the patient gave a persuasive story that the tenant was still there. The other informant then reported that the tenant had, in fact, moved out some time ago, and that the patient still believed she lived with her and was the cause of several things going in wrong in the house.

Obsessions, compulsions, and *phobias* are also surveyed in this section of the MSE. *Obsessions* are recurrent, intrusive thoughts that the patient attempts to resist. The most common obsession is doubting that something has been done (eg, the door has been locked, the hands have been sufficiently cleaned). Typical obsessions involve a potential dangers, cleanliness, or orderliness. To check for obsessions, the examiner asks questions such as, "Are there times when you have repetitive thoughts that you cannot control? For example, do you think that the door is not locked or that the stove is not off, or that things are dirty and need cleaning, or that something will go wrong? Do these thoughts make you anxious? Or do they make you want to do things, such as check? How easily can you stop those thoughts?"

Compulsions are repetitive behaviors (eg, hand washing, touching the wall) that the patient feels driven to perform but regards as unreasonable and attempts to resist. Compulsions usually occur in response to obsessions and are followed by a reduction in anxiety. To inquire about compulsions, the examiner might ask, "Do have to do certain things over and over again, or a certain number of times, such as checking, washing your hands, or making sure something bad has not happened to a loved one? What makes you want to do these things? How anxious are you before you do them and how do you feel afterwards? What happens if you try to stop yourself?" In the context of certain neurologic diseases (eg, Parkinson's disease), repetitive behaviors such as gambling, hoarding of objects, or rummaging have been described. (See Chapter 8.)

Occasionally patients with neurologic diseases experience *phobias*—fears that the patients themselves regard as excessive. Patients with phobias try to avoid the feared object or situation; when they cannot do that they try to escape from what they fear. Thus, for example, someone with a phobia of crossing bridges will try to avoid doing so; when this is impossible, the person will cross the bridge as quickly as he or she can. Phobias usually precede the onset of a neurologic disease, and some phobias (eg, fear of spiders, snakes) are quite common in the general population. Phobias should be distinguished from a fear that arises in response to a delusion, from the anxiety that occurs in the context of generalized anxiety disorder, and from the anxiety that is experienced when a compulsion cannot be expressed. The examiner might ask about phobias by using questions such as, "Are there any situations that you are afraid of and try very hard to avoid because they make you anxious, such as riding an elevator, crossing a bridge, or being in crowds?" A fear of small, enclosed spaces (*claustrophobia*) often makes it hard for patients to have brain imaging studies.

Insight and Judgment

Insight refers to patients' awareness of their circumstances, including their neurologic condition, family relationships, and other important matters. Insight is often impaired or lacking in patients with cortical—especially frontal lesions. This lack of awareness is a consequence of the underlying brain damage rather than a psychologic denial because it is uncommon in subcortical disorders. The inability to recognize neurologic or cognitive deficit such as paralysis, memory loss, or aphasia is called *nosoagnosia*. Insight is assessed by asking questions such as, "Do you think there is something wrong with your health?" or "Is your memory functioning OK or are you having difficulty with it?" Lack of insight can explain what seem to be foolish, dangerous, or unusual behaviors, and it can explain why patients do not follow medical advice. For example, a patient with poor insight into amnesia, apraxia, or mania should not be expected to grasp the significance of what he or she is being told about the deficit and should not be castigated for failing to correct its manifestations.

Judgment refers to a person's ability to assess a situation, consider the facts and issues, and draw an appropriate conclusion. It can be assessed by asking questions about the patient's neurologic disease. Thus, for example, someone with epilepsy might be asked: "If you notice that the medication is making you drowsy, what will you do?" Judgment is also assessed from the history provided by the family and through the course of the interview by observing the way in which the patient approaches the examiner.

Cognition

Because cognitive impairment is a common feature of neurologic conditions that affect the brain, every neurologic patient should undergo a thorough assessment of cognition. The extent of cognitive assessment can vary, however, depending on the purposes of the examiner and the setting in which the examination is being carried out. A neuropsychologist would be expected to carry out an in-depth extensive inventory of a patient's cognitive abilities that would take several hours. A physician assessing a patient with neurologic disease might use a brief, global assessment at the bedside to monitor the patient's course.

The nature and extent of the cognitive assessment should be based on the patient's background. Individuals who have always been very bright or were well educated need to be asked more complex questions to identify and assess cognitive deficits than do people with less intelligence and education.

In the context of neurologic disease, cognitively impaired patients are commonly encountered who may be reluctant to answer direct questions that test their cognitive capacity. One way around the problem is to ask questions in the course of taking a history. Thus, for example, orientation to year can be determined during the personal history. "Where were you born? What year was that? Do you know what year it is now? How old does that make you?" For cognitively impaired patients, resistance to the MSE can sometimes be overcome by the examiner's emphasizing that the assessment is being carried out to identify abilities as well as impairments ("Let's see how well you do with this question") and by acknowledging that some questions are difficult ("I'm going to ask you a more difficult one now. Let's see how good you are at math. Take 7 away from 100."). Sometimes it is useful to say that the information is being gathered for the benefit of the patient ("I know this is hard, but if I know what problems you have, I'll be better able to help you."). Helping a patient with a difficult question is often reassuring. For example, if a person answers the question, "Do you know where we are now" with, "I can't remember" and is upset, the examiner can be supportive by responding, "Well, let me help you. Do you know what city are we in?" Even in the best of hands, however, a small number of patients are unwilling to undergo this part of the psychiatric evaluation.

The mini-mental state examination. It is useful to have a standard method of cognitive examination with which one starts and then to supplement it as appropriate for individual patients. The most widely used bedside cognitive examination is the

Mini-Mental State Examination (MMSE) (Folstein, Folstein, and McHugh, 1975). The major strengths of this examination are its brevity and broad coverage of cognitive functions. Its chief limitations are an inability to identify mild cognitive impairment, which is called the *ceiling effect;* its dependence on language (as are almost all general cognitive function tests), which results in artificially low scores in patients who have an aphasia; and its inability to discriminate the degree of impairment in severely impaired individuals, which is called the *basement effect.* As with all general cognitive assessments, patients with little education do less well than those with more. Despite these limitations, the MMSE is a most useful tool for detecting changes in cognitive ability that may be indicative or delirium, dementia, or other cognitive syndromes.

There are several published methods of administering and scoring the MMSE, including the original one published in 1974 that had several limitations that have since been addressed. What is presented below is the approach most often used by the Division of Geriatric Psychiatry and Neuropsychiatry at Johns Hopkins University. Consistency of scoring is important because it allows for an individual patient's performances to be compared over time and for the comparison of the capacities of different individuals.

Table 1–4 shows MMSE median score norms by age and education. The first two items assess orientation to time and place. Questions include, "Can you tell me where we are now?" and "What city and state are we in?" One point is given for each correct answer. When testing for orientation to time (year, month, season, day of the week, and date), the first question asked may depend on whether the person appears, based on the initial conversation, to have a significant cognitive impairment. If disorientation is likely, the clinician might ask if the patient knows the month and introduce the questioning in a non-threatening fashion (eg, "Have you been keeping up with the

Table 1.4. Median Mini-Mental State Examination Scores by Age and Educational Level

| Age | *Years of Education* | | | |
	0–4	5–8	9–12	12+
18–24	23	28	29	30
25–29	25	27	29	30
30–34	26	26	29	30
35–39	24	27	29	30
40–44	23	27	29	30
45–49	23	27	29	30
50–54	22	27	29	30
55–59	22	27	28	29
60–64	22	27	28	29
65–69	22	27	28	29
70–74	21	26	28	29
75–79	21	26	28	29
80–84	19	25	26	28
85+	20	24	26	28

Source: *Adapted with permission from* Crum, R.M., Anthony, J.C., Basset, S.S., Folstein, M.F. (1993). Population-based norms for the Mini-Mental State Examination by age and educational level. *Journal of the American Medical Association* 269: 2386–91.

date? Do you know what month it is?"). Every question should be asked, whether or not a person is doing well.

The next item tests registration, that is, the ability to immediately repeat back items being committed to memory. This is the first part of memory testing. Three words are given to remember in the following manner: "I'd like to test your memory by asking you to remember three words. Please listen carefully and repeat these three words after me." It is good to use the same three words for the assessment of each new patient. This has the benefit of preventing embarrassment should the examiner forget the words. This item is scored by counting the number of words the person is able to correctly repeat *the first time.* If a patient misstates a word, he or she should not receive a point for it. If the patient asks for the words to be repeated, the examiner should first ask the patient to repeat as many words as he or she can remember, because the score for registration measures how many words an individual reports on the first try. The examiner then repeats the three words until the patient is able to say all three or it is clear that he or she cannot register all of them. Difficulty in registering the words can indicate a hearing problem or a language problem. If not previously alerted to the possibility of a hearing problem, the examiner should note this as a possibility and perform a hearing assessment at some point.

The next item—a choice between serial seven subtractions or spelling "world" backward—serves two functions: first it distracts the patient from the three words he or she was just asked to repeat; and second, it is a test of attention and concentration. We prefer to use the serial sevens subtraction task for patients with an eighth grade or higher education. The patient is asked to subtract 7 from 100 and then to continue subtracting 7 from the answer for a series of five subtractions. A patient who is able to subtract 7 from 100 correctly should be able to do all the subsequent subtractions. One point is scored for each correct subtraction even if the previous subtraction was incorrect (so that "93, 87, 80, 73, 66" is given four out of a total of five points). If it is clear that patients have memorized answers from prior examinations, the subtraction can be altered, and they can be asked instead to subtract 7s beginning from 101 or 103. This is one item that many clinicians do not expect older persons to perform correctly. Experience and research demonstrate that individuals with an eighth grade education or better can perform serial sevens without error. The speed of performance may slow down with age, so the examiner should allow ample time for completion of the task.

When a patient does not complete the first subtraction—and it should be noted whether that is because the patient refuses or tries but cannot perform a subtraction—or when the patient has less than an eighth grade education, the patient might be given the easier task of being asked to spell backward a five-letter word with three consonants in a row (usually "world," with "spray" as a backup). To determine whether the patient has the ability to spell the word, it is best to ask him or her to spell it forward and then to spell it backwards. For the occasional patient who misspells the word forward, his or her incorrect spelling in reverse is used as the correct sequence. When scoring backward spelling, a point is given for each response that matches the correct position in the sequence, "d-l-r-o-w." For example, "d-l-o-r-w" would score three out of five points, whereas "d-r-o-l-w" and "l-r-d-o-w would score two.

After the concentration task, the patient is asked if he or she can remember any of the three words that he was asked to remember. This tests *recall*. It is important to give the patient adequate time. Some patients may take 30 seconds to recall all three words. One point is given for each word correctly recalled. The words must be spontaneously remembered to receive a point. For words that cannot be recalled (and thus scored as zero points), the examiner might want to determine whether giving a cue or hint or asking the patient to chose the correct word from a list of words, some of which were not in the original three, improves performance. These additional questions can provide useful information but are not scored on the MMSE. A patient who cannot benefit from cues is more likely to have cortical pathology affecting her memory, whereas one whose memory benefits from cuing is more likely to have subcortical pathology. In giving cues, the clinician might start with a category (eg, "One was an animal"). If the patient is still unable to remember, he or she can then be given a choice such as "Was it a puppy, a pony, or a kitten?" The MMSE does not have a set time interval after which items are recalled, but 5 minutes seems an appropriate time to wait.

Several aspects of language are assessed in the MMSE. Asking the person to name two familiar objects—a pen and a watch—tests *naming*. A point is given for each correct response. Visually impaired individuals can be asked to name a pencil and a key that are placed in their palm. Examiners might also want to assess naming in more depth by asking the patient to name other common objects, such as a button, an eraser, a lapel, the stem of a watch, shoelaces, or the buckle of a belt. Points are not given on the examination for naming these other objects, but repeated failures suggest a naming deficit.

Repetition is assessed by testing the ability to repeat the phrase, "no ifs, ands, or buts." The phrase must be repeated exactly, including all the "s" at the end of the words. The patient is allowed only one attempt. One point is given for a correct repetition. An alternate phrase that might be used as an additional repetition task but not scored is "Methodist, Protestant, Episcopal." These phrases are difficult for individuals of some ethnic backgrounds or for individuals for whom English is not native. If there is a question about this being a problem, the sentence, "Today is a (sunny) day in the month of May" might be used in its place. It is necessary that the patient say each and every word correctly. Repetition is a good screen for whether a person has language problems. It requires intact comprehension, intact registration, and intact expression of language. Repetition can be adversely affected by hearing impairment. If this is present it should be noted, but the item is still scored as not performed correctly.

The next item addresses the ability to *read a sentence and carry out the action*. The sentence "Close your eyes" is the one used in the MMSE. The patient is asked to read the sentence to himself or herself and then carry out the action. The print should be large enough so that those with visual problems can easily read it. Some patients are able to say the sentence but not carry out the action. A point is not given in this case.

Following a three-step command requires the patient to comprehend that the examiner wants him to do something, that he or she can hear what is said, and that he or she is able to carry out the three distinct steps. This tests several cognitive abilities but is most indicative of the ability called *praxis*—the ability to carry out learned motor movements. The three-step command on the MMSE asks the patient to take a piece of paper in the right hand, fold it in half, and then place it on the floor. A point is given for each step done correctly. The reliability of this item is surprising to some people. Patients who are able to do only one or two steps when first asked to complete the task will usually be able to do only the same number of steps when asked to do it a second time.

Next, the patient is asked to *write a sentence* of his or her choosing. One point is given if it is a complete sentence (ie, with a subject and verb) that is grammatically correct. Some patients say they do not know what to write. In this instance they can be encouraged to "write anything that comes to mind." When a patient is still not able to write a simple sentence, the examiner might suggest one, for example, "today is a (warm or cold) day," changing the adjective depending on the temperature. This is useful because it reveals the patient's handwriting, but a point is given only if the patient spontaneously writes a complete, grammatically correct sentence.

Finally, the patient is asked to *copy a design with two interlocking pentagons.* A point is given if each figure has five sides and five angles and if the overlap is a four-sided figure. This assesses visuospatial function and praxis.

The significance of the total score on the MMSE depends on the presence or absence of noncognitive impairments (eg, blindness, dominant arm weakness), which may account for the loss of certain points, as well as on the patient's estimated premorbid cognitive abilities, which reflect such factors as his or her age, education, and occupation. In general, a MMSE score of less than

24 is indicative of cognitive impairment. For blind individuals, a score of 27 is probably normal, because they would be unable to complete three items due to blindness. A score of 25 would be abnormal for a person with a high premorbid ability, such as a college graduate. Median scores for the MMSE by age and education normative groups are provided in Table 1–4 to help the physician interpret a given score.

The expanded cognitive examination. The MMSE adequately tests orientation, memory, praxis, language, attention, and calculation. However, other aspects of cognition (Table 1–3) such as consciousness, fund of knowledge, and executive function are not assessed well by the MMSE. Because successful performance on the MMSE does not necessarily indicate the absence of a cognitive impairment, particularly in patients who premorbidly were quite high functioning intellectually, a more in-depth cognitive examination is sometimes indicated. For these reasons, some physicians might choose to use in their day-to-day practice the Modified MMSE (3MS), which quantifies cognitive functioning on a broader, 100-point scale and overcomes certain limitations of the MMSE, such as the ceiling effect (Teng and Chui, 1987).

Formulation and Differential Diagnosis

The final part of the evaluation is the formulation and differential diagnosis. The formulation is concerned with describing the pertinent psychiatric phenomena and appreciating the context and person in which they occur, whereas the differential diagnosis attempts to explain the psychiatric phenomena as consequences of one or more conditions. In developing the formulation, the physician organizes the history, physical examination, MSE, and any pertinent laboratory studies in a coherent and systematic fashion. The first step is to decide the aspects of the person's background most relevant to the problem at hand (eg, education, work history, and prior personality). The second step is to decide the relevant aspects of the neurologic condition, including its causes, course, current severity and treatment. The third step is to synthesize the psychiatric phenomena elicited from the history and examination into a coherent whole that then allows for the consideration of possible causes of the patients condition.

An example of such a formulation is: "This is a 48-year-old married woman, who is a college school graduate and who has taught high school for many years. She has a family history of depression in her otherwise healthy older sister. She is happily married and the mother of two preteen children. Premorbidly she was a cheerful, emotionally stable, active person, who tended to be rather preoccupied with cleanliness, had high standards for herself, and was always on time. She always liked being with people and had many close friends. She has no prior medical or psychiatric history. Three years ago, she was diagnosed with multiple sclerosis (MS) after developing optic neuritis and sensory loss in her left leg. These symptoms remitted after several months, but she suffered two relapses and was started on interferon-beta. After her last remission she developed intermittent crying, feelings of failure, trouble sleeping, anorexia, and lack of pleasure at being with her children. On MSE she was sad, with a reduced vital sense and strong feelings of guilt, but no other abnormalities. The MMSE score was 29/30, with one point lost on orientation to date."

Once the central psychiatric features of a case are summarized, it is helpful to ask whether they seem best explained as something the patient *has* (eg, major depression); something the patient *is* (eg, dependent or passive), something the patient *does* (eg, feigning a symptom), or something the patient *encounters* (eg, a disability that has demoralized her) (McHugh and Slavney, 1998). This approach to understanding a psychiatric case is derived from a methodologic approach to clinical reasoning. Thus, thinking that the patient *has* something is thinking in terms of a disease (in this case MS) that has directly produced the psychiatric features (eg, major depression), just as it has led to neurologic features (eg, optic neuritis). Alternatively, the psychiatric features (eg, emotional distress) might be understood as the interaction of the patient's premorbid personality traits (eg, having high standards), and circumstances in her life that play to her vulnerabilities (eg, that she cannot be the mother she would like to be), thus, something the patient *is*. Or, the psychiatric complaints might be the consequence of the patient engaging in a behavior (eg, taking on the sick role) in a way that is affecting her functioning and mental state; this is the outcome of something the patient is *doing*. Finally, the formulation could be that the patient's psychiatric complaints are the understandable emotional reaction of a person with wishes, desires, and hopes for herself (eg, to see her children have children) who now has encountered a chronic and perhaps fatal disease; this is the consequence of something the patient has *encountered.*

The formulation lays the foundation for *explaining* the psychiatric phenomena that have been elicited by the examiner. In this case, the problem seems to be that the patient has developed depressive symptoms several years after the onset of MS, although not during a time when she was disabled. This makes it unlikely that the MS was demoralizing her. It is also unlikely that she had been saddened by other events in her life, because she was happily married, had healthy children, and liked her job. Neither were the depressive symptoms accompanied by features suggestive of delirium, dementia, anxiety disorder, or schizophrenia, nor did they appear to be consistent with the patient's premorbid personality, because she seems to have been able to deal well with adversity in the past. Rather, her psychiatric symptoms are most consistent with a major

depression caused by the effects of MS, or its treatment—
interferon-beta—on her brain.

In this formulation, the central features of the psychiatric
disturbances are identified as being in the affective realm of
mental life, rather than in the cognitive, perceptual, or behavioral realms, and their etiology is considered. It is concluded that
the disturbance is best explained as a consequence of the effects
of a brain disease or its treatment. Alternative formulations,
such as thinking of this a psychologic reaction to having a disease or disability or viewing this patient as someone with a
vulnerable personality who is having difficulty coping with the
neurologic illness, are not consistent with the presentation.

With this approach, the physician can develop and resolve
a differential diagnosis of the patient's psychiatric symptoms.
More than one of these methods of explanatory reasoning might
be relevant for a given patient, who may, for example, both *have*
something and have *encountered* something. In the case described above, the patient might also have developed transient
distress and demoralization when she first developed blindness,
consistent with the severity of that disability. Or she may have
developed a psychogenic paralysis—something she *does*—during
a time of stress, in the absence of an MS exacerbation. The aggregate of this reasoning can then be expressed in the language
of the fourth edition of the *Diagnostic and Statistical Manual*
(DSM-IV) (APA, 1994) or the tenth edition of the *International
Classification of Diseases* (ICD-10) (WHO, 2004). The most common diagnostic options available to physicians in DSM and ICD
are presented in Table 1–5.

DSM-IV encourages multiaxial diagnosis, which encourages
the development of therapeutic interventions targeted at all
salient features of a case (eg, diseases, personality traits, adjustment problems). Ideally then, the physician should generate
a diagnosis as appropriate on Axis I (clinical syndromes), Axis II
(mental retardation, personality disorders), Axis III (medical

Table 1.5. Diagnostic Groups for Psychiatric Conditions in Patients with Neurologic Disease

---

Delirium
Dementia
Psychiatric disorder due to a general medical condition
  (eg, the neurologic disease)
Psychiatric disorder due to the effects of a substance
  or medication (eg, treatment for the neurologic disease)
Substance use disorders
Mood, anxiety, and other affective disorders
  Major depression
  Minor depression
  Obsessive-compulsive disorder
  Panic disorder
  Generalized anxiety disorder
Somatoform disorders
Personality disorders
Adjustment disorders
Schizophrenia and related psychotic disorders

---

conditions), Axis IV (psychosocial stressors), and Axis V (level of psychosocial functioning). Such an approach represents good clinical practice, for it acknowledges that several factors may contribute to the patient's illness and response to treatment.

In addition, it is important to appreciate that on DSM-IV Axis I—clinical syndromes—certain conditions "trump" others in the differential diagnosis. The physician should attempt to assign a single diagnosis on this axis, if possible, rather than to assign several Axis I diagnoses at once, based on the presence of individual symptoms. For example, because almost any psychiatric symptoms can be explained by delirium if the patient is delirious, then it is prudent to avoid making other diagnoses (eg, dementia, major depression, schizophrenia) until the delirium is resolved and it is clear that the symptoms indicative of other disorders persist. Similarly, in the presence of dementia, mental symptoms other than cognitive ones are initially best considered associated with the dementia. The same approach is preferred if the psychiatric condition is related to the use of medications, illicit substances, or another medical condition ("psychiatric disorder due to ..." in the DSM-IV). In the presence of depressive symptoms, if delusions are evident, a diagnosis such as "major depression, with psychotic features" would be appropriate. An adjustment disorder diagnosis is best reserved for patients for whom an obvious stressor has precipitated emotional distress or behavioral change. However, such a diagnosis should be made only *in the absence* of other psychiatric conditions such as major depression or schizophrenia (ie, the presence of major depression "trumps" a diagnosis of adjustment disorder), because stressors are often precipitants for the other conditions as well. The diagnosis of schizophrenia, given its serious prognostic implications, should be approached as a diagnosis of exclusion and probably is best made by a psychiatrist. The same is true of a diagnosis of a personality disorder. A diagnosis of a somatoform disorder (eg, conversion disorder, somatization disorder), appropriately made at times by nonpsychiatric physicians for patients with conditions such as "hysteria," pseudoseizures, or psychogenic pain, has important implications for patients and their treatment. Such a diagnosis is best made in collaboration with a psychiatrist.

References

[APA] American Psychiatric Association (1994). *Diagnostic and Statistical Manual of Mental Disorders* (4th ed.). Washington, DC: American Psychiatric Association.

Crum, R.M., Anthony, J.C., Basset, S.S., Folstein, M.F. (1993). Population-based norms for the Mini-Mental State Examination by age and educational level. *Journal of the American Medical Association* 269: 2386–91.

Folstein, M.F., Folstein, S.E., McHugh, P.R. (1975). Mini-Mental State: a practical method for grading the cognitive state of patients for the clinician. *Journal of Psychiatric Research*, 12: 189–98.

McHugh, P.R., Slavney, P.R. (1998). *The Perspectives of Psychiatry* (2nd ed.). Baltimore, MD: Johns Hopkins University Press.

Teng, E.L., Chui, H.C. (1987). The Modified Mini-Mental State (3MS) examination. *Journal of Clinical Psychiatry*, 48: 314–18.

[WHO] World Health Organization (2004). *ICD-10: International Statistical Classification of Diseases and Related Health Problems: 10th Revision* (2nd ed.). Geneva, Switzerland: World Health Organization.

2

Overview of Psychiatric Symptoms and Syndromes

PETER V. RABINS
PHILLIP R. SLAVNEY

T his chapter provides an overview of psychiatric symptoms and syndromes that can be seen with neurologic diseases. Our goal is not to discuss every psychiatric disorder that might occur but to focus on those that are the most common.

Demoralization

Important characteristics of this condition include:

- Intermittently sad mood
- Identifiable precipitant
- Absence of major depression

Just as grief is a normal response to loss, demoralization is a normal response to adversity. When bad things happen, our spirits fall. Because adversity is common with neurologic diseases, so is demoralization. Thus, patients may become demoralized when they learn they have a neurologic disease (eg, amyotrophic lateral sclerosis, Alzheimer's disease, Huntington's disease), when they experience the symptoms of such a disease (eg, blindness, aphasia, pain), or when they develop the side effects of treatment for the disease (eg, weight gain from prednisone, dyskinesias from levodopa). Demoralization is not linked to any particular group of neurologic diseases, but it tends to be more common in those that are chronic, progressive, painful, debilitating, or disfiguring.

Demoralized patients are almost always sad, but they may also be frustrated, irritable, pessimistic, or anxious. These unpleasant emotions are directly related to the patient's situation and diminish as that situation improves. Someone who is demoralized by pain cheers up when the pain is relieved. Even when patients are demoralized by circumstances that cannot be reversed, their mood often improves when they discover that they are not powerless in the face of adversity. In this way, patients who become demoralized when they are told that they have a terminal illness may feel better as they start to focus on what they can do with the time left to them, and patients who become demoralized by the onset of a paraplegia may brighten as they begin to make progress in rehabilitation. This direct relationship between the patient's mood and his or her situation helps distinguish the sadness of demoralization from that of major depression, because in the latter condition the patient's mood remains low despite improving circumstances.

Other features of a demoralized state also help differentiate demoralization from major depression. Patients who are demoralized may voice what seem like suicidal thoughts (eg, "If this pain doesn't go away soon, you might as well shoot me"), but such statements are expressions of frustration, not of an intention to die. Demoralized patients want to live; they just want the suffering to end. They can see hope somewhere in their situation, and they turn to their physicians for help. In patients with major depression, suicidal thoughts (eg, "My life is over, I'm just burdening my family, I'm going to save them all this trouble and expense") are often accompanied by feelings of hopelessness and guilt, so that death seems the best way, or even the only way, to end the suffering. Demoralized patients respond positively to encouragement that time will bring improvement or that new approaches might help, whereas depressed patients often dismiss such statements. Although delusions and hallucinations are uncommon in major depression, they never occur in demoralization. Sometimes, of course, it is difficult to decide whether a patient is demoralized or depressed, and in such cases a psychiatric consultation is indicated.

The best treatment for demoralization is to remove the cause of the patient's suffering. If that is impossible or requires a long time to accomplish, continuing encouragement by the physician and others is essential. Antidepressants do not relieve normal sadness; if they did, they would be the most abused drugs in the world. In clear-cut cases of demoralization, then, antidepressants have no role in treatment. When it is difficult to decide whether the patient is demoralized, depressed, or both, a trial of antidepressant medication should be considered, although it must be remembered that such drugs have side effects (see Chapter 15) and that prescribing an antidepressant does not lessen the physician's responsibility to help the patient combat demoralization.

Major Depression

Important characteristics of this condition include:

- Persistently sad mood
- Diminished self-attitude and self-confidence
- Diminished energy and impaired sleep
- Episodic course

In normal happiness and sadness (including demoralization), the brain's mood-regulating system responds appropriately to events in the patient's life. In mania and major depression, the mood-regulating system appears to be disconnected from such events, so that emotions occur and are sustained without much relationship to the patient's situation. An example of this disconnection in major depression can be seen in the phenomenon of anhedonia—a state in which patients lose the capacity to enjoy events that would ordinarily bring pleasure. In neurologic diseases, this dysregulation of mood and related phenomena (eg, self-attitude, outlook, sleep, appetite, energy level, libido) can be caused by the disease itself or as a side effect of treatment. Thus, for example, the initial manifestation of Huntington's disease can be mania or depression, and both mania and depression can be produced by corticosteroid medication.

In neurologic patients with major depression, mood is sad (and perhaps irritable or anxious), even when the neurologic disease is improving or is in remission. Such patients have a diminished self-attitude and a pessimistic outlook. At times, these gloomy thoughts are delusional in nature, and patients can believe (for example) that their suffering is deserved punishment for unforgivable sins or that they are doomed to die, even though their illness is not a fatal one. Depressed patients can act on such delusions, and in a hopeless, guilty state may take their lives. Hallucinations are less common than delusions in major depression, but they, too, are negative in character, so patients can hear voices criticizing them or see their relatives being tortured. Such mood-congruent hallucinations may reinforce a depressed patient's impetus to suicide.

In addition to disturbances in mood, cognition, and perception, patients with major depression have abnormal sleep, diminished appetite, low energy, slowed thinking and movements, and little interest in sex. Sleep is usually reduced, but even when increased it is not refreshing. Because neurologic diseases and their treatments can themselves disturb sleep, appetite, energy level, psychomotor activity, and libido, abnormalities in these vital functions are by no means pathognomonic of major depression. Before insomnia, anorexia, and the like can be seen as evidence of major depression, then, other causes must be excluded. This exercise in differential diagnosis is especially important when major depression is being considered as the explanation for a patient's psychomotor retardation or lack of motivation (eg, refusal to participate in physical therapy). In many such cases that are referred for psychiatric evaluation, the patient is found to be delirious, not depressed.

The treatment of major depression associated with specific neurologic diseases is discussed in subsequent chapters,

whereas more general information about antidepressants, electroconvulsive therapy (ECT), and psychotherapy is reviewed
in Chapters 15, 21, and 22, respectively. Many nonpsychiatric
physicians are comfortable treating patients with mild or moderate depression, but psychiatric referral is needed when patients remain sad despite antidepressant treatment, when they
are delusional or hallucinated, or when they acknowledge suicidal thoughts.

Mania

Important characteristics of this condition include:

- Persistently elevated mood
- Elevated self-attitude and self-confidence
- Increased energy and diminished need for sleep
- Episodic course

The clinical manifestations of mania are generally the opposite of those in major depression. The patient's mood is often
euphoric or excited, although sometimes it is irritable or—very
briefly—sad. Whereas the mood in major depression is persistent, in mania it is labile. The manic patient's self-attitude is
grandiose and may be delusionally so. Thus, manic patients can
believe that they are geniuses, millionaires, or world-class mu-
sicians, and sometimes they experience hallucinations (eg,
voices praising them) that seem to validate such beliefs. Like
patients with major depression, patients with mania can act on
their delusions, so that those who think they have unlimited
wealth may bankrupt themselves.

The grandiose self-attitude and optimistic outlook seen in
mania often interfere with treatment; manic patients can believe that there is nothing wrong with them and that, in any

event, they know more than their physicians do. This confident stance is strengthened by the patient's sense of physical well-being, with reduced need for sleep, increased libido, and increased energy. In mild mania (hypomania), an increase in energy makes patients more productive; in severe mania, it makes them less productive, because they are so hyperactive and distractible that they cannot complete any but the simplest task. An increased speed of movement is accompanied by an increased speed of thinking, and with a parallel result: in severe mania the patient's thoughts can be so rapid and disjointed (thought-disordered) that coherent conversation is impossible.

The treatment of mania associated with specific neurologic diseases is discussed in subsequent chapters, and more general information about neuroleptics and mood stabilizers is reviewed in Chapters 17 and 18, respectively. In many ways, mania is more difficult to treat than depression, and the threshold for psychiatric referral should be lower. Whereas even moderate depressions can be treated on an outpatient basis by nonpsychiatric physicians, only the mildest of manias can.

It is not known how the brain produces normal moods, let alone mania and depression, or why mania is less common than depression. Even more mysterious is how mania and depression can alternate in the same person—sometimes on a daily basis. Studying the neurologic diseases that cause mania and depression may produce greater understanding of these matters.

Anxiety

Important characteristics of this condition include:

- Pervasive feelings of tension, apprehension, and worry
- Physical symptoms such as palpitations, sweating, and hyperventilation

The term anxiety is used in general discourse to refer to a state of worry. Clinically, it refers to a group of disorders in which feelings of tension and worry and the physical experiences associated with these emotions occur so frequently, persistently, or to such a severe degree that they impair function and cause distress. The following paragraphs will describe the several anxiety syndromes as distinct conditions. However, it should be noted that they sometimes overlap or co-occur, and that they can occur secondarily to major depression, demoralization, and other psychiatric syndromes as well. Individual symptoms of excessive worry without a clear or actual stimulus, generalized muscle tension, or vague "nervousness" are also seen secondarily to other psychiatric syndromes.

Generalized anxiety is a state in which feelings of tension and anxiety are persistent and lack a clear trigger or precipitant. Difficulty falling asleep, mildly diminished appetite, and diminished concentration may be reported. The feelings of tension may be localized to the epigastrium, abdomen, or muscles throughout the body. Similar complaints can be seen in hyperthyroidism.

Panic disorder is an episodic experience of fearfulness and apprehension that usually lasts several or many minutes, is associated with palpitations, shortness of breath and/or the experience of being unable to "catch my breath," tremulousness, and perioral or fingertip tingling. The episodes are generally stereotyped, that is, they are quite similar from episode to episode, can be triggered by specific plans (eg, planning to go outside) or settings, and are frightening. Panic attacks need to be distinguished from other episodic disorders, including seizures, the release of catecholamines by a pheochromocytoma, and cardiac arrhythmias.

Phobias (phobic disorder) is the experience of excessive fearfulness and apprehension that is triggered by a specific event (eg, public speaking), setting (eg, tight spaces, going outside, going into a crowded market) or object (eg, snakes, spiders) and that is recognized by the person as excessive, unreasonable, or an overreaction, and that actually interferes with function. They should be distinguished from objects or events that cause dislike or upset but do not interfere with everyday life. For example, a dislike of heights or a feeling of anxiety about standing at an edge is not a phobia if the reaction does not interfere with everyday existence. What is an example of interference is living in a tall building but not being able to use the elevator because of a phobia of enclosed spaces.

Any of the anxiety disorders can occur secondarily with major depression. A secondary anxiety state can be recognized by its occurrence episodically only when episodes of depression occur.

The anxiety disorders respond to cognitive-behavioral therapy (CBT) and to pharmacotherapy about equally. The combination of the two is often more effective than either alone. If the anxiety disorder or symptom is secondary to depression, the treatment should primarily target the major depression, but symptomatic relief of the anxiety in the short term may be appropriate if the associated distress is significant.

Obsessive-Compulsive Disorders and Symptoms

Important characteristics of these conditions include:

- Repetitive thoughts (obsessions) that are distressing and resisted
- Repetitive actions (compulsions) that are distressing and resisted

As reviewed in Chapter 1, obsessions are repetitive thoughts (eg, "Did I lock the door?" "Are my hands clean?"), whereas compulsions are repetitive actions (eg, checking a lock three times or washing one's hands for 15 minutes). Obsessions are more common than compulsions, and when compulsions are seen they are usually linked to obsessions.

In obsessive-compulsive disorder (OCD), these experiences are not only recurrent but also stereotyped and intrusive. The person experiencing obsessions and compulsions recognizes them as excessive but ultimately cannot resist thinking about them or doing them. This attempt to resist is initially experienced as increasingly distressing and ultimately impossible, although in chronic cases the stress and resistance can fade. When a compulsion is enacted, there is a temporary release of tension. OCD is diagnosed when the obsessions or compulsions interfere with function or cause significant distress.

The course of OCD is often variable. Symptoms can worsen without any explanation, but sometimes an exacerbation of an underlying neurologic disorder such as Tourette's syndrome or an associated psychiatric disorder such as major depression is associated with a worsening of symptoms.

Obsessional *traits* are characteristic aspects of a person that include perfectionism, rigidity, inflexibility, and slowness. Associated behaviors include extreme neatness, repetitive checking or touching (for example, of light switches), and excessive orderliness, but these do not interfere with daily function or cause significant distress.

The symptoms of OCD may be difficult to treat. Selective serotonin reuptake inhibitors (SSRIs) are the mainstay of pharmacologic therapy, but CBT can also be helpful. Neurologists may wish to give a patient with obsessions and compulsions a trial of an SSRI, but if this is unsuccessful, referral to a psychiatrist is indicated.

Conversion Disorder

Important characteristics of this condition include:

- Behavior suggesting a neurologic disorder
- Desire to be in the sick role

The first question about patients with conversion disorder is: does their neurologic complaint represents something they have (eg, paralysis) or something they do (eg, behave as if they are paralyzed)? This question arises because there is a discrepancy between what the patients report and what their physicians observe: a discrepancy between symptoms and signs.

Once it is established that patients with conversion disorder are acting as if they have a neurologic disease when they do not, a second question arises: why are they doing it? Perhaps the most useful answer is that patients with conversion disorder want to be regarded as sick so that others will treat them differently. Thus, for example, dependent, inarticulate people who are repeatedly criticized by their spouses can discover that when they are sick, the spouses relent. Such people may then use the sick role to help them deal indirectly with a problem that seems impossible to solve directly. (Among individuals who utilize the sick role for purposes other than health care, a distinction is made between those with conversion disorder, who unconsciously deceive themselves, and those with malingering and factitious disorder, who consciously deceive others.)

Neurologists most often see patients with conversion disorder during a consultation to exclude a neurologic disease. Sometimes, however, patients under the care of neurologists develop conversion disorder. Although such patients are already entitled to the sick role because of their neurologic disease, they discover that when they are more symptomatic, they are better able to cope with a difficult relationship or situation. This discovery leads them to use the manifestations of their neurologic disease as a template for behavior that alters their circumstances. Conversion disorder can occur with any neurologic disease because it depends more on the nature of the patient's personality and situation than it does on the type of the neuropathology. However, it may be more common in diseases with an episodic course (eg, epilepsy, multiple sclerosis), perhaps because the behavior can stopped when its purpose is accomplished and still give the appearance of having been an authentic relapse. When patients begin to act in this way, it is often difficult for them to give up the behavior until they have both a face-saving way of doing so and a better solution to the problem that provoked it.

Once it is clear that the problem is psychologic rather than physiologic, the neurologist's task is to help the patient accept the psychiatric sick role in addition to the neurologic one. Patients are often reluctant to do this, but if the neurologist emphasizes that (1) the goal is to help the patient feel better and function better, (2) a psychiatric consultation may reveal sources of stress that are affecting the patient's health, and (3) the neurologist will continue to care for the patient, many neurologic patients with conversion disorder will agree to psychiatric treatment. It is important for the neurologist and psychiatrist to stay in contact while this occurs to reduce the risk that either will misinterpret an actual worsening of the patient's neurologic disease as further evidence of conversion disorder.

Delirium

Important characteristics of this condition include:

- Decline in cognitive function
- Reduced level of consciousness and impairedattention
- Disturbed sleep–wake cycle

Delirium (also known as *acute brain syndrome; acute confusional state; encephalopathy;* intensive care unit, or *ICU, psychosis;* or *toxic psychosis*) is a syndrome whose fundamental features are disturbances in consciousness, attention, and cognition. In addition to these phenomena, abnormalities in perception, behavior, and mood often occur. Because delirium can affect so many psychologic functions, it should be considered in the differential diagnosis of acute or subacute changes in the mental state or behavior of any patient with a disease of the central nervous system, especially if the patient is old or very ill.

The disturbances in consciousness and attention seen in delirium usually take one of two forms: a hypoactive-hypoalert state, or a hyperactive-hyperalert one. Although these states are superficially quite different, both are characterized by the "clouding" of consciousness and difficulty in focusing and sustaining attention that are central to the concept of delirium.

In the hypoactive-hypoalert form of delirium, patients are inert and drowsy. They seem indifferent to their environment, speak little, and cannot attend for more than a few seconds. This state may wax and wane over the course of the day, but it is not abolished by sleep or rest. Unless patients with the hypoactive-hypoalert form of delirium are examined—rather than merely observed—their psychomotor retardation and constricted affect may lead to the mistaken conclusion that they are profoundly depressed or have catatonic schizophrenia. Even a brief assessment of their cognitive function (as with the Mini-Mental State Examination) reveals deficits in orientation, concentration, memory, language, and praxis—deficits that are absent in affective disorders and schizophrenia. Although patients with dementia also have abnormalities in multiple cognitive domains, they are alert and lack the clouded consciousness seen in delirium.

In the hyperactive-hyperalert form of delirium, patients are restless and aroused. Although they are very awake, they are not very aware of their surroundings. This diminished aware-ness is a different type of clouded consciousness than that seen in the hypoactive-hypoalert form of delirium, but it can be so severe that patients are oblivious to people and events around them. Here, the problem with attention is not generating it, but sustaining it. Even when patients interact with others they may be so distractible that they are incoherent. Communication is further impaired when the patients are so agitated that they cannot sit or stand still. Unless a cognitive assessment is per-formed, the patients' abnormal behavior can be mistakenly at-tributed to mania or paranoid schizophrenia. Such diagnostic errors are more common when delirious patients are halluci-nated or delusional.

In addition to disturbances in consciousness, attention, and cognition, delirious patients often have abnormalities in per-ception, belief, and mood. Although these latter phenomena are not specific for delirium, they are common and often very distressing.

Perceptual abnormalities take the form of illusions and hallucinations (see Chapter 1). These may occur in any sensory modality, but visual ones are the most frequent. Patients may, for example, perceive an intravenous line as a snake (an illu-sion) or see dead relatives in the room (an hallucination). De-pending on their content, such perceptual abnormalities can leave patients baffled, frightened, or (rarely) comforted.

Whereas an illusion is an abnormal perception, a delusion is an abnormal belief (see Chapter 1). The most common type of delusion in delirium is persecutory in nature, so that patients can believe that they are being spied on (eg, through the tele-vision set) or that members of their family are in danger of being murdered. Such delusions are accompanied by anxiety and, sometimes, by agitation.

A final abnormality that characterizes both the hypoactive-hypoalert and hyperactive-hyperalert forms of delirium is a disturbance in the sleep–wake cycle. Typically, delirious patients cannot sleep at night and are drowsy during the day. Further, delirium often begins at night and is worse at that time. Patients with a mild delirium may be disturbed only at night and report their illusions and hallucinations as bad dreams the next morning.

Given certain conditions, anyone can develop delirium, just as anyone can have a generalized seizure. Delirium and generalized seizures are innate responses of the brain to a variety of pathophysiologic processes and are not an indication of a particular cause. Furthermore, in both cases, the process responsible for the disorder can be intrinsic to the brain or extrinsic to it.

When considering the causes of delirium, it is helpful to think in terms of vulnerabilities and precipitants. Among neurologic patients, the most common vulnerabilities are old age and brain disease (eg, Alzheimer's disease, Parkinson's disease, cerebrovascular disease). Patients who have such vulnerabilities should be monitored closely for the development of delirium when they are exposed to one or more of its many possible precipitants. These precipitants include intoxication with medications (eg, anticholinergics, opioids, corticosteroids); withdrawal from medications (eg, benzodiazepines, barbiturates); metabolic abnormalities (eg, hyponatremia, uremia); infection (eg, urinary tract infection, pneumonia, encephalitis); head trauma; and status epilepticus.

Most of these precipitating causes tend to produce the hypoactive-hypoalert form of delirium, except for withdrawal from alcohol, benzodiazepines, and barbiturates, which produces the hyperactive-hyperalert form known as delirium tremens. In general, the hypoactive-hypoalert form is associated with a generalized slowing of the electroencephalogram (EEG), whereas the hyperactive-hyperalert form is associated with an excess of low-voltage fast activity. In both cases, the degree of abnormality on the EEG is proportional to the severity of the delirium. Although low-voltage fast activity can be seen in schizophrenia or mania, diffuse slowing is not found in either of those disorders or in major depression.

The most important thing in the treatment of delirium is to recognize it, because when an affective disorder, schizophrenia, or a conversion disorder is mistakenly thought to be responsible for a delirious patient's abnormal mental state and behavior, the process causing the delirium can worsen and become more difficult to treat. Delirium, of course, has a morbidity of its own; delirious patients can injure themselves (eg, by pulling out catheters, by falling while trying to escape from hallucinations) and injure staff members (eg, by striking nurses who they think are molesting, rather than repositioning, them).

Among the principles informing the treatment of delirium are protecting the patient, optimizing the environment, and controlling the signs and symptoms (Slavney, 1998). Protecting the patient should begin with having someone at the bedside (especially at night) to reassure and reorient the patient. Although this level of care may not be needed in mild cases, when patients are agitated, hallucinated, or delusional, a staff member at the bedside reduces the need for neuroleptic medication and physical restraint.

Optimizing the environment includes measures such as having the patient in a single room, placing a clock and calendar where the patient can see them, and turning off the television set to reduce the risk that the patient will misinterpret stimuli (eg, thinking that gunshots are coming from the corridor, rather than the television).

The most prominent signs and symptoms of the hypoactive-hypoalert form of delirium—obtundation, confusion, and poor concentration—cannot themselves be treated with medication, although they will quickly abate when the delirium is due to an intoxication for which there is an antidote (eg, physostigmine for atropine poisoning) or to a metabolic state that can be quickly corrected (eg, hypoglycemia). The most prominent signs and symptoms of the hyperactive-hyperalert form—agitation, hallucinations, and delusions—are more effectively treated with neuroleptic medications than with benzodiazepines. Haloperidol, which can be given intravenously if necessary, is especially useful in this regard, although it should be given with great caution if the patient's QT interval is prolonged because it can (although rarely) produce torsades de pointes. In general, the only situations in which benzodiazepines are preferable to neuroleptics are when neuroleptics are potentially dangerous (eg, when the patient has had the neuroleptic malignant syndrome) and in delirium tremens from alcohol, benzodiazepine, or barbiturate withdrawal, where benzodiazepines are the cornerstone of treatment and neuroleptics are given to help control hallucinations and delusions. (See Chapter 17 and 19 for more information about neuroleptics and benzodiazepines, respectively.)

Dementia

Important characteristics of this condition include:

- Global decline in cognitive function
- Normal level of consciousness

The dementia syndrome is characterized by three elements: adult onset, two or more cognitive impairments, and normal levels of consciousness and alertness. Onset in adulthood distinguishes dementia from lifelong mental retardation. The criterion of multiple cognitive impairments distinguishes it from focal cognitive syndromes such as the amnestic syndrome and aphasia. The requirement of normal levels of consciousness and alertness distinguishes it from delirium.

The definition does not include irreversibility or progression as essential, although most degenerative dementias (eg, Alzheimer's disease, dementia with Lewy bodies, frontotemporal dementia) have both qualities. A number of potentially reversible causes of dementia have been identified. The most common are medication-induced cognitive decline, hypothyroidism, major depression, and normal pressure hydrocephalus; these account for 1% to 2% of cases presenting for evaluation. The workup, therefore, includes a thorough physical, neurologic, and psychiatric examination; metabolic and hematologic laboratory studies; and brain neuroimaging. However, many potentially reversible cases do not improve after treatment. Nonprogressive dementias include those following head trauma and stroke.

Psychiatric symptoms are common in dementia irrespective of type. They include apathy (approximately 30%), agitation (approximately 25%), depression (approximately 20%), delusions (approximately 20%), and hallucinations (approximately 15%). In one community-based epidemiologic study, 60% of individuals with dementia had an identifiable psychiatric symptom cross-sectionally and 90% experienced at least one symptom at some time during the dementia. Lack of insight is also very common, even at the start of the illness, as are catastrophic reactions—sudden emotional outbursts usually precipitated by minor environmental stressors.

More than 75 diseases can cause the symptoms of dementia, so the differential diagnosis is extensive. Alzheimer's disease is most prevalent, accounting for approximately 60% of cases. Other common causes are vascular dementia (about 15%), mixed vascular dementia and Alzheimer's disease (about 10%), Lewy body dementia (about 15%), and frontotemporal dementia (about 5%).

The term "pseudodementia" was used in the past to refer to the dementia syndrome sometimes seen in major depression. It was thought to be "pseudo" because it was reversible—this at a time when the definition of dementia included irreversibility The dementia of depression is a "real" dementia in that it meets the defining characteristics of the syndrome. The term "pseudodementia" has also been used like the word "pseudoseizure" to indicate the presence of a conversion disorder, factitious disorder, or malingering.

The treatment of dementia focuses on five general elements: evaluation with subsequent discussion of the diagnosis and prognosis, pharmacologic treatment of the cognitive disorder and psychiatric symptoms (see Chapters 9 and 10), treatment of coexisting medical illnesses, nonpharmacologic and pharmacologic treatment of psychiatric symptoms such as hallucinations, and family support and referral to a support organization such as the Alzheimer's Disease Association. Referral to a psychiatrist should be made when the differential diagnosis includes depression, when the psychiatric symptoms are severe, when the psychiatric symptoms have not responded to two or three treatment trials, or when family discord is a prominent issue.

Catastrophic Reaction

Important characteristics of this condition include:

- Sudden expressions of negative emotion out of proportion to the precipitating stimulus
- Presence of an identifiable brain disease

Patients with cognitive impairments are vulnerable to outbursts of anger, anxiety, frustration, or sadness when they are faced with a task they cannot master or a situation that overwhelms them. These explosions of affect are called *catastrophic reactions*, and they can occur in patients with dementias, delirium, traumatic brain injuries, cerebrovascular accidents, and mental retardation.

Catastrophic reactions can be triggered not only by everyday situations (eg, when a caregiver impatiently asks a patient to do several things at once), but also by clinical ones (eg, when a physician conducts a bedside cognitive assessment). Catastrophic reactions usually last minutes, rather than hours, and they almost always respond to interpersonal interventions (eg, suspending the cognitive assessment, reassuring the patient, reducing noise and distractions in the environment).

When treating a patient who is vulnerable to catastrophic reactions, the goal should be to prevent their occurrence. The most important thing in this regard to make sure that everyone who interacts with the patient knows about this potential and acts accordingly. Thus, for example, caregivers should make only one request of patients at a time, and physicians who detect that patients are becoming distressed should immediately stop what they are doing and give the patients a chance to compose themselves.

Schizophrenia and Other Psychotic Disorders

Important characteristics of this condition include:

- Hallucinations, delusions, and/or thought disorder
- Dilapidation of social, occupational, and interpersonal function over time
- Absence of prominent mood symptoms
- Chronic course

The disorder referred to as schizophrenia is characterized by abnormalities in the content and form of thought, abnormalities in sensory experience, and a dilapidation over time in social and interpersonal functioning. In contrast to depression and de-moralization, the symptoms discussed in this section are alien to usual human experience and so more difficult to understand in the abstract, that is, without reference to clinical experience or case examples.

The abnormalities in the content of thought that are common in schizophrenia are delusions and first-rank symptoms as described in Chapter 1. No specific type of delusion is necessary, but delusions of persecution (sometimes referred to as "paranoid delusions") are most common. Grandiose delusions without mood elevation or elation are common as well. First-rank symptoms seen in schizophrenia that reflect abnormalities of thought content include delusional perception, or the sudden "realization" that an actual perception proves the accuracy of a delusion or an hallucination. Other abnormalities of thought include the belief that one's thoughts can be read by others, that thoughts or sensations are being beamed or projected into the person's brain or body, that thoughts are being withdrawn from a person's mind, or that observed phenomena such as a television refer directly to the person or have a special meaning that can only be understood by the patient.

The abnormalities in the form of thought manifest as a unique type of speech referred to as "thought disorder." In this form of thought, the ideas contained in sentences are not connected in a manner that can be understood in the context of usual speech. For example, "the sky is blue so I will go to the bank" might be connected in the patient's mind because the bank building is blue, but the two clauses are not recognized as linked in usual conversation. Thought disorder can usually be distinguished from aphasia by an absence of paraphasic errors, by intact repetition, naming and following multistep commands, and by the presence of connecting words (absent in nonfluent aphasia) and both nouns and verbs (diminished in fluent aphasia).

The abnormal sensory experiences are hallucinations, most commonly in the auditory realm. The content of these hallucinations are classically multiple voices talking about the person in the third person and commenting on his or her actions (eg, "look at her brush her teeth. I'll bet she's going to get sick") and are reported by the patient as coming from outside the head and through the ears just are "real" voices do.

The social and interpersonal dilapidation takes place over time. For this reason, many standardized diagnostic criteria include a length of illness criterion as a defining feature. For example, *Diagnostic and Statistical Manual*, fourth edition requires 6 months of symptoms as well as evidence of social, occupational or functional decline (APA, 1994). This reflects the original conceptualization of schizophrenia as "dementia praecox" by Emil Krapelin in the late 1890s.

The definition of schizophrenia also includes an exclusionary criterion. Both mood disorders (major depression and bipolar disorder) and cognitive disorder (delirium and dementia) must be excluded for a diagnosis of schizophrenia to be made. Depressive symptoms are sometimes present in patients with schizophrenia but either take the form of demoralization or clearly began after the symptoms of schizophrenia were established. The purpose of these exclusions is to rule out other causes of hallucinations and delusions that can be attributed directly to a structural brain lesion or to mood disorder that has a different treatment and time course. When delusions and hallucinations are seen in the mood disorders they are mood-congruent, that is, they can be seen to reflect the underlying mood-disordered state of the patient. Mood-congruent depressive delusions are often self-blaming or hopeless (eg, "the world is coming to an end because I am such a horrible person"— congruent with the depressed mood and diminished self-attitude of major depression) or grandiose (eg, "I can drive 110 miles an hour and not get hurt because I am the son of God"—

congruent with the elated mood and elevated self-concept of mania).

Schizophrenia-like disorders can be seen in association with several neurologic illnesses. In these cases, the criteria of the schizophrenic syndrome are met, even though a structural brain lesion is present.

Hallucinations or delusions can also be seen in association with structural brain disease of almost any sort. They are often referred to as psychotic phenomena and are distinguished from schizophrenia by a temporal association with the brain lesion, lack of thought disorder and dilapidation seen in schizophrenia, non–first-rank nature (ie, they are in sensory modalities other than auditory, or if they are auditory, they are not in the first or second person and are reported to come from inside the head).

The treatment of schizophrenia is primarily psychopharmacologic, but social and occupational therapies are an important component. Hallucinations and delusions that occur in the context of structural brain disease also respond to pharmacotherapy, but drug side effects are often a clinical challenge in such cases.

References

[APA] American Psychiatric Association (1994). *Diagnostic and Statistical Manual of Mental Disorders* (4th ed.). Washington, DC: American Psychiatric Association. p. 285.

Slavney, P.R. (1998). *Psychiatric Dimensions of Medical Practice: What Primary-Care Physicians Should Know about Delirium, Demoralization, Suicidal Thinking, and Competence to Refuse Medical Advice.* Baltimore, MD: Johns Hopkins University Press. pp. 39–51.

PART II

PSYCHIATRIC ASPECTS OF NEUROLOGIC DISEASES

3

Stroke

HOCHANG BEN LEE

JOHN R. LIPSEY

W ith an annual incidence of more than 600,000 cases, thromboembolic stroke is the third leading cause of death in the United States after heart disease and cancer (Kochanek et al., 2004). The number of stroke survivors has increased to 4.5 million adults nationally as the management of acute stroke continues to improve (AHA, 2002). Psychiatric syndromes are common complications of stroke and are associated with psychologic distress, increased impairment, poor rehabilitation outcomes, and excess morbidity. The purpose of this chapter is to describe clinically important poststroke psychiatric disorders and suggest appropriate treatment.

Vascular Cognitive Impairment and Dementia

Cognitive deficits are the most common psychiatric complication of stroke and affect nearly all stroke survivors. The type of cognitive disturbance depends on the location of the brain injury. Left hemisphere strokes frequently cause aphasia. Right hemisphere strokes cause substantial (but often underrecognized) cognitive impairments such as diminished insight, decreased attention, impaired spatial reasoning, and neglect syndromes. Furthermore, depending on the location of a stroke, other functions such as motivation, memory, judgment, and impulse control may also be affected.

A large stroke or a series of small strokes affecting both hemispheres may lead to the global cognitive impairment of dementia. When a series of strokes is involved, the cognitive decline develops in a stepwise manner. This *vascular dementia* or *multi-infarct dementia* may be difficult to distinguish from Alzheimer's disease. Autopsy studies of patients diagnosed with vascular dementia have often demonstrated the presence of Alzheimer's disease pathology. As many as 25% of all dementia cases are attributable to a combined neuropathology of Alzheimer's disease and multiple infarcts (Massoud et al., 1999).

In addition to strategies such as speech and language therapy, physical and occupational therapy, and cognitive rehabilitation, pharmacologic treatment may improve cognitive deficits in some stroke patients. The parallels between vascular dementia and Alzheimer's disease, as well as the evidence that reduced cholinergic function may play a role in both (Gottfries et al., 1994) have encouraged the use of acetylcholinesterase inhibitors (eg, donepezil) in vascular dementia. These drugs have shown modest benefits in such patients (Roman et al., 2005), and their use is described in Chapter 20.

Poststroke Depression

Although demoralization in the context of stroke-related impairment of cognitive capacity, physical function, social role, and independence is understandable, depression severity in patients with acute stroke is not strongly correlated with such impairment variables (Robinson et al., 1983). Depressive syndromes more severe and sustained than the sadness associated with demoralization occur frequently, and these mood disorders require specific treatment.

Major depression occurs in approximately 25% of hospitalized patients with acute stroke (Robinson et al., 1983; Astrom, Adolfsson, and Asplund, 1993) and is clinically almost indistinguishable from major depression in non–brain-injured patients (Lipsey et al., 1986). Frequent symptoms (in addition to sustained depression) include lack of energy, self-doubt, poor concentration, anorexia, sleep disturbance, pessimism, and anhedonia. Suicidal ideas may occur in 20% of such cases.

Somewhat less severe clinical depressions are also seen following stroke. These conditions (referred to as *minor depressions* or *dysthymic depressions*) have a narrower range of symptoms and occur in another 20% of acute stroke inpatients (Robinson et al., 1983). However, nearly 50% of these patients develop the full syndrome of major depression within the next 6 months (Robinson, Starr, and Price, 1984).

Left untreated, acute poststroke major depressions last approximately 1 year (Robinson, Bolduc, and Price, 1987). Minor depressions are more persistent: at 2-year follow-up, 70% of patients with such illnesses can be diagnosed with major or minor depression (Robinson, Bolduc, and Price, 1987). Thus, poststroke depressions are not only common and severe but long in duration.

In addition to psychologic suffering, poststroke depressions create other burdens for patients and their families. Major depression amplifies cognitive impairments following stroke and impedes cognitive recovery (Robinson et al., 1986). Moreover, untreated poststroke depressions hinder recovery in activities of daily living as measured 2 years following stroke (Parikh et al., 1990). Effects on mortality are even more striking: at 15-month or 10-year follow-up, patients with poststroke depression are between 3.5 and 8 times more likely to die than patients without depression (Morris, Robinson, and Samuels, 1993; Morris et al., 1993). The causes of poststroke depression remain unknown, and its anatomical correlates have been controversial in research studies. Left frontal cortical and left basal ganglia strokes are associated with the highest frequency of major depression during the acute poststroke period (Robinson et al., 1984; Starkstein, Robinson, and Price, 1987; Astrom, Adolfsson, and Asplund, 1993; Morris et al., 1996). Moreover, depression severity correlates directly and strongly with the proximity of these left-sided stroke lesions to the frontal pole (Robinson et al., 1984; Starkstein, Robinson, and Price, 1987). This correlation is much stronger than those between impairment variables (cognitive and physical) and depression (Robinson et al., 1983; Robinson et al., 1984), thus supporting the conclusion that poststroke major depression is more than a psychologic response to the consequences of medical illness.

Although some studies have not found a relationship between left frontal stroke lesions and depression in the first 2 months following stroke (House et al., 1990; Gainotti, Azzoni, and Marra, 1999), interstudy differences in the timing of psychiatric evaluation may account for the discrepancy in some investigations. That is, the frequency of depression in left hemisphere stroke is no greater than in right hemisphere stroke if evaluations are done at 3 or more months poststroke.

Given the severity and persistence of poststroke depressions and their adverse effects on rehabilitation, effective treatment is essential, whatever the location of the inciting brain injury. Two randomized, placebo-controlled studies of the tricyclic antidepressant (TCA) nortriptyline and one such study of the selective serotonin reuptake inhibitor (SSRI) citalopram have demonstrated the efficacy of these agents in the treatment of poststroke depression.

The first study (Lipsey et al., 1984) compared nortriptyline to placebo in the treatment of poststroke depression. Nortriptyline was slowly increased from 20 mg at bedtime to 100 mg at bedtime over 6 weeks. All patients on active medication achieved steady state serum nortriptyline levels within the accepted therapeutic range for treatment of major depression (50 to 140 ng/ml, drawn 10 to 14 hours after the last dose). Although patients assigned to placebo showed initial improvement, by 3 weeks those on active medication surpassed them, and by 6 weeks the nortriptyline group had a significantly greater recovery from depression.

Another 6-week study (Andersen, Vestergaard, and Lauritzen, 1994) demonstrated the superiority of citalopram over placebo in poststroke depression. Patients were treated with citalopram 20 mg daily (10 mg daily if over age 65) initially, and the dose could be doubled at 3 weeks if necessary. The citalopram group showed significantly greater improvement from the third week of treatment onward.

A most recent 12-week study (Robinson et al., 2000) compared patients randomly assigned to fluoxetine, nortriptyline, or placebo. Fluoxetine doses were slowly increased from 10 mg to 40 mg daily, and nortriptyline doses were slowly increased from 25 mg to 100 mg at bedtime. In this study, nortriptyline-treated patients had a significantly greater treatment response (63%) than those treated with fluoxetine (9%) or placebo (24%), and the latter two groups were not significantly different in their longitudinal response to treatment. Moreover, fluoxetine treatment was associated with a mean weight loss of 15 pounds over 12 weeks. It is possible that the dose of fluoxetine used in this study was excessive for elderly stroke patients and that lower doses may have been more effective.

Based on the above studies, a reasonable treatment approach for sustained poststroke depression is a trial of citalopram or nortriptyline. Citalopram is easier to use first in most patients because of its generally milder side effect profile. Patients may be started on 20 mg daily (10 mg in the elderly), with subsequent dose escalation to 40 mg daily over the next 3 or 4 weeks for patients who are not improving.

For patients for whom citalopram is ineffective or cannot be tolerated, a trial of nortriptyline is warranted if there are no contraindications to treatment with a TCA (eg, cardiac arrhythmia, heart block, ischemic heart disease, significant orthostatic hypotension, narrow-angle glaucoma, or urinary outlet obstruction). We choose nortriptyline over other TCAs because it usually causes less orthostatic hypotension, sedation, and anticholinergic effects than other drugs of its class. Moreover, it has a well established range of effective serum levels.

After obtaining a pretreatment electrocardiogram, we begin nortriptyline at 25 mg at bedtime for a week, and then obtain a 12-hour postdose serum level and follow-up orthostatic blood pressure measurement. Bedtime doses of nortriptyline may be increased by 10 to 25 mg per week as indicated by weekly serum levels, vital signs, treatment response, and tolerance of side effects. We aim to get most patients to the midpoint of the therapeutic range of serum levels (50 to 140 ng/ml), and few patients require more than 75 mg to 100 mg per day to achieve this. Side effects are minimized by raising doses slowly and monitoring steady state serum levels as doses increase.

Whichever agent is selected to treat depression, it is important to recognize that poststroke patients respond no more rapidly than patients without neurologic disorder. Although patients may improve in a few areas over the first 1 or 2 weeks of treatment (eg, better sleep, reduced anxiety), many patients do not begin to substantially improve until the third or fourth week. Full recovery, if it is reached, often takes 6 to 8 weeks, and a few patients require 10 or 12 weeks of treatment. Thus, patients need to be informed about the likely course of improvement so that they do not become inappropriately discouraged by the inevitable delay that precedes recovery.

Poststroke depression cases failing to respond to treatment should be seen by psychiatric consultants. Patients with delusional ideas accompanying their depression, and those with persistent wishes for death or suicidal ideas should also be promptly referred to psychiatrists. Furthermore, patients who develop medical complications of depression-related immobility and anorexia (eg, skin breakdown, aspiration, recurrent infections, deep venous thrombosis) must be seen by psychiatrists without delay so that effective treatment may proceed as rapidly as possible. Such treatments may include augmentation of antidepressants with lithium or neuroleptics, or consideration for electroconvulsive therapy. Many such patients require psychiatric admission.

Finally, all patients treated for depression must be carefully monitored for the development of suicidal thoughts or plans. Many patients do not report suicidal thoughts unless specifically asked about them at follow-up visits, and suicidal intentions or acts may emerge early in treatment when the patients' energy levels may improve before their moods. That is, a hopeless or self-critical patient with sustained depression may develop suicidal impulses as the energy to drive suicidal impulses increases. Family members of depressed patients must be educated about such risks during early treatment, and they and the patient must have ready access to communication with the physician.

Poststroke Mania

Mania is a rare complication of stroke, presenting in less than one percent of such patients (Robinson et al., 1988). When it occurs, the clinical phenomena (euphoria, grandiosity, excessive energy and activity) are the same as those seen in patients without brain injury. Frequent correlates of poststroke mania include right hemisphere lesion location and a family history of mood disorder (Robinson et al., 1988).

No systematic study of the treatment of poststroke mania has been completed. Case reports and general clinical experience suggest that lithium and valproic acid, the most effective mood stabilizers in idiopathic bipolar disorder, are also effective in stroke patients. Valproic acid may cause less gait disturbance and tendency to delirium in this population, but the tolerance for either agent shows great individual variability. Manic patients should be referred to psychiatrists. Their need for frequent monitoring when acutely ill, and their tendency toward impulsive action makes them appropriate cases for specialty care.

Poststroke Anxiety Disorders

Panic symptoms are a rare complication of stroke. Generalized anxiety, however, occurs in approximately 25% of patients after acute stroke (Castillo et al., 1993). In these patients, sustained anxiety and worry are accompanied by symptoms such as restlessness, fatigue, diminished concentration, sleep disturbance, muscle tension, and irritability. Almost 50% of patients with poststroke anxiety suffer from comorbid major depression, and another 25% have minor depression. Although the median duration of poststroke anxiety is only a few months, patients comorbid for anxiety and major depression have longer depressions and less improvement in activities of daily living than stroke patients with major depression alone.

No systematic treatment study of poststroke anxiety has been reported. Both TCAs and SSRIs are effective for generalized anxiety in general psychiatric populations. Given the diagnostic overlap between depression and anxiety in poststroke cases, both classes of drugs should be considered. Citalopram and nortriptyline may be used as they are in the treatment of poststroke depression. Occasionally, patients with generalized anxiety have an initial exacerbation of symptoms as antidepressants are begun. In that event, initial doses should be reduced (to 10 mg daily for citalopram and 10 mg at bedtime for nortriptyline) and subsequent dose escalations made more slowly.

Benzodiazepines, are generally poorly tolerated by stroke patients, whose vulnerabilities include their age, gait abnormalities, and tendency to easily become sedated or delirious.

Pathologic Laughing and Crying

Pathologic laughing and crying is a disorder of emotional expression seen in a wide variety of neurologic diseases, including stroke, amyotrophic lateral sclerosis, multiple sclerosis, Alzheimer's disease, brain tumors, gelastic epilepsy, and central nervous system infection. In patients suffering from the most severe form of pathologic laughing and crying, the vocal, respiratory, secretory, and vasomotor features of normal laughing and crying are preserved. However, the emotional displays are provoked by nonspecific or inappropriate stimuli may even develop spontaneously and are not associated with a congruent mood change. The laughter or crying comes on suddenly, is sensed by the patient as uncontrollable and irresistible, resolves slowly, and has a severity and duration that are stereotypical rather than varying with the stimulus. At times, laughter and crying are combined within a single episode.

A variety of terms have been used to describe this state of severely disinhibited affective display, including *organic emotionalism, emotional incontinence,* and *pseudobulbar affect.* The last term, however, implies a clinicopathologic correlation that is not uniform among the afflicted patients. Although pseudobulbar palsy has been associated with pathologic laughing and crying, some patients with pseudobulbar palsy have normal emotional expression. Likewise, many cases of pathologic laughing and crying are not associated with the pseudobulbar state.

In clinically less severe forms of pathologic laughing and crying, patients' disinhibited emotional expressions may not be totally inappropriate; rather, they are excessive in degree and duration to the stimulus that provoked them. For instance, a modestly sentimental experience provokes waves of tears, or a mildly amusing situation elicits irrepressible laughter. In these situations, patients may experience a mood change that is somewhat congruent to their affective response. The emotional expressions, however, remain pathologic in their excess, stereotypical nature, and resistance to usual control.

In the first year after acute stroke, 10%–20% of patients patients exhibit pathologic laughing or crying over 1 year follow-up (House et al., 1989). The condition occurs with unilateral or bilateral hemispheric lesions and may persist for many months. Bouts of laughter or crying, or a combination of the two, may occur many times a day, but crying episodes are experienced far more frequently than laughter. Episodes of either type, especially if frequent, impede conversation, embarrass the patient, impair family and social connections, and lead some patients to avoid social interactions altogether. Similarly, patients may find it difficult and embarrassing to participate in rehabilitation. At mealtimes, episodes may provoke aspiration, especially in patients with concurrent swallowing dysfunction.

Many stroke patients suffer from major depression and pathologic crying concurrently, whereas others may have only one of the disorders. Each condition may exacerbate the other, but the two syndromes are distinct—one is a disorder of mood itself, the other a disorder of affective expression.

Effective treatment of pathologic laughing and crying is imperative if the adverse effects for patients are to be avoided. Fortunately, successful treatments have been demonstrated in two well-controlled studies of stroke patients.

In the first such study (Andersen, Vestergaard, and Riis, 1993), 16 patients who had suffered strokes approximately 6 months earlier were treated with citalopram or placebo in a double-blind crossover design. None of the patients had major depression. All of the patients had pathologic crying episodes, and three had additional episodes of pathologic laughter. Citalopram was used at a dose of 20 mg daily for 3 weeks (10 mg daily for patients over 65 years). Citalopram treatment resulted in rapid and substantial reduction of symptoms compared to placebo, and in half of the patients a 50% reduction in the frequency of crying episodes occurred within the first 24 hours. After 3 weeks of treatment with citalopram, eight patients were completely free of bouts of crying. Relapse was rapid with discontinuation of active treatment.

The second study (Robinson et al., 1993) compared nor-triptyline (N = 14) to placebo (N = 20) in patients 8 to 16 months poststroke. Treatment assignment was double-blind. In contrast to the above study using citalopram, 19 of the patients had major depression in addition to pathologic affective display. Almost all of the patients had pathologic crying; only two had pathologic laughing. Nortriptyline dosage was slowly increased from 20 mg at bedtime to 100 mg at bedtime over 6 weeks. All patients were evaluated every 2 weeks using the Pathological Laughter and Crying Scale (Robinson et al., 1993), an instrument that quantifies these episodes based on duration, degree of voluntary control, inappropriateness in relation to emotions, degree of resultant distress, and relation of episodes to external events. Patients treated with nortriptyline showed significantly greater improvement than placebo-treated patients by 4 weeks. By the sixth week, the nortriptyline patients had a mean decrease of 90% on the Pathological Laughing and Crying scale, compared to a mean decrease of 30% in the placebo group. Response to treatment was independent of depression status.

Given these study results, we generally treat pathologic laughing and crying in stroke patients with citalopram (or another SSRI) as the initial treatment. Improvement on such agents is often rapid, and required dosage may be somewhat lower than that needed for the treatment of depression. Citalopram may be started at 20 mg daily (10 mg daily in the elderly) and increased only as needed by 10 mg per week. Doses greater than 40 mg daily are seldom required.

For patients whose pathologic laughing and crying does not respond to citalopram (and who have none of the contraindications noted above for treatment with TCAs), we use nortriptyline in the manner described above for the treatment of poststroke depression. However, if patients improve adequately on relatively lower serum levels than needed to treat major depression, we do not escalate the dose. Of course, if patients suffer from major depression and pathologic laughing and crying concurrently, the doses of any antidepressant must be adequate for the treatment of major depression. Patients whose illnesses fail to improve on the treatments described above should be evaluated by a psychiatrist.

Recently, Brooks et al. (2004) completed a double-blind study comparing dextromethorphan plus low-dose quinidine to dextromethorphan alone and quinidine alone in the treatment of pathologic laughing and crying among patients with amyotrophic lateral sclerosis. (Quinidine was used to increase available dextromethorphan blood levels.) The combination of dextromethorphan and quinidine reduced episodes of laughing and crying by 50% compared to treatment with either agent alone. Further experience will determine whether such treatment is equivalent to antidepressants in stroke patients with pathologic laughing and crying.

References

[AHA] American Heart Association (2002). *Heart Disease and Stroke Statistics—2003 Update.* Dallas, TX: American Heart Association.

Andersen, G., Vestergaard, K., Lauritzen, L. (1994). Effective treatment of poststroke depression with the selective serotonin reuptake inhibitor citalopram. *Stroke* 25: 1099–1104.

Andersen, G., Vestergaard, K., Riis, J. (1993). Citalopram for post-stroke pathological crying. *Lancet* 342: 837–9.

Astrom, M., Adolfsson, R., Asplund, K. (1993). Major depression in stroke patients: a 3-year longitudinal study. *Stroke* 24: 976–82.

Brooks, B.R., Thisted, R.A., Appel, S.H., Bradley, W.G., Olney, R.K., Berg, J.E., Pope, L.E., Smith, R.A. (2004). Treatment of pseudobulbar affect in ALS with dextromethorphan/quinidine. *Neurology* 63: 1364–70.

Castillo, C.S., Starkstein, S.E., Federoff, J.P., Price, T.R., Robinson, R.G. (1993). Generalized anxiety disorder following stroke. *Journal of Nervous and Mental Disease* 181: 100–6.

Gainotti, G., Azzoni, A., Marra, C. (1999). Frequency, phenomenology and anatomical-clinical correlates of major post-stroke depression. *British Journal of Psychiatry* 175: 163–7.

Gottfries, C.G., Blennow, K., Karlsson, I., Wallin, A. (1994). The neurochemistry of vascular dementia. *Dementia* 5: 163–7.

House, A., Dennis, M., Molyneux, A., Warlow, C., Hawton, K. (1989). Emotionalism after stroke. *British Medical Journal* 298: 991–4.

House, A., Dennis, M., Warlow, C., Hawton, K., Molyneux, K. (1990). Mood disorders after stroke and their relation to lesion location: a CT scan study. *Brain* 113: 1113–30.

Kochanek, K.D., Murphy, S.L., Anderson, R.N., Scott, C. (2004). Deaths: final data for 2002. National Vital Statistics Report Rep 53: 1–115.

Lipsey, J.R., Robinson, R.G., Pearlson, G.D., Rao, K., Price, T.R. (1984). Nortriptyline treatment of post-stroke depression: a double-blind study. *Lancet* 1 (8372): 297–300.

Lipsey, J.R., Spencer, W.C., Rabins, P.V., Robinson, R.G. (1986). Phenomenological comparison of poststroke depression and functional depression. *American Journal of Psychiatry* 143: 527–9.

Massoud, F., Devi, G., Stern, Y., Lawton, A., Goldman, J.E., Liu, Y., Chin, S.S., Mayeux, R. (1999). A clinicopathological comparison of community-based and clinic-based cohorts of patients with dementia. *Archives of Neurology* 56: 1368–73.

Morris, P.L., Robinson, R.G., Samuels, J. (1993). Depression, introversion and mortality following stroke. *The Australian and New Zealand Journal of Psychiatry* 24: 443–9.

Morris, P.L., Robinson, R.G., Andrezejewski P, Samuels, J., Price, T.R. (1993). Association of depression with 10-year post-stroke mortality. *American Journal of Psychiatry* 150: 124–9.

Morris, P.L., Robinson, R.G., Raphael, B., Hopwood, M.J. (1996). Lesion location and poststroke depression. *Journal of Neuropsychiatry and Clinical Neurosciences* 8: 399–403.

Parikh, R.M., Robinson, R.G., Lipsey, J.R., Starkstein, S.E., Federoff, J.P., Price, T.R. (1990). The impact of post-stroke depression on recovery in activities of daily living over a 2-year follow-up. *Archives of Neurology* 47: 785–9.

Robinson, R.G., Starr, L.B., Price, T.R. (1984). A two-year longitudinal study of mood disorders following stroke: prevalence and duration at six months follow-up. *British Journal of Psychiatry* 144: 256–62.

Robinson, R.G., Bolduc, P.L., Price, T.R. (1987). Two-year longitudinal study of post-stroke mood disorders: diagnosis and outcome at one and two years. *Stroke* 18: 837–43.

Robinson, R.G., Starr, L.B., Kubos, K.L., Price, T.R. (1983). A two-year longitudinal study of post-stroke mood disorders: findings during the initial evaluation. *Stroke* 14: 736–41.

Robinson, R.G., Kubos, K.L., Starr, L.B., Rao, K., Price, T.R. (1984). Mood disorders in stroke patients: importance of lesion location. *Brain* 107: 81–93.

Robinson, R.G., Bolla-Wilson, K., Kapan, E., Lipsey, J.R., Price, T.R. (1986). Depression influences intellectual impairment in stroke patients. *British Journal of Psychiatry* 148: 541–7.

Robinson, R.G., Boston, J.D., Starkstein, S.E., Price, T.R. (1988). Comparison of mania and depression after brain injury: causal factors. *American Journal of Psychiatry* 145: 172–8.

Robinson, R.G., Parikh, R.M., Lipsey, J.R., Starkstein, S.E., Price, T.R. (1993). Pathological laughter and crying following stroke: validation of a measurement scale and a double-bind treatment study. *American Journal of Psychiatry* 150: 286–93.

Robinson, R.G., Schultz, S.K., Castillo, C., Kopel, T., Kosier, J.T., Neman, R.M., Curdue, K., Petracca, G., Starkstein, S.E. (2000). Nortriptyline versus fluoxetine in the treatment of depression and in short-term recovery after stroke: a placebo-controlled double-blind study. *American Journal of Psychiatry* 157: 351–9.

Roman, G.C., Wilkinson, D.G., Doody, R.S., Black, S.E., Salloway, S.P., Schindler, R.J. (2005). Donepezil in vascular dementia: combined analysis of two large-scale clinical trials. *Dementia and Geriatric Cognitive Disorders* 20: 338–44.

Starkstein, S.E., Robinson, R.G., Price, T.R. (1987). Comparison of cortical and subcortical lesions in the production of poststroke mood disorders. *Brain* 110: 1045–59.

4

Traumatic Brain Injury

VANI RAO

Traumatic brain injury (TBI) is a significant cause of disability in the United States, with an incidence of about 1.5 million cases per year (National Institutes of Health Consensus Development Panel, 1999). It is associated with both neurologic and psychiatric consequences. Although the neurologic problems usually stabilize with time, the psychiatric disorders often continue to remit and relapse. Factors associated with the development of psychiatric disorders include older age, arteriosclerosis, and chronic alcoholism, all of which interfere with the reparative process within the central nervous system. Other contributors to psychiatric disability include a pre-TBI history of psychiatric illness, illicit drug abuse, and lack of social support. Because post-TBI psychiatric disturbances interfere with rehabilitation and cause emotional and financial burden for patients and caregivers, early diagnosis and treatment are important.

Post-TBI psychiatric disturbances are best classified according to their clinical presentation. These disturbances are discussed below and their pharmacologic and nonpharmacologic treatment strategies are recommended.

Mood Disorders

The mood disturbances most commonly associated with TBI are major depression, mania, anxiety, and apathy.

Major Depression

Major depression is seen in about 25% of people with TBI. Symptoms of major depression include persistent sadness; guilt; feelings of worthlessness; hopelessness; suicidal thoughts; anhedonia; and changes in patterns of sleep, appetite, and energy. Sometimes these symptoms may be associated with psychotic features such as delusions and hallucinations. It is important to remember that changes in sleep, appetite, or energy are not specific to the syndrome of major depression and may be due to the brain injury itself, or to the noise, stimulation, or deconditioning associated with hospitalization. If due to the latter conditions, gradual improvement occurs with time in most patients. Sadness in excess of the severity of injury and poor participation in rehabilitation are strong indicators of the presence of major depression. The presence of poor social functioning pre-TBI and left dorsolateral frontal and/or left basal ganglia lesion have been associated with an increased probability of developing major depression following brain injury (Jorge et al., 1993a; Jorge et al., 2004). Major depression should be differentiated from demoralization, primary apathy syndrome, and pathologic crying (Table 4–1).

Pharmacotherapy for post-TBI depression includes antidepressants, psychostimulants, and electroconvulsive therapy (ECT). Selective serotonin reuptake inhibitors (SSRIs) are the antidepressants of choice. Commonly used SSRIs include escitalopram, citalopram, and sertraline. Second-line antidepressants include venlafaxine, a serotonin/norepinephrine reuptake inhibitor, and mirtazapine, a presynaptic alpha-2 adrenergic/serotonin antagonist (Table 4–2). Drugs with anticholinergic potential such as tricyclic antidepressants (eg, amitriptyline, nortriptyline) and bupropion should only be used after a trial of the first- and second-line agents. The maximum dose of bupropion should not exceed 150 mg because higher doses are associated with increased risk of seizures. Psychostimulants (eg, methylphenidate) and dopaminergics (eg, amantadine) can be helpful to augment the effect of antidepressants. ECT is a highly effective mode of treatment for patients with TBI whose depression is refractory to antidepressants. In patients with TBI who have major depression with psychotic features, neuroleptics (eg, risperidone, olanzapine, quetiapine, aripiprazole) should be used in addition to antidepressants. If there is no

Table 4.1. Differential Diagnosis of Major Depression in TBI Patients

Signs and Symptoms	Major Depression	Demoralization	Apathy	Pathologic Crying
Depressed mood	Pervasive and persistent	Transient; related to physical and psychosocial changes associated with traumatic brain injury (TBI)	Not present	May be present
Changes in sleep, appetite, energy, concentration	Usually present	Transient	Often absent	Often absent
Decrease in self-worth	Often persistent and associated with guilt	Often absent	Not present	Often absent
Feeling of hopelessness	Most often present and persistent	Transient; related to physical and psychosocial changes associated with TBI	If present, transient	Not present
Suicidal thoughts	Often present	Often absent	Not present	Often absent
Lack of interest in usual activities	Often present	Transient	Always present; severe	Often absent
Initiation of activities	Decreased	Transient	Markedly decreased	Normal
Tearfulness	May be present	Transient; related to physical and psychosocial changes associated with TBI	Not present	Always present
Treatment	Medication and psychotherapy	Psychotherapy	Medications and psychotherapy	Medication and education

Table 4.2. Dosages (Total Daily) and Indications for Medications Commonly used to Treat Post-Traumatic Brain Injury Psychiatric Disturbances

Dosage	Indication
SELECTIVE SEROTONIN REUPTAKE INHIBITORS Escitalopram 5–20 mg Citalopram 10–40 mg Sertraline 50–150 mg	Major depression Pathologic crying Impulsivity/irritability
SEROTONIN-NOREPINEPHRINE REUPTAKE INHIBITOR Venlafaxine 25–225 mg	Major depression Pathologic crying Impulsivity/irritability
PRESYNAPTIC ALPHA-2 ADRENERGIC/SEROTONIN ANTAGONIST Mirtazapine 15–30 mg	Major depression Pathologic crying Insomnia
SEROTONIN ANTAGONIST AND REUPTAKE INHIBITOR Trazodone 50–200 mg	Insomnia
DOPAMINE AGONISTS Amantadine 50–200 mg Bromocriptine 2.5–20 mg	Apathy Inattention Impulsivity Major depression
PSYCHOSTIMULANTS Methylphenidate 2.5–20 mg	Apathy Inattention Impulsivity Major depression
ANTICONVULSANTS Valproate 125–1000 mg Carbamazepine 100–400 mg	Mania Impulsivity Aggression
ATYPICAL ANTIPSYCHOTICS Risperidone 0.25–4 mg Olanzapine 2.5–20 mg Quetiapine 12.5–200 mg Aripiprazole 5–30 mg	Psychotic phenomenon Severe agitation or aggression (brief period only)
CHOLINESTERASE INHIBITORS Donepezil 5–10 mg Galantamine 8–16 mg Rivastigmine 3–12 mg	Memory problems Inattention Apathy
BETA BLOCKERS Propranolol 60–520 mg	Aggression

improvement in depressive or psychotic symptoms after a single trial of an antidepressant and a neuroleptic, patients should be referred to a psychiatrist for further treatment.

Psychotherapy for depression includes supportive therapy (ie, providing education and hope), interpersonal therapy (focusing on social interactions with the goal of improving communication skills and self-esteem), and cognitive-behavioral therapy (ie, identifying distorted thinking patterns and establishing new patterns by directing attention to incorrect assumptions patients make about themselves and others). Supportive psychotherapy can begin in the neurologist's office, and patients can be referred to mental health professionals for other types of psychotherapy, if necessary.

Mania

Mania after TBI is less common than major depression but much more common than in the general population. The characteristic features of mania are elevated mood, increased energy, decreased need for sleep, irritability, agitation, aggression, impulsivity, and even violent behavior. Very often, manic symptoms are associated with psychotic symptoms such as grandiose delusions, persecutory delusions, and auditory hallucinations. There is no consistency in the literature regarding the relationship between lesion location and the development of mania after TBI.

Mania should be differentiated from personality changes associated with TBI. In a single cross-sectional evaluation, it may be difficult to differentiate a manic episode from the disinhibited or impulsive personality change associated with TBI. Hence there is a need to obtain collateral information from family members and caregivers regarding the duration and chronicity of symptoms. The key differentiating feature is that mania is episodic and personality change is persistent.

It is important to make this distinction because treatment differs. Anticonvulsants (eg, valproate, carbamazepine) are the preferred drugs for the treatment of mania, whereas dopamine agonists (eg, amantadine) and stimulants (eg, methylphenidate) are often used for the treatment of post-TBI personality changes (Table 4–2). If the latter drugs are used in mania, they can worsen manic symptoms. Lithium carbonate, a mood stabilizer, is considered a second-line agent for the treatment of mania, because patients with TBI are often sensitive to its neurotoxic side effects. Neuroleptics (eg, risperidone, olanzapine, quetiapine, aripiprazole) should be considered the first-line of drugs when patients present with symptoms of acute agitation, restlessness, and psychosis. In general, patients with mania should be referred immediately to a psychiatrist because symptoms can increase in severity rather rapidly, either requiring aggressive outpatient treatment or immediate hospitalization. Psychotherapy for the patient with mania is not effective unless the illness is very mild. However, support, education, and hope should be provided to caregivers, because they are often overwhelmed and stressed.

Anxiety

Anxiety disorders are common in patients with TBI and can present as generalized anxiety disorder, panic disorder, phobic disorders, post-traumatic stress disorder, and obsessive-compulsive disorder. The most common presentation is that of generalized anxiety disorder associated with persistent worry, tension, and fearfulness. More often than with lesions elsewhere, anxiety disorder is associated with right hemispheric cortical lesions (Jorge et al., 1993b).

Medication treatment for persistent anxiety often includes use of SSRIs. An important treatment point is avoidance of chronic use of benzodiazepines, because they tend to cause memory impairment, motor incoordination, and sometimes paradoxical excitation. However, SSRIs take at least a few weeks to be effective, so benzodiazepines such as lorazepam (0.25–2 mg/day) can be used in patients with moderate to severe anxiety for 1 to 2 weeks. In addition to medications, patients with anxiety disorders also do well with cognitive-behavioral therapy. The goal of the cognitive component is to change unhealthy and harmful thinking patterns that prevent anxious persons from overcoming fears. The goal of the behavioral component is to alleviate anxiety by exposing patients to anxiety-provoking situations in a controlled and structured setting. Patients with anxiety disorders who do not improve on medications or are unwilling to take medications should be referred to mental health professionals experienced in cognitive-behavioral techniques.

Apathy

Apathy is common after TBI. Symptoms include loss of interest in day-to-day activities, poor engagement in interpersonal relationships, lack of initiation in starting new activities, reduced motivation in participating in rehabilitation, and diminished emotional responsiveness (Marin and Wilkosz, 2005). Apathy may be due to the brain injury or to associated depression, delirium, or dementia. With apathy caused by brain injury itself, the dsyphoric symptoms of major depression (eg, sadness, guilt, hopelessness, and suicidal thoughts) are not seen. Damage to the mesial frontal lobe and its subcortical structures has been implicated in the genesis of apathy.

Stimulants (eg, methylphenidate), and dopaminergic agents (eg, amantadine, bromocriptine) have been found to be useful in the treatment of post-TBI apathy (Table 4–2). Cholinesterase inhibitors (eg, donepezil, galantamine, rivastigmine) can also be considered; they have found to be efficacious in the treatment of apathy related to dementia. Caregiver education about apathy is very important because caregivers often consider apathetic patients to be lazy. Caregivers should be educated and helped to tread the fine line between gently encouraging the patient to become involved in activities and pushing the patient too hard, because this can lead to agitation and other behavior problems. An occupational therapy assessment of motor and processing skills is often helpful to understand the patient's cognitive and functional capabilities. Occupational therapists can often help patients and caregivers to devise and maintain a daily routine.

Cognitive Impairments

TBI is associated with impairments in one or more of the cognitive domains of arousal, attention, concentration, memory, language, and executive function. Cognitive impairments can be seen in all stages of recovery after injury. The acute stage, immediately after the injury, is characterized by a period of unconsciousness that can vary in duration from a few seconds to days, depending on the severity of injury. The next stage is characterized by a mixture of cognitive and behavioral abnormalities such as poor concentration, inattention, inability to learn new information, agitation, confusion, disorientation, and alteration in psychomotor activity. These first two stages last anywhere from minutes to a few days. During the early recovery stage, there is a 6- to 12-month period of rapid recovery of cognitive function, followed by stabilization for another 6 to 12 months. The last phase is characterized by permanent cognitive sequelae and may include problems in one or more cognitive domains. This phase has also been described as dementia due to head trauma.

The cognitive deficits are caused by the cumulative effects of focal and diffuse brain damage. Cognitive outcome depends on a number of factors: degree of diffuse axonal injury, duration of loss of consciousness, clinical evidence of brainstem dysfunction at the time of injury, and presence and size of focal hemispheric injury (Novack et al., 2001).

Treatment of post-TBI cognitive impairments is multidisciplinary and includes neurologists, physiatrists, psychiatrists, and psychologists working together. Medication treatment includes use of dopaminergics (eg, amantadine) and psychostimulants (eg, methylphenidate) to treat attention problems and cholinesterase inhibitors (eg, donepezil, rivastigmine, galantamine) to treat short-term memory problems (Table 4–2).

In addition to medications, nonpharmacologic approaches such as cognitive rehabilitation are beneficial. Cognitive rehabilitation is an effective mode of treatment for post-TBI cognitive deficits, although it is still unclear what TBI and demographic factors enhance cognitive rehabilitation outcomes (Cicerone et al., 2005). The goal of cognitive rehabilitation is to improve functioning by strengthening learned patterns of behavior and establishing new patterns of compensatory activity in specific cognitive domains. Cognitive rehabilitation can be initiated in the neurologist's office by encouraging patients to maintain a timetable for each day, to improve concentration by reducing distractions (eg., turning off the radio or television while working on a task), and to use external aides (eg, day-planner, personal digital assistant) to help remember appointments and events. Neurologists can also educate patients who have executive function deficits not to act on their impulses, but to stop and think about the situation. To this end, telling patients to use a "stop–think–act" formula is helpful. These kinds of compensatory techniques are really common-sense approaches to improved functioning and may seem very simple. However, after TBI, patients with cognitive deficits are often not aware of their problems and require repeated education and reminders. If these approaches fail, patients can be referred to outpatient rehabilitation programs for comprehensive assessment and treatment of cognitive deficits. Information on TBI rehabilitation day programs can be obtained by contacting the local chapter of the Brain Injury Association of America.

Behavior Disorders

Behavioral problems are very commonly seen after TBI and can interfere with the rehabilitative process. Common behavior problems include inability to control a sudden desire to do or say something, aggression, social inappropriateness, impulsivity, decreased motivation, and poor judgment with consequent unsafe behaviors. They can occur in isolation or together and can range in severity from outbursts of yelling to severe physically violent behavior. Post-TBI behavior problems have been called by various diagnostic terms such as *frontal-temporal lobe syndrome, personality changes due to TBI,* and *organic personality syndrome.*

Catastrophic reaction is an emotional-behavioral problem that more commonly occurs in TBI patients with significant cognitive deficits. Common precipitants include failure to comprehend or perform a task, real or perceived threat, and stressful or demanding situations. It is characterized by outbursts of yelling or screaming, crying or laughing uncontrollably, hand-wringing, making false accusations, and sometimes even physically aggressive behavior (eg, pushing people, throwing objects). Catastrophic reactions can occur very suddenly and can be frightening to the caregiver.

Evaluation of behavior problems include assessing the type of behavior and its severity and duration; the presence of mood changes, psychotic phenomena, and seizures; the ability of the person to be redirected; and associated triggers. Family members and caregivers are good collateral informants and are often able to provide relevant history on the behavior problems; hence they should always be interviewed. If the behavioral problem is due to depression, mania, or a schizophrenia-like psychosis, appropriate treatment of these disorders should be initiated. However, in a cross-sectional examination or in an acute situation, it may not be possible to evaluate the behavior problem completely and or to diagnose a psychiatric disorder such as mania. In this case, an immediate psychiatric consultation should be obtained, with the goal of admission to a psychiatric unit. Mild nondisruptive behavior problems can be managed in an outpatient setting. Medication treatment includes use of dopaminergics, psychostimulants, SSRIs, high-dose beta-blockers (eg, propranolol), and mood stabilizers (Table 4–2). Family members and caregivers should also be educated about strategies such as environmental and behavioral modification (eg, reducing stimuli, redirection of inappropriate behavior, reinforcement of appropriate behavior). However, if these techniques are ineffective, patients should be referred to mental health professionals who have experience in this area.

Catastrophic reactions do not respond well to medications. However, if the patient is becoming increasingly agitated, low-dose benzodiazepines (eg, lorazepam, 0.25–0.5 mg) or low-dose atypical antipsychotics (eg, risperidone, 0.25–5.0 mg; quetiapine, 25–50 mg; or olanzapine, 2.5–5.0 mg) can be used to treat the acute agitation. Identification and avoidance of triggers are the key factors in the management of catastrophic reactions. When they do occur, caregivers should be educated about staying calm, reassuring the patient, redirecting the patient's attention, and removing the patient from the stressful situation.

Schizophrenia-like Psychosis

Psychotic phenomena (ie, hallucinations, delusions, thought disorder) are more common in patients with TBI than in the general population. Psychotic phenomena can occur in the settings of delirium, dementia, mania, or depression, as well as in isolation from these syndromes in a disorder that resembles schizophrenia. Risk factors associated with the development of a schizophrenia-like psychosis after TBI include positive family history of schizophrenia, mild TBI, occurrence of brain injury in the adolescent period, and presence of mild neurologic dysfunction at birth (Fujii and Ahmed, 2001). Common presentations include hallucinations, delusions, and thought disorder occurring together, or the isolated occurrence of persecutory delusions, thought disorder, or auditory hallucinations. Both right and left hemispheric injuries have been implicated in the etiology of schizophrenia-like psychosis after TBI. In the pharmacologic treatment of this disorder, "atypical" neuroleptics (eg, risperidone, olanzapine, quetiapine, aripiprazole) are the drugs of choice (Table 4–2). Animal studies reveal that "typical" neuroleptics such as haloperidol delay neuronal recovery (Feeney, Gonzales, and Law, 1982). If no improvement occurs after use of neuroleptics, anticonvulsants (eg, valproate, carbamazepine) can be tried in case the psychotic phenomenon are manifestations of subclinical seizures (Fujii and Ahmed, 2002). Similarly, even though this seems counterintuitive, dopaminergics (eg, amantadine) have been found to be useful in people with psychotic symptoms associated with severe frontal lobe injury.

Other Psychiatric Disturbances

In addition to the previously mentioned conditions, two other psychiatric disorders are often seen in patients with TBI: postconcussive syndrome (PCS) and sleep disturbance. PCS refers to a cluster of phenomena that are more often seen after mild TBI than after moderate or severe TBI. The syndrome includes physical, cognitive, and emotional symptoms such as headaches, dizziness, fatigue, increased sensitivity to noise and other stimuli; memory lapses; poor concentration; sadness; anger; anxiety; and irritability. About 80% to 90% of people with PCS spontaneously recover within the first three months, whereas about 10% to 15% have residual symptoms that can last for 1 or more years. Diffuse axonal injury from acceleration and deceleration forces is thought to be the cause. In most people with this disorder, the neurologic examination is essentially normal. There is no specific medication treatment for PCS. However, it is important to provide education and support to the patient and caregivers. If symptoms persist beyond 3 months or cause interference with daily activities, careful evaluation must be done to rule out other neurologic (eg, chronic subdural hematoma, vestibular dysfunction) or psychiatric (eg, major depression, generalized anxiety disorder) conditions.   ˈ

Sleep problems, including excessive daytime sleepiness and sleeplessness at night, are common after TBI. Careful evaluation is necessary to rule out disorders (eg, delirium, major depression) that can disrupt sleep. Patients with an isolated sleep disturbance should be educated about sleep hygiene: maintaining regular sleeping hours; avoiding late afternoon and nighttime caffeine, alcohol, and tobacco; avoiding exercise and stimulating activities before bedtime; and minimizing daytime napping. If this is not effective, medications such as trazodone can be used for the treatment of sleeplessness (Table 4–2). Excessive daytime sleepiness is best managed by nonpharmacologic treatment modalities such as maintaining a structured timetable for the day and following sleep hygiene rules. If the sleep problem is persistent and resistant to treatment, patients should be referred for sleep studies to rule out causes such as sleep apnea.

General Guidelines for the Treatment of Psychiatric Sequelae of Traumatic Brain Injury

Treatment of TBI-associated psychiatric disorders is complex and challenging. The approach should be multidisciplinary, with the neurologist working in close collaboration with the other physicians and with physical therapists, occupational therapists, nurses, and social workers. A treatment plan should be formulated as soon as the psychiatric diagnosis is made, with the goals of improving quality of life, maximizing productivity, and minimizing disability. Treatment often includes a combination of pharmacotherapy and psychotherapy for the patient, plus support and education of caregivers. The treatment plan should take into take into account the nature and severity of the TBI, the neurologic and psychiatric disturbances, and the patient's social circumstances and resources. The plan should be flexible, changing with the needs of the patient and family. Psychiatric consultation should be obtained when disturbances are severe or dangerous (eg, marked reduction of food and fluid intake, aggression to self or others) or when there is poor or no response after a first trial of medications.

The general principles regarding pharmacotherapy, psychotherapy, and caregiver support and education are outlined below.

Pharmacotherapy

Table 4–2 describes the indications and dosages of medications commonly used to treat post-TBI psychiatric disturbances. In general, patients with TBI are very sensitive to medications; hence one should follow the golden rule of "start low and go slow." Other principles include minimizing the number of medications; avoiding, if possible, medications that may have a deleterious effect on the central nervous system (eg, phenytoin, haloperidol, barbiturates, benzodiazepines); monitoring serum levels of medications; and discussing indications, risks, and benefits of medications with patients and family members.

Psychotherapy

Psychotherapy is very important in the rehabilitation of patients with post-TBI psychiatric disorders. Supportive psychotherapy should include recommendations on nutrition, regular exercise, and the importance of maintaining a routine. Patients and caregivers should be encouraged to attend brain injury support groups and to maintain contact with local and national brain injury associations. As discussed above, if other types of psychotherapy are warranted, patients should be referred to experienced mental health professionals. To identify such experienced personnel, calling brain injury rehabilitation programs in the area or the local chapter of the Brain Injury Association of America is a good starting place.

Caregiver Support and Education

A caregiver may be a family member, a friend, or a professional care provider. Who ever it is, addressing caregiver's needs is important because caregivers often experience major depression and anxiety as a result of caring for a person with TBI (Marsh et al., 1998). In addition, other problems such as financial difficulties, role changes, social isolation, and impaired family functioning are also common. Support of caregivers is therefore an essential component of treatment of the brain-injured patient. The general approach to caregiver support and education includes education about the nature and sequelae of the injury;

provision of emotional support; psychiatric care if symptoms of anxiety or low mood are persistent; encouragement to use resources such as local and national brain injury associations; and discussion of the importance of respite care.

References

Cicerone, K.D., Dahlberg, C., Malec, J.F., Langenbahn, D.M., Felicetti, T., Kneipp, S., Ellmo, W., Kalmar, K., Giacino, J.T., Harley, J.P., Laatsch, L., Morse, P.A., Catanese, J. (2005). Evidence-based cognitive rehabilitation: updated review of the literature from 1998 through 2002. *Archives of Physical Medicine and Rehabilitation* 86: 1681–92.

Feeney, D., Gonzales, A., Law, W. (1982). Amphetamine, haloperidol and experience interact to affect rate of recovery after motor cortex injury. *Science* 217: 855–7.

Fujii, D.E., Ahmed, I. (2001). Risk factors in psychosis secondary to traumatic brain injury. *Journal of Neuropsychiatry and Clinical Neurosciences* 13: 61–9.

Fujii, D., Ahmed, I. (2002). Characteristics of psychiatric disorder due to traumatic brain injury: an analysis of case studies in the literature. *Journal of Neuropsychiatry and Clinical Neurosciences* 14: 130–40.

Jorge, R.E., Robinson, R.G., Arndt, S.V., Forrester, AW., Geisler, F., Starkstein, SE. Comparison between acute- and delayed-onset depression following traumatic brain injury (1993a). *Journal of Neuropsychiatry and Clinical Neurosciences*. 5(1): 43–9

Jorge, R.E., Robinson, R.G., Starkstein, S.E., Arndt, S.V. (1993b). Depression and anxiety following traumatic brain injury. *Journal of Neuropsychiatry and Clinical Neurosciences* 5: 369–74.

Jorge, R.E., Robinson, R.G., Moser, D., Tateno, A., Crespo-Facorro, B., Arndt, S. (2004). Major depression following traumatic brain injury. *Archives of General Psychiatry* 61(1): 42–50.

Marin, R.S., Wilkosz, P.A. (2005). Disorders of diminished motivation. *The Journal of Head Trauma Rehabilitation* 20: 377–88.

Marsh, N.V., Kersel, D.A., Havill, J.H., Sleigh, J.W. (1998). Caregiver burden at 1 year following severe traumatic brain injury. *Brain Injury* 12: 1045–59.

National Institutes of Health Consensus Development Panel on Rehabilitation of Persons with Traumatic Brain Injury (1999). Rehabilitation of persons with traumatic brain injury. *Journal of the American Medical Association* 282: 974–83.

Novack, T.A., Bush, B.A., Meythaler, J.M., Canupp, K. (2001). Outcome after traumatic brain injury: pathway analysis of contributions from premorbid, injury severity, and recovery variables. *Archives of Physical Medicine and Rehabilitation* 82: 300–5.

5

Headaches and Chronic Pain

MICHAEL R. CLARK

Pain has been defined as "an unpleasant sensory and emotional experience associated with actual or potential tissue damage, or described in terms of such damage" (Lindblom et al., 1986). Table 5–1 contains definitions of terms commonly used to describe pain sensations (Merskey et al., 1986). Pain is the most common reason a patient presents to a physician for evaluation. The U.S. Center for Health Statistics found that 32.8% of the general population suffers from chronic pain symptoms (Magni et al., 1993). Many factors can influence patients' reports of pain, including medical and psychiatric disorders, social circumstances, disease states, personality traits, memory of past pain experiences, and personal interpretations of the meaning of pain (Clark and Treisman, 2004). There

Table 5.1. Definitions Relating to Pain Sensations

- Allodynia–pain from a stimulus that does not normally provoke pain
- Deafferentation pain–pain resulting from loss of sensory input into the central nervous system
- Dysesthesia–an unpleasant, abnormal sensation that can be spontaneous or evoked
- Hyperalgesia–an increased response to a stimulus that is normally painful
- Hyperesthesia–increased sensitivity to stimulation that excludes the special senses
- Hyperpathia–pain characterized by an increased reaction to a stimulus, especially a repetitive stimulus, and an increased painful threshold to that stimulus
- Hypoesthesia–diminished sensitivity to stimulation that excludes the special senses
- Nociception–detection of tissue damage in skin and deeper structures and the central propagation of this information via A delta and C fibers in the peripheral nerves
- Paresthesia–an abnormal sensation, spontaneous or evoked, that is not unpleasant
- Sensitization–lowered threshold and prolonged or enhanced response to stimulation

Source: Merskey et al 1986.

is no simple algorithm for determining whether the cause of pain is psychologic or neurologic (Clark and Chodynicki, 2005). The clinical evaluation of patients complaining of pain should be comprehensive and incorporate the patient's descriptions of pain (ie, location, intensity, duration, precipitants, ameliorators); observations of pain-related behaviors (eg, limping, guarding, moaning); descriptions of problems performing activities; and neurologic and psychiatric examinations (Clark and Cox, 2002).

Selected Chronic Pain Conditions

Post-Herpetic Neuralgia

Post-herpetic neuralgia (PHN) is defined as pain persisting or recurring at the site of shingles at least 3 months after the onset of the acute varicella zoster viral rash. PHN occurs in about 10% of patients with acute herpes zoster. More than 50% of patients older than 65 years of age with shingles develop PHN, and it is more likely to occur in patients with cancer, diabetes mellitus, and immunosuppression. During the acute episode of shingles, characteristics such as more severe pain and rash, presence of sensory impairment, and higher levels of emotional distress are associated with developing PHN (Schmader, 2002). Most cases gradually improve, with only about 25% of patients with PHN experiencing pain 1 year after diagnosis. Approximately 15% of patients referred to pain clinics suffer from PHN. Early treatment of varicella zoster with low-dose amitriptyline (25–100 mg QD) can reduce the prevalence of pain at 6 months by 50% (Bowsher, 1997). In addition to tricyclic antidepressants (TCAs) such as amitriptyline, anticonvulsants (eg, sodium valproate, 125–500 mg BID) and opioids (eg, sustained-release oxycodone, 10–120 mg QD) are the most common effective treatments for

PHN and may have potential for its prevention (Dworkin and Schmader, 2003).

Peripheral Neuropathy Pain

The pain of a peripheral neuropathy can be any or all of the following: constant, paroxysmal, evoked, burning, lancinating, or electrical (Mendell and Sahenk, 2003). These phenomena are primarily the result of axonal degeneration, segmental demyelination, and ectopic impulse generation. When a peripheral nerve is damaged, central sensitization amplifies and sustains neuronal activity, which increases pain. Pharmacologic treatments for the pain of peripheral neuropathy are similar to those utilized in the treatment of PHN.

Parkinson's Disease

Pain is the most common sensory manifestation of Parkinson's disease and is reported by half of patients with that condition (Starkstein, Preziosi, and Robinson, 1991). The pain is typically described as a cramping and aching in the lower back and extremities, not associated with muscle contraction or spasm. These pains often decrease when the patient is treated with levodopa, suggesting a central origin or central sensitization. Optimizing dopaminergic transmission for the improvement of primary motor functions typically improves pain. However, in some patients, pain remains an independent symptom that should be treated with the agents described above for neuropathic pain conditions.

Central Post-Stroke Pain

Approximately 5% of patients who have suffered a stroke experience intractable pain (Bowsher, 1995). Patients typically have hemibody sensory deficits and pain associated with dysesthesias, allodynia, and hyperalgesia. Lesions are usually present in the thalamus, although other sites are often involved. Pharmacological treatment is usually not effective for such pain, although TCAs, serotonin-norepinephrine reuptake inhibitors (SNRIs; e.g., venlafaxine, duloxetine), anticonvulsants, and opioids should be tried to improve this refractory illness.

Migraine and Chronic Daily Headache

Over their lifespans, 18% of women and 6% of men suffer from migraine (Lipton, Stewart, and Von Korff, 1997). The peak incidence of migraine occurs between the third and sixth decades of life and then decreases with age. Calcium channel blockers (eg, verapamil, 80–160 mg TID–QID), beta-blockers (eg, atenolol, 50–100 mg BID), antidepressants (eg, nortriptyline, 25–150 mg QD), and anticonvulsants (eg, valproate, 125–500 BID) are the treatments with the best-documented efficacy. Multidisciplinary treatment consisting of modalities such as stress management, supervised exercise, dietary education, and massage therapy significantly improve outcomes (Lemstra, Stewart, and Olszynski, 2002).

Headache is the most common pain condition reported by the U.S. workforce as the reason for lost productivity (Stewart et al,. 2003). Chronic daily headache affects about 5% of the population and includes several conditions: migraine, chronic tension-type headaches, and hemicrania continua (Lake and Saper, 2002). Patients with chronic daily headache are at risk for overuse medication with resulting rebound headache, psychiatric comorbidity such as depression and anxiety, functional disability, and stress-related headache exacerbations. The traditional prophylactic agents such as those described above should be tried for the treatment of chronic daily headaches. Abortive medications (eg, sumatriptan) typically used in the treatment of migraine should be avoided because of rebound pain and dependence. Combined medication and cognitive-behavioral psychotherapy are more effective than either treatment alone.

Low Back Pain

Low back pain (LBP) is one of the most common and costly physical complaints in terms of lost productivity and health care expenditures (Stewart et al., 2003). Poor functional status 4 weeks after seeking treatment is the most powerful predictor of pain chronicity. Both economic and social rewards are associated with higher levels of disability and depression (Ciccone, Just, and Bandilla, 1999). Patients with LBP who are not working and involved in litigation have higher scores on measures of pain, depression, and disability than those who have returned to work (Suter, 2002). Anxiety, depression, and mental stress attributed to the patient's occupation predict lower rates of return to work in patients undergoing lumbar surgeries than those without such psychiatric symptoms (Trief, Grant, and Fredrickson, 2000). Although treatment of chronic LBP often produces symptom reduction, there is conflicting evidence about its ability to improve functional status, particularly returning to work. Even conservative interventions such as education, exercise, massage, and transcutaneous electrical stimulation produce inconsistent results (Pengel, Maher, and Refshauge, 2002). Multidisciplinary (eg, medicine, psychology, physical therapy, occupational therapy) rehabilitation programs usually offer the best outcomes (Karjalainen et al., 2003). For treatment to succeed, the patient's self-perceived level of disability must be decreased.

Complex Regional Pain Syndrome (Causalgia and Reflex Sympathetic Dystrophy)

The term *complex regional pain syndrome* (CRPS) has replaced *reflex sympathetic dystrophy* (CRPS type I) and *causalgia* (CRPS type II) (Stanton-Hicks et al., 1995). The symptoms of CRPS are not limited to a single peripheral nerve but usually involve an extremity. Type I is precipitated by a specific noxious trauma or immobilization of the affected area and is characterized by a spontaneous burning pain usually associated with hyperalgesia or allodynia to cutaneous stimuli. Pain is usually accompanied by evidence of vascular and sudomotor dysfunction in the affected region. Motor changes such as tremor, weakness, and limitations in movement are common. Type II is distinguished

Table 5.2. Commonly Used Antidepressant Medications for Chronic Pain

Generic Name (brand)	Daily Dose
HETEROCYCLIC TERTIARY AMINES (TCAS)	
Amitriptyline (Elavil)	50–300 mg
Imipramine (Tofranil)	50–300 mg
Doxepin (Sinequan)	50–300 mg
HETEROCYCLIC SECONDARY AMINES (TCAS)	
Nortriptyline (Pamelor)	50–150 mg
Desipramine (Norpramin)	75–300 mg
SEROTONIN-NOREPINEPHRINE REUPTAKE INHIBITORS	
Venlafaxine (Effexor)	75–450 mg
Duloxetine (Cymbalta)	30–120 mg

Table 5.3. Commonly Used Anticonvulsant Medications for Chronic Pain

Generic Name (brand)	Daily Dose
Carbamazepine (Tegretol)	100–1200 mg
Oxcarbazepine (Trileptal)	150–1200 mg
Divalproex sodium (Depakote)	125–1000 mg
Lamotrigine (Lamictal)	25–400 mg
Topiramate (Topamax)	25–400 mg
Gabapentin (Neurontin)	100–3600 mg
Pregabalin (Lyrica)	50–600 mg
Tiagabine (Gabitril)	2–32 mg

from type I by the presence of nerve injury; this is the only difference between the types.

Patients with CRPS progress through three clinical stages. Stage 1 (acute, early) is characterized by an inflammatory onset with constant aching or burning pain. Stage 2 (dystrophic, intermediate) is notable for cool, pale, and cyanotic skin. Stage 3 (atrophic, late) manifests as atrophy and wasting of multiple soft tissues, fixed joint contractures, and osteoporosis. When pain is relieved by blockade of the efferent sympathetic nervous

Table 5.4. Commonly Used Opioid Medications for Chronic Pain

Generic Name (brand)	Daily Dose
ORAL	
Morphine (Avinza, MS Contin, Kadian)	15–300 mg
Oxycodone (OxyContin)	10–200 mg
Methadone (Dolophine)	10–100 mg
TRANSDERMAL	
Fentanyl (Duragesic)	12.5–100 μg/h

system, the diagnostic modifier, *sympathetically maintained pain (SMP)*, is added, and the patient usually complains of hyperalgesia to cold stimuli.

Patients with CRPS often exhibit emotional distress and psychiatric disorders. Affective (46%), anxiety (27%), and substance abuse disorders (14%) are most common (Rommel et al., 2001). Treatment for CRPS usually combines regional sympathetic blocks with oral sympatholytics (eg, clonidine); physical therapies that increase activity, range of motion, and strength; adjuvant analgesic medications (eg, antidepressants, anticonvulsants, opioids, see Tables 5–2 to 5–4); electrical stimulation of peripheral nerves or spinal cord; and even surgical sympathectomy.

Orofacial Pain

Trigeminal neuralgia (tic douloureux) is a chronic pain syndrome with severe, unilateral, paroxysmal, recurrent, lancinating pain in the distribution of the trigeminal nerve that most commonly involves the mandibular division. Sensory or motor deficits are not usually present. Pain can be spontaneous or evoked by nonpainful stimuli to trigger zones: activities such as talking or chewing; or environmental conditions such as cold air or water. Between episodes, patients are typically pain-free. Pain syndromes involving the intermedius branch of the facial nerve or the glossopharyngeal nerve are less common and present with pain that can involve the ear, posterior pharynx, tongue, or larynx.

The majority of patients with classical trigeminal neuralgia show evidence of trigeminal nerve root compression by blood vessels (85%), mass lesions, or other diseases (eg, multiple sclerosis, herpes zoster, PHN) that cause demyelination and hyperactivity of the trigeminal nucleus (Love and Coakham, 2001). Pharmacological treatment includes anticonvulsants (Table 5–3), antidepressants (Table 5–2), baclofen (15–60 mg/day), topical lidocaine, and opioids (Table 5–4). When pharmacologic treatments fail, a variety of surgical procedures such as microvascular decompression, percutaneous gangliolysis, and stereotactic radiosurgery may be undertaken.

Cluster headache occurs predominantly in men, with an onset before age 25. The episodes of pain, described as excruciating, surround one eye, last minutes to hours, and are associated with autonomic symptoms (eg, tearing, rhinorrhea, erythema). Short-lasting, unilateral, neuralgiform pain with conjunctival injection and tearing (SUNCT) syndrome is a rare condition that commonly affects older males, and the Tolosa-Hunt syndrome presents with pain in the ocular area accompanied by ipsilateral paresis of cranial nerves III, IV, V_1, and VI. When no clear diagnosis can be made, the diagnosis of *atypical facial pain* is used. These patients more commonly exhibit psychiatric disorders (eg, depression, addiction, personality disorders) that amplify their pain, distress, and disability (Kapur, Kamel, and Herlich, 2003). The treatments for these atypical headache syndromes are generally the same as those used in the treatment of migraine, but they also include oxygen inhalation and steroids for symptomatic treatment of cluster headache as well as lithium, 150–600 mg/day. Sphenopalatine ganglion neural blockade may be effective in refractory patients.

Burning mouth syndrome (BMS) is characterized by pain in oral and pharyngeal cavities, especially the tongue, often associated with dryness and taste alterations. Most cases are idiopathic and are accompanied by depression and anxiety (Drage and Rogers, 2003). The disorder mainly affects middle-aged, postmenopausal women, and the oral mucosa is usually normal. Psychological factors such as severe life events (eg, divorce, death of a family member, life-threatening illness) have been associated with the condition. Potential underlying etiologies include nutritional/hormonal deficiencies (e.g., estrogen, iron, folate, vitamin B_{12}), maladaptive oral habits (eg. bruxism), and medications (eg, anticholinergics, antibiotics, corticosteroids). Treatment with TCAs (eg, nortriptyline, 50–150 mg/day; desipramine, 100–300 mg/day), selective serotonin reuptake inhibitors (SSRIs) (eg, fluoxetine, 20–80 mg/day; sertraline, 50–300 mg/day; escitalopram, 10–40 mg/day), anticonvulsants (eg, pregabalin, 150–600 mg/day; gabapentin, 300–1800 mg/day), or nutritional (eg, B-complex vitamins) or hormonal supplements (eg, estrogen, progesterone) has been effective for some patients with BMS (Zakrzewska, Glenny, and Forssell, 2001).

Psychiatric Comorbidity

Somatization Disorder

The diagnosis of somatization disorder is rarely made in patients with chronic pain. Most patients with multiple medically unexplained symptoms have subsyndromal forms of somatization disorder, depressive disorders, or anxiety disorders (Dickinson et al., 2003). Such patients are likely to catastrophize the severity of their symptoms, to believe that the cause of their pain is a mystery, to express feelings of losing control, and to think that physicians believe that their pain is imaginary. Patients with chronic pain and medically unexplained symptoms are at risk for iatrogenic consequences of excessive diagnostic tests, inappropriate medications, and unneeded surgery. The treatment of these patients starts with the recognition that they are legitimately suffering. The plan of care should validate patients' distress, reformulate the diagnosis as a disorder that requires psychologic treatments, limit potentially dangerous evaluations and interventions (eg, exploratory surgery, toxic medications), remove any reinforcing factors of patients' distress and illness behaviors (eg, visiting Internet sites and chat rooms, taking unnecessary medications, seeking excessive consultations), and treat psychiatric diagnoses (eg, major depression, generalized anxiety disorder, panic disorder).

Medication Abuse and Dependence

The prevalence of medication dependence (addiction) in patients with chronic pain ranges from 3% to 19% (Nicholson, 2003). The core criteria for a medication use disorder (Table 5–5) in patients with chronic pain include: (1) loss of control in the use of the medication, (2) excessive preoccupation with the medication despite adequate analgesia, and (3) adverse consequences associated with the medication use (American Academy of Pain Medicine, 2001; Savage et al., 2003). Risk factors for addiction to prescribed medications include patients' belief that they are addicted, an increase in their analgesic dose or frequency, and a preference for a certain route of administration (eg, intravenous versus intramuscular). The presence of aberrant behaviors (eg, misusing medications, obtaining medications from multiple sources, reporting prescriptions as lost or stolen) must be demonstrated to diagnose addiction, because physical dependence and tolerance alone are expected physiologic phenomena associated with chronic treatment.

Determining whether patients with chronic pain are abusing prescribed controlled medications (eg, opioids, benzodiazepines) is a routine but challenging issue. Patients with chronic pain who develop problems with their opioid medication generally have a history of substance abuse, and the onset of that abuse usually predates the chronic pain disorder (Brown et al., 1996). However, inaccurate reporting of medication use by patients complicates the assessment of addiction. In patients with chronic pain who developed new substance use disorders, the problem most commonly involves the medications pre-

Table 5.5. Definitions Relating to Medication Use (American Academy of Pain Medicine, the American Pain Society and the American Society of Addiction Medicine 2001; Savage *et al.* 2003)

Term	Definition
Abuse	Harmful use of a specific psychoactive substance
Addiction	A chronic neurobiologic disease, with genetic, psychosocial, and environmental factors influencing its development and manifestations. It is characterized by behaviors that include one or more of the following: impaired control over drug use, compulsive use, continued use despite harm, and craving.
Misuse	Any use of a prescription drug that varies from accepted medical practice
Physical dependence	A state of adaptation that is manifested by a drug class–specific withdrawal syndrome that can be produced by abrupt cessation, rapid dose reduction, decreasing blood level of the drug, and/or administration of an antagonist
Psychologic dependence	A subjective sense of need for a specific psychoactive substance, either for its positive effects or to avoid negative effects associated with its abstinence
Tolerance	A state of adaptation to the presence of a drug in the body such that increased doses are required to produce the pharmacologic effects initially resulting from smaller doses

American Academy of Pain Medicine, American Pain Society, American Society of Addiction Medicine. (2001). Definitions related to the use of opioids for the treatment of pain. *Wisconsin Medical Journal* 100: 28–9; Savage, S.R., Joranson, D.E., Covington, E.C., Schnoll, S.H., Heit, H.A., Gilson, A.M. (2003). Definitions related to the medical use of the opioids: evolution towards universal agreement. *Journal of Pain and Symptom Management* 26: 655–67.

scribed by their physicians (Long et al., 1988). Patients with preexisting substance use disorders have increased rates of chronic pain and are at the greatest risk for stigmatization and undertreatment with appropriate medications (Rosenblum et al., 2003).

The prevention of opioid abuse should begin with a treatment agreement for all patients to clarify the conditions under which opioids will be prescribed. The agreement should explicitly describe all the conditions under which the use of opioids will be considered inappropriate and include the consequences that will result if abuse is detected. Such consequences include tapering opioid medications and discharge from care (Fishman et al., 2002). A single physician should direct therapy and prescribe small quantities, perform random pill counts, and not refill lost supplies. External sources of information such as urine toxicology testing, interviews with the patient's relatives, conversations with pharmacists and other physicians, data from prescription monitoring programs, and review of past medical records can improve detection of medication use disorders. Patients who deny using illicit substances that are detected on urine toxicology screens are more likely to be younger, to be receiving workers' compensation benefits, and to have a previous diagnosis of polysubstance abuse (Katz and Fanciullo, 2002).

Major Depression

In World Health Organization data from 14 countries on five continents, 69% (range, 45%–95%) of patients with depression presented with only somatic symptoms, of which pain complaints were most common (Simon et al., 1999). These somatic symptoms are usually medically unexplained and associated with high levels of health care utilization and patient dissatisfaction with care. Depressive disorder doubles the risk of developing new-onset chronic musculoskeletal pain, headache, LBP, and chest pain (Larson, Clark, and Eaton, 2004). As for the converse association, the Canadian National Population Health Survey found that the incidence of major depression is doubled in subjects who report a long-term medical condition such as back problems and migraine (Patten, 2001). In patients with medically unexplained symptoms such as back pain, 67% have a history of recurrent major depression compared with less than 20% of medically ill control groups (Sullivan and Katon, 1993).

Depression in patients with chronic pain is associated with greater pain intensity; more pain persistence; feelings that life is out of control; use of passive-avoidant coping strategies (eg, praying pain will stop, decreasing physical activity); noncompliance with treatment; application for early retirement; and greater interference with daily activities from pain, including more pain behaviors observed by others (Magni et al., 1993). Depression is a better predictor of disability than pain intensity or duration. Thus, for example, the presence of preoperative depression in patients undergoing lumbar diskectomy predicts poorer surgical outcome at 1-year follow-up, and primary care patients with musculoskeletal pain complicated by depression use more medications, especially sedative-hypnotics, than patients without depression (Mantyselka et al., 2002).

The symptoms of impaired self-attitude, hopelessness, suicidal ideation, and neurovegetative phenomena (eg, early morning awakening, diurnal mood variation) are more likely to indicate a major depression than a state of demoralization that occurs in most patients living with chronic pain. Patients suffering from chronic pain syndromes including migraine, chronic abdominal pain, and orthopedic pain syndromes have increased rates of suicidal ideation, suicide attempts, and suicide completion (Magni et al., 1998). Cancer patients with pain and depression, but not pain alone, are significantly more likely to take steps to end their lives (Emanuel et al., 1996). Although TCAs and SNRIs are superior to SSRIs in the treatment of neuropathic pain, this distinction does not exist in the treatment of major depression. Antidepressants should be prescribed at the doses usually recommended for the treatment of major depression (eg, fluoxetine, 20–40 mg/day; citalopram, 20–80 mg/day; bupropion, 150–300 mg/day; nortriptyline, 50–150 mg/day; venlafaxine, 75–225 mg/day; duloxetine, 40–120 mg/day).

Anxiety, Fear, and Catastrophizing

Almost 50% of patients with chronic pain report anxiety symptoms (eg, nervousness, worry, tension) and as many as 30% of patients have an anxiety disorder such as panic disorder or generalized anxiety disorder (Dersh, Polatin, and Gatchel, 2002). Fear of pain, movement, reinjury, and other negative consequences that result in the avoidance of activities promote the transition to and sustaining of chronic pain and its associated disabilities (Vlaeyen and Linton, 2000). Fear-avoidance beliefs are one of the most significant predictors of failure to return to work in patients with chronic low back pain. If the avoidance provides any short-term benefits such as reducing anticipatory anxiety or relieving the patient of unwanted responsibilities, then disability is reinforced. Catastrophic thinking about pain is marked by symptom magnification, rumination about symptoms, and feelings of helplessness. Pain-related cognitions like catastrophizing and fear-avoidance beliefs predict poor coping and adjustment to chronic pain better than objective factors such as disease status, physical impairment, or occupational descriptions. Treatment for anxiety disorders usually requires a combination of medications (ie, antidepressants and benzodiazepines) and psychotherapy (see below).

Pharmacologic Treatment of Chronic Pain

Unfortunately, medications are often underutilized and under-dosed in the treatment of patients with chronic pain. In one study of neuropathic pain, 73% of patients complained of inadequate pain control, but 72% had never received anticonvulsants, 60% had never received TCAs, 41% had never received opioids; 25% of patients had never received any of these medications (Gilron et al., 2002). Physicians still attempt to alleviate pain with simple analgesics and fail to appreciate the advantages of adjuvant medications.

Opioids

The analgesic effects of opioids typically decrease the distressing affective component of pain more than the physical sensation of pain. An exception to this is in neuropathic pain, where studies of neuropathic pain show that opioids decrease pain intensity instead of counteracting the unpleasantness of pain (Dellemijn and Vaneste, 1997). For example, continuous-release morphine decreases the pain intensity of patients with PHN significantly more than TCAs (Raja et al., 2002). Long-acting opioid preparations should be used for long-term treatment of chronic pain conditions (Table 5–4).

The treatment of nonmalignant chronic pain with opioids remains a subject of considerable debate because of physicians' concerns about regulatory pressure; medication abuse by patients; and criminal prosecution of physicians for causing addiction, drug trafficking, and insurance fraud (Ballantyne and Mao, 2003). Successful treatment of chronic pain with opioids requires the assessment and documentation of improvements in function and analgesia without accompanying adverse side effects and medication-related aberrant behaviors. The Federation of State Medical Boards, the American Academy of Pain Medicine, the American Pain Society, and the American Geriatric Society have produced guidelines for the treatment of chronic pain (American Geriatric Society Panel on Chronic Pain in Older Persons, 1998). If opioid therapy is unsuccessful, the medication should be gradually tapered and discontinued.

The development of tolerance to opioids is uncommon in clinical practice (Freye and Latasch, 2003). A return of, or even an increase in, pain can be the result of disease progression; new injury; comorbid psychiatric disorders; or medication effects such as toxicity, withdrawal, or opioid-induced hyperalgesia. If tolerance develops, suggested strategies include simultaneous administration of other agents (eg, opioid agonists with differing receptor affinities; ultra–low-dose opioid antagonists; calcium channel blockers; alpha-2 agonists; cyclooxygenase-2 inhibitors; N-methyl-D-aspartate [NMDA] receptor antagonists such as ketamine, dextromethorphan, memantine, and amantadine); opioid rotation to a more potent agonist; and intermittent cessation of certain agents (eg, opioids, benzodiazepines) (Bolan, Tallarida, and Pasternak, 2002). Similarly, augmentation of analgesia may occur by using opioids that possess NMDA antagonist actions such as methadone or those that inhibit monoamine reuptake such as methadone, tramadol, and levorphanol.

Antidepressants

The analgesic effect of antidepressants is probably mediated by the blockade of reuptake of norepinephrine and serotonin, increasing their availability in the spinal cord to enhance the activation of descending inhibitory neurons. However, antidepressants may produce antinociceptive effects through a variety of other pharmacologic mechanisms (Ansari, 2000). Typically, the analgesic effects of antidepressants are independent of improvement in mood.

Antidepressants, particularly the TCAs, are commonly prescribed for chronic pain syndromes, including diabetic neuropathy, trigeminal neuralgia, postherpetic neuralgia, central pain, headaches, and oral-facial pain (Clark, 2000). Nortriptyline is better tolerated than amitriptyline with equivalent efficacy (Dworkin and Schmader, 2003). Noradrenergic activity is often associated with better analgesic effects than serotonergic activity alone. The efficacy of SSRIs in chronic pain syndromes has been poor and inconsistent.

The SNRIs venlafaxine and duloxetine inhibit the presynaptic reuptake of both serotonin and norepinephrine without the side effects and potential toxicity of the TCAs. Relatively higher doses of venlafaxine (eg, 225–375 mg/day) are generally recommended to achieve analgesic action for neuropathic pain. Duloxetine more potently blocks 5-HT and norepinephrine transporters than venlafaxine (Bymaster et al., 2001). Duloxetine is an effective treatment for major depression and significantly reduces associated painful physical complaints at doses of 60–120 mg per day (Detke et al., 2002). Duloxetine decreases the pain of fibromyalgia and painful diabetic neuropathy without depression (Arnold et al., 2005; Goldstein et al., 2005).

Anticonvulsants

Anticonvulsants (Table 5–3) are effective for trigeminal neuralgia, diabetic neuropathy, PHN, and migraine recurrence (Wiffen et al., 2000). Carbamazepine is the most widely studied anticonvulsant effective for neuropathic pain. Valproic acid is used in the prophylaxis of migraine and cluster headache but is also effective in the treatment of neuropathic pain (Gallagher, Mueller, and Freitag, 2002). Gabapentin can reduce neuropathic pain in multiple sclerosis, migraine, PHN, spinal cord injury, human immunodeficiency virus (HIV)-related neuropathy, reflex sympathetic dystrophy, diabetic peripheral neuropathy, and postamputation phantom limb pain (Serpell and the Neuropathic Pain Study Group, 2002). Patients are more likely to benefit from gabapentin if they had experienced allodynia as a feature of their neuropathic pain (Gustorff et al., 2002). Topiramate, tiagabine, pregabalin, and lamotrigine are newer anticonvulsants that have also been shown to be effective for the same spectrum of chronic pain disorders as the older anticonvulsants (Marson et al., 1997). Pregabalin is similar to gabapentin but with greater potency and linear bioavailability

(Chen, Xu, and Pan, 2001). Topiramate offers the advantages of low protein binding, minimal hepatic metabolism, a long half-life, and the unusual side effect of weight loss.

Benzodiazepines

Benzodiazepines (BZs) are commonly prescribed for insomnia and anxiety in patients with chronic pain, but there is little evidence of their utility (King and Strain, 1990). Only a limited number of chronic pain conditions such as trigeminal neuralgia, phantom limb pain, tension headache, and temporomandibular disorders improve when treated with BZs (Dellemijn and Fields, 1994). Although BZs can be helpful in some chronic pain conditions, they should generally be avoided because they can have many negative consequences. Dependence, with a potentially fatal withdrawal syndrome, is the most serious of these, but there are others of concern. Thus, for example, the use of BZs in patients with chronic pain is associated with increased rates of healthcare visits, domestic instability, depression, disability days, and cognitive impairment (Buffett-Jerrott and Stewart, 2002). BZs have also been associated with exacerbation of pain, interference with opioid analgesia, and development of tolerance (Freye and Latasch, 2003; Nemmani and Mogil, 2003).

Psychologic Treatment

Psychological treatment for chronic pain was pioneered by Fordyce using a behavioral model (Fordyce et al., 1973). In treatment, productive behaviors are targeted for reinforcement and pain behaviors (eg, grimacing, guarding, taking analgesics) for extinction. For patients with chronic pain, behavioral treatment can decrease pain intensity and improve behavioral outcomes (van Tulder et al., 2001). The cognitive-behavioral model of chronic pain assumes that individual perceptions and evaluations of life experiences affect emotional and behavioral reactions to these experiences. If patients believe that pain, depression, and disability are inevitable and uncontrollable, then they experience more negative emotional responses, increased pain, and even more impaired physical and psychosocial functioning.

The components of cognitive-behavioral therapy (CBT) such as relaxation and cognitive restructuring to minimize distressing thoughts and feelings interrupt this cycle of disability (Turner, 1982; Turner and Chapman, 1982). CBT has produced significant improvements in pain intensity, pain behaviors, physical symptoms, depression, coping, physical functioning, treatment-related and indirect socioeconomic costs, and rates of returning to work (Hiller, Fichter, and Rief, 2003).

Referral for Specialty Treatment

Patients should be referred for additional consultations when their level of disability, associated pain behaviors, and emotional distress is beyond that expected for their condition. In other words, when patients complain of multiple medically unexplained somatic symptoms, are not coping well with their illness, are misusing medications, or are beginning to use increasing amounts of health care resources without improvement, the neurologist should seek additional input about their treatment.

Patients should be referred to a psychiatrist in several situations. First, immediate referral to a psychiatrist should occur if the patient reports suicidal thoughts, especially if they are accompanied by hopelessness. Second, a psychiatrist should evaluate the patient when there is diagnostic uncertainty, complicated medical comorbidity, or another psychiatric condition such as substance abuse, depression, or a personality disorder. Third, a psychiatrist may be able to design pharmacologic treatments for patients who have failed to respond completely to initial medication trials.

Psychologic treatments are important for patients suffering with chronic pain disorders. Mental health professionals other than psychiatrists specialize in psychologic treatments and should be utilized by the neurologist when referral to a psychiatrist is not required. Specifically, referral should occur when patients have mild to moderate symptoms but do not want to take medications, when they have residual symptoms (eg, anxiety, insomnia) that could benefit from relaxation techniques, and when they have difficulty coping with the impact of the illness on their lives and relationships. Many different types of psychotherapy are practiced by many different types of mental health professionals.

Psychologists with a special interest in behavioral medicine or expertise in pain management provide CBT. These techniques offer specific applications for chronic pain disorders such as anxiety management; cognitive restructuring that recognizes, challenges, and formulates alternatives to anxious thoughts; applied relaxation and electromyography biofeedback; and behavioral methods such as graded exposure and systematic desensitization. Social workers and nurse therapists are more likely to specialize in interpersonal relationships and emotion-focused psychotherapy. These target the themes of patients' difficulties in managing negative emotions, feelings of loss, and needing to maintain interpersonal control in relationships. After patients have identified the emotional components of their distress as well as their associated meanings, treatment shifts to learning how to manage troubling emotions.

Multidisciplinary Treatment

The multidisciplinary pain center offers a full range of treatments for the most difficult pain syndromes in a setting that encourages patients to take an active role in improving their functional status and reinforces positive changes in behavior. Specifically, interventions are designed to change maladaptive behavior such as inactivity and social withdrawal, alter maladaptive cognitions such as catastrophizing and passive expectations of medical care, adopt active and positive coping skills, identify and stop conditioned illness behavior, and increase emotional control and stability while decreasing affective distress and depression.

Multidisciplinary pain programs improve patient functioning globally and in a number of specific areas (eg, pain intensity, depression, disability, pain-related cognitions, coping responses) (Jensen, Turner, and Romano, 2001). Quality of life improves with multidisciplinary pain treatment and is associated with lower levels of pain, distress, and interference with performing daily activities.

Ultimately, the goal of treating patients with chronic pain is to end their disability and return them to productive activities. One of the most important predictors of returning to work is the patient's own intention of doing so. For example, good job availability, high satisfaction, low dangerousness, fewer physical demands, and absence of related litigation are factors more likely to increase the odds of a patient's return to work (Fishbain et al., 1999). In the longest follow-up study (13 years) of an inpatient pain management program, 50% of the patients were employed, compared with only 10% at the time of admission (Maruta et al., 1998).

References

American Academy of Pain Medicine, American Pain Society, American Society of Addiction Medicine. (2001). Definitions related to the use of opioids for the treatment of pain. *Wisconsin Medical Journal* 100: 28–9.

American Geriatric Society Panel on Chronic Pain in Older Persons. (1998). The management of chronic pain in older persons. *Journal of the American Geriatrics Society* 46: 635–51.

Ansari, A. (2000). The efficacy of newer antidepressants in the treatment of chronic pain: a review of current literature. *Harvard Review of Psychiatry* 7: 257–77.

Arnold, L.M., Rosen, A., Pritchett, Y.L., D'Souza, D.N., Goldstein, D.J., Iyengar, S., Wernicke, J.F. (2005). A randomized, double-blind, placebo-controlled trial of duloxetine in the treatment of women with fibromyalgia with or without major depressive disorder. *Pain* 119:5–15.

Ballantyne, J.C., Mao, J. (2003). Opioid therapy for chronic pain. *New England Journal of Medicine* 349: 1943–53.

Bolan, E.A., Tallarida, R.J., Pasternak, G.W. (2002). Synergy between mu opioid ligands: evidence for functional interactions among mu opioid receptor subtypes. *Journal of Pharmacology and Experimental Therapeutics* 303: 557–62.

Bowsher, D. (1995). The management of central post-stroke pain. *Postgraduate Medical Journal* 71: 598–604.

Bowsher, D. (1997). The effects of pre-emptive treatment of postherpetic neuralgia with amitriptyline: a randomized, double-blind, placebo-controlled trial. *Journal of Pain and Symptom Management* 13: 327–31.

Brown, R.L., Patterson, J.J., Rounds, L.A., Papasouliotis, O. (1996). Substance use among patients with chronic pain. *Journal of Family Practice* 43: 152–60.

Buffett-Jerrott, S.E., Stewart, S.H. (2002). Cognitive and sedative effects of benzodiazepine use. *Current Pharmaceutical Design* 8: 45–58.

Bymaster, F.P., Dreshfield-Ahmad, L.J., Threlkeld, P.G., Shaw, J.L., Thompson, L., Nelson, D.L., Hemrick-Luecke, S.K., Wong, D.T. (2001). Comparative affinity of duloxetine and venlafaxine for serotonin and norepinephrine transporters in vitro and in vivo, human serotonin receptor subtypes, and other neuronal receptors. *Neuropsychopharmacology* 25: 871–80.

Chen, S.R., Xu, Z., Pan, H.L. (2001). Stereospecific effect of pregabalin on ectopic afferent discharges neuropathic pain induced by sciatic nerve ligation in rats. *Anesthesiology* 95: 1473–9.

Ciccone, D.S., Just, N., Bandilla, E.B. (1999). A comparison of economic and social reward in patients with chronic nonmalignant back pain. *Psychosomatic Medicine* 61: 552–63.

Clark, M.R. (2000). Pharmacological treatments for chronic non-malignant pain. *International Review of Psychiatry* 12: 148–56.

Clark, M.R., Chodynicki, M.P. (2005). Pain Management. In J. Levenson (Ed.), *Textbook of Psychosomatic Medicine*. Washington, DC: American Psychiatric Publishing. pp. 827–67.

Clark, M.R., Cox, T.S. (2002). Refractory chronic pain. *Psychiatric Clinics of North America* 25: 71–88.

Clark, M.R., Treisman, G.T. (2004). Perspectives on pain and depression. *Advances in Psychosomatic Medicine* 25: 1–27.

Dellemijn, P.L., Fields, H.L. (1994). Do benzodiazepines have a role in chronic pain management? *Pain* 57: 137–52.

Dellemijn, P.L., Vanneste, J.A. (1997). Randomised double-blind active-placebo-controlled crossover trial of intravenous fentanyl in neuropathic pain. *Lancet* 349:753–758.

Dersh, J., Polatin, P.B., Gatchel, R.J. (2002). Chronic pain and psychopathology: research findings and theoretical considerations. *Psychosomatic Medicine* 64: 773–86.

Detke, M.J., Lu, Y., Goldstein, D.J., McNamara, R.K., Demitrack, M.A. (2002). Duloxetine 60 mg once daily dosing versus placebo in the acute treatment of major depression *Journal of Psychiatric Research* 36: 383–90.

Dickinson, W.P., Dickinson, L.M., deGruy, F.V., Candib, L.M., Main, D.S., Libby, A.M., Rost, K. (2003). The somatization in primary care study: a tale of three diagnoses. *General Hospital Psychiatry* 25: 1–7.

Drage, L.A., Rogers, R.S. III (2003). Burning mouth syndrome. *Dermatologic Clinics* 21: 135–45.

Dworkin, R.H., Schmader, K.E. (2003). Treatment and prevention of postherpetic neuralgia. *Clinical Infectious Diseases* 36: 877–82.

Emanuel, E.J., Fairclough, D.L., Daniels, E.R., Clarridge, B.R. (1996). Euthanasia and physician-assisted suicide: attitudes and experiences of oncology patients, oncologists, and the public. *Lancet* 347: 1805–10.

Fishbain, D.A., Cutler, R.B., Rosomoff, H.L., Khalil, T., Steele-Rosomoff, R. (1999). Prediction of "intent," "discrepancy with intent," and "discrepancy with nonintent" for the patient with chronic pain to return to work after treatment at a pain facility. *Clinical Journal of Pain* 15: 141–50.

Fishman SM, Mahajan G, Jung S, Wilsey, B.L. (2002). The trilateral opioid contract: bridging the pain clinic and the primary care physician through the opioid contract. *Journal of Pain and Symptom Management* 24: 335–44.

Fordyce, W., Fowler, R., Lehmann, J., Delateur, B.J., Sand, P.L., Trieschmann, R.B. (1973). Operant conditioning in the treatment of chronic pain. *Archives of Physical Medicine and Rehabilitation* 54: 399–408.

Freye, E., Latasch, L (2003). Development of opioid tolerance—molecular mechanisms and clinical consequences. *Anästhesiologie, Intensivmedizin, Notfallmedizin, Schmerztherapie* 38: 14–26.

Gallagher, R.M., Mueller, L.L., Freitag, F.G. (2002). Divalproex sodium in the treatment of migraine and cluster headache. *Journal of the American Osteopathic Association* 102: 92–4.

Gilron, I., Bailey, J., Weaver, D.F., Houlden, R.L. (2002). Patients' attitudes and prior treatments in neuropathic pain: A pilot study. *Pain Research and Management* 7: 199–203.

Goldstein, D.J., Lu, Y., Detke, M,J., Lee, T.C., Iyengar, S. (2005) Duloxetine vs. placebo in patients with painful diabetic neuropathy. *Pain* 116: 109–18.

Gustorff, B., Nahlik, G., Spacek, A., Kress, H.G. (2002). Gabapentin in the treatment of chronic intractable pain. *Schmerz* 16: 9–14.

Hiller, W., Fichter, M.M., Rief, W. (2003). A controlled treatment study of somatoform disorders including analysis of healthcare utilization and cost-effectiveness. *Journal of Psychosomatic Research* 54: 369–80.

Jensen, M.P., Turner, J.A., Romano, J.M. (2001). Changes in beliefs, catastrophizing, and coping are associated with improvement in multidisciplinary pain treatment. *Journal of Consulting and Clinical Psychology* 69: 655–62.

Kapur, N., Kamel, I.R., Herlich, A. (2003). Oral and craniofacial pain: diagnosis, pathophysiology, and treatment. *International Anesthesiology Clinics.* 41: 115–50.

Karjalainen, K., Malmivaara, A., van Tulder, M., Roine, R., Jauhiainen, M., Hurri, H., Koes, B. (2003). Multidisciplinary biopsychosocial rehabilitation for subacute low back pain among working age adults. *Cochrane Database of Systematic Reviews* CD002193.

Katz, N., Fanciullo, G.J. (2002). Role of urine toxicology testing in the management of chronic opioid therapy. *Clinical Journal of Pain* 18: S76–82.

King, S.A., Strain, J.J. (1990). Benzodiazepine use by chronic pain patients. *Clinical Journal of Pain* 6: 143–7.

Lake, A.E. III, Saper, J.R. (2002). Chronic headache: new advances in treatment strategies. *Neurology* 59: S8–13.

Larson, S.L., Clark, M.R., Eaton, W.W. (2004). Depressive disorder as a long-term antecedent risk factor for incident back pain: a thirteen year followup study from the Baltimore epidemiological catchment area sample. *Psychological Medicine* 34: 1–9.

Lemstra, M., Stewart, B., Olszynski, W.P. (2002). Effectiveness of multidisciplinary intervention in the treatment of migraine: a randomized clinical trial. *Headache* 42: 845–54.

Lipton, R.B., Stewart, W.F., Von Korff, M. (1997). Burden of migraine: societal costs and therapeutic opportunities. *Neurology* 48: S4–9.

Long, D.M., Filtzer, D.L., BenDebba, M., Hendler, N.H. (1988). Clinical features of the failed-back syndrome. *Journal of Neurosurgery* 69: 61–71.

Love, S., Coakham, H.B. (2001). Trigeminal neuralgia: pathology and pathogenesis. *Brain* 124: 2347–60.

Magni, G., Rigatti-Luchini, S., Fracca, F., Merskey, H. (1998). Suicidality in chronic abdominal pain: an analysis of the Hispanic Health and Nutrition Examination Survey (HHANES). *Pain* 76: 137–44.

Magni, G., Marchetti, M., Moreschi, C., Merskey, H., Luchini, S.R. (1993). Chronic musculoskeletal pain and depressive symptoms in the National Health and Nutrition Examination. I. Epidemiologic follow-up study. *Pain* 53:163–168.

Magni, G., Rigatti-Luchini S., Fracca, F., Merskey, H. (1998). Suicidality in chronic abdominal pain: an analysis of the Hispanic Health and Nutrition Examination Survey (HHANES). *Pain* 76: 137–144.

Mantyselka, P., Ahonen, R., Viinamaki, H., Takala, J., Kumpusalo, E. (2002). Drug use by patients visiting primary care physicians due to nonacute musculoskeletal pain. *European Journal of Pharmaceutical Sciences* 17: 210–16.

Marson, A.G., Kadir, Z.A., Hutton, J.L., Chadwick, D.W. (1997). The new antiepileptic drugs: a systematic review of their efficacy and tolerability. *Epilepsia* 38: 859–80.

Maruta, T., Malinchoc, M., Offord, K.P., Colligan, R.C. (1998). Status of patients with chronic pain 13 years after treatment in a pain management center. *Pain* 74: 199–204.

Mendell, J.R., Sahenk, Z. (2003). Clinical practice. Painful sensory neuropathy. *New England Journal of Medicine* 348: 1243–55.

Lindblom, U., Merskey, H., Mumford, J.M., Nathan, P.W., Noordenbos, W., Sunderland, S. (1986). Pain terms: a current list with definitions and notes on usage. *Pain* 3: S215–21.

Nemmani, K.V., Mogil, J.S. (2003). Serotonin-GABA interactions in the modulation of mu- and kapp-opioid analgesia. *Neuropharmacology* 44: 304–10.

Nicholson, B. (2003). Responsible prescribing of opioids for the management of chronic pain. *Drugs* 63: 17–32.

Patten, S.B. (2001). Long-term medical conditions and major depression in a Canadian population study at waves 1 and 2. *Journal of Affective Disorders* 63(3): 5–41.

Pengel, H.M., Maher, C.G., Refshauge, K.M. (2002). Systematic review of conservative interventions for subacute low back pain. *Clinical Rehabilitation* 16: 811–20.

Raja, S.N., Haythornthwaite, J.A., Pappagallo, M., Clark, M.R., Travison, T.G., Sabeen, S., Royall, R.M., Max, M.B. (2002). Opioids versus antidepressants in postherpetic neuralgia: a randomized, placebo-controlled trial. *Neurology* 59: 1015–21.

Rommel, O., Malin, J.P., Zenz, M., Janig, W. (2001). Quantitative sensory testing, neurophysiological and psychological examination in patients with complex regional pain syndrome and hemisensory deficits. *Pain* 93: 279–93.

Rosenblum, A., Joseph, H., Fong, C., Kipnis, S., Cleland, C., Portenoy, R,K. (2003). Prevalence and characteristics of chronic pain among chemically dependent patients in methadone maintenance and residential treatment facilities. *Journal of the American Medical Association* 289: 2370–8.

Savage, S.R., Joranson, D.E., Covington, E.C., Schnoll, S.H., Heit, H.A., Gilson, A.M. (2003). Definitions related to the medical use of opioids: evolution towards universal agreement. *Journal of Pain and Symptom Management* 26: 655–67.

Schmader, K.E. (2002). Epidemiology and impact on quality of life of postherpetic neuralgia and painful diabetic neuropathy. *Clinical Journal of Pain* 18: 350–4.

Serpell, M.G., and the Neuropathic Pain Study Group (2002). Gabapentin in neuropathic pain syndromes: a randomised, double-blind, placebo-controlled trial. *Pain* 99: 557–66.

Simon, G.E., Von Korff, M., Piccinelli, M., Fullerton, C., Ormel, J. (1999). An international study of the relation between somatic symptoms and depression. *New England Journal of Medicine* 341: 1329–35.

Stanton-Hicks, M., Janig, W., Hassenbusch, S., Haddox, J.D., Boas, R., Wilson, P. (1995). Reflex sympathetic dystrophy: changing concepts and taxonomy. *Pain* 63: 127–133.

Starkstein, S.E., Preziosi, T.J., Robinson, R.G. (1991). Sleep disorders, pain, and depression in Parkinson's disease. *European Neurology* 31: 352–5.

Stewart, W.F., Ricci, J.A., Chee, E., Morganstein, D., Lipton, R. (2003). Lost productive time and cost due to common pain conditions in the US workforce. *Journal of the American Medical Association* 290: 2443–54.

Sullivan, M., Katon, W. (1993). Somatization: the path between distress and somatic symptoms. *American Pain Society Journal* 2: 141–9.

Suter, P.B. (2002). Employment and litigation: improved by work, assisted by verdict. *Pain* 100: 249–57.

Trief, P.M., Grant, W., Fredrickson, B. (2000). A prospective study of psychological predictors of lumbar surgery outcome. *Spine* 25: 2616–21.

Turner, J.A. (1982). Psychological interventions for chronic pain: a critical review. II. Operant conditioning, hypnosis, and cognitive-behavioral therapy. *Pain* 12: 3–46.

Turner, J.A., Chapman, C.R. (1982). Psychological interventions for chronic pain: a critical review. I. Relaxation training and biofeedback. *Pain* 12: 1–21.

van Tulder, M.W., Ostelo, R., Vlaeyen, J.W., Linton, S.J., Morley, S.J., Assendelft, W.J. (2001). Behavioral treatment for chronic low back pain: a systematic review within the framework of the Cochrane Back Review Group. *Spine* 26: 270–81.

Vlaeyen, J.W., Linton, S.J. (2000). Fear-avoidance and its consequences in chronic musculoskeletal pain: a state of the art. *Pain* 85:3 17–32.

Wiffen, P., Collins, S., McQuay, H., Carroll, D., Jadad, A., Moore, A. (2000). Anticonvulsant drugs for acute and chronic pain. *Cochrane Database Systematic Review* 3: CD001133.

Zakrzewska, J.M., Glenny, A.M., Forssell, H. (2001). Interventions for the treatment of burning mouth syndrome. Cochrane Database Systematic Review 3: CD002779.

6

Multiple Sclerosis

ADAM I. KAPLIN

KATHERINE A.L. CARROLL

Multiple sclerosis (MS) is characterized by demyelination, axonal injury, inflammation, and gliosis (scarring) and can involve the brain, spinal cord, and optic nerves. The course of MS is characterized either by episodes of exacerbation separated by periods of relative quiescence (relapsing-remitting) or by relentless progression, but it typically involves insults that are multiphasic and multifocal (ie, disseminated in time and location throughout the neuraxis). By conservative estimates, at least 350,000 individuals in the United States have MS (Anderson et al., 1992). MS is usually diagnosed between the ages of 20 and 40 years and is twice as common in women as men. In Western societies, MS is second in frequency only to trauma as a cause of neurologic disability in early to middle adulthood.

MS can vary from a benign illness with minimal impairment to a rapidly evolving and incapacitating disease requiring profound lifestyle adjustments. The disability is manifest both as physical/sensory impairments and as neuropsychiatric disorders.

Demoralization

Although the functional impairment and disability that can occur in MS is a source of distress as it would be in any physically impairing illness, the unpredictable course makes it particularly difficult for many patients to cope. It is more difficult to adapt to acute rather than gradual changes, and MS exacerbations usually start without warning and evolve over days to weeks. Moreover, its unpredictable and variable course can make MS a challenging illness to diagnose, so patients often undergo a frustrating course of multiple evaluations before finally receiving the correct diagnosis.

Sometimes an individual's capacity to adapt is overwhelmed by the stresses with which he is confronted, and he becomes discouraged, bewildered, and overwhelmed. This is a state called demoralization. Demoralization has been defined (Frank and Frank, 1991) as a state of helplessness, hopelessness, confusion, subjective incompetence, isolation, and diminished self-esteem. The subjective experience of demoralization involves feeling incapable of meeting both internal and external expectations, feelings of being trapped and powerless to change or escape, and feelings of being unique and therefore not understood. The combined effect usually leads to frustration, bewilderment, and isolation. To combat the feelings of failure and being overwhelmed, as well as the sense of isolation, which collectively represent demoralization, people must be taught how to achieve remoralization. This is generally accomplished through the development of problem-focused coping skills, individual and group support and education, and cognitive reframing to help examine unrealistic or faulty assumptions. Ultimately, with time, but only in the absence of a supervening depression, patients with MS usually come to adapt to living their lives under the altered circumstances that their illness imposes.

A study of the subjective experiences and psychosocial consequences of MS in patients whose average time since diagnosis was 9 years found that the acute adaptation is often difficult but that most patients identify beneficial as well as detrimental effects of their illness on their lives (Mohr et al., 1999). A minority of patients (20%) reported that MS led to a deterioration in their relationships; most often, this was expressed as concerns that they were not as good a mate or that their partners were angry or irritated more often. Thirty percent reported feeling demoralized, with feelings of sadness, loss of independence, or uncertainty about the future. Notably, the majority of patients (60%) spontaneously reported benefits as a result of contracting their disease. Their relationships seemed closer; they felt they were more compassionate and communicative; and they gained a better appreciation of, and perspective on, life.

Major Depression and Suicide

Epidemiology and Presentation

From its earliest characterization, depression was among the first symptoms recognized as being associated with MS. Jean-Martin Charcot (1825–1893), who provided the first accurate and comprehensive clinicopathologic description of MS, described severe depression in his first case presentation, Mlle. V., a 31-year-old woman who ceased eating and had to be fed by a stomach pump to keep her alive.

The point prevalence of major depression among clinic patients with MS is 15% to 30%, and lifetime prevalence is 40% to 60% (Caine and Schwid, 2002). This rate is three to ten times that in the general population. Furthermore, depression is more common in MS than in many other chronic illnesses, including other neurologic disorders.

The application of standard criteria for diagnosing depression in MS patients can be challenging because the somatic signs and symptoms seen in MS are similar to some symptoms of depression. For example, sleep disorder is common in both conditions, but is manifest in depression as early morning awakening, whereas difficulty initiating or maintaining sleep is more prevalent in MS-associated insomnia. Diurnal variation in patient's mood and energy level is common in depression, with patients progressively improving during the course of the day, whereas in MS, patients commonly report worsening fatigue in the latter half of the day. We suggest that debilitating fatigue that almost always interferes with a patient's activities be considered a symptom made worse by an underlying depression until proven otherwise.

Cognitive impairment in depression is often variable and characterized by variable performance, inattention, and a tendency on the part of patients to highlight their difficulties and put forth poor effort. In contrast, cognitive impairment in MS is typically stable, and patients tend to conceal their difficulties and provide full efforts during testing. With experience, these different qualities overlap, and symptoms of cognitive impairment in depression and in MS can become apparent to the clinician practiced in mental status examination. Finally, suicidal thoughts are the result of depression until proven otherwise and should prompt an urgent assessment by a trained physician or mental health professional.

An important step in correctly diagnosing major depression is resisting the temptation to attribute all distress to a reaction to environmental stressors. Although it might seem self-evident that depression is a "normal" response to the diagnosis of a progressive unpredictable neurodegenerative disease such as MS, the presence or severity of depression in MS does not correlate with the degree of physical disability (Patten and Metz, 1997; Feinstein, 2002; McGuigan and Hutchinson, 2006). Moreover, in amyotrophic lateral sclerosis (ALS), a relentlessly progressive neurodegenerative disease that almost inevitably results in death from respiratory insufficiency or aspiration within 3 to 5 years of symptom onset, the prevalence of major depression in late-stage disease is rare (<10%); depressive symptoms generally do not increase as death approaches (Rabkin et al., 2005). Thus, stress alone is not sufficient to precipitate major depression, although it may play a role in its genesis in vulnerable individuals.

The importance of recognizing major depression in patients with MS is demonstrated by the finding that depression has a greater impact than physical disability, fatigue, or cognitive impairment in MS patients' self-reported quality of life (Provinciali et al., 1999; Fruehwald et al., 2001; Benedict et al., 2005). In addition, depression has a significant impact on daily function, interpersonal relationships, cognition, and fatigue. The level of depression in patients with MS is the most significant determinant of quality of primary relationships as rated both by patients and significant others. Depression is also associated with increased time lost from work, disruption of social support, and decreased adherence to neuromedical treatment regimens for MS.

Depression can also exacerbate the symptoms directly attributable to neuronal dysfunction. The cognitive impairments of MS and depression can be additive, and disabling fatigue, a common symptom in MS, is six times more likely in patients with clinically significant depressive symptoms. Moreover, treatment of depression leads to reduction of fatigue in MS patients in proportion to the improvement in mood (Mohr, Hart, and Goldberg, 2003).

Suicidal ideation, defined as a desire to kill oneself, has a cumulative lifetime prevalence of 30% in patients with MS, and 6%–12% of patients with MS make a suicide attempt. This is a rate 7.5 times that of the age-matched general population. In a large study of outpatient MS clinics, suicide was the third leading cause of death (accounting for 15% of all deaths during a 16-year period), close behind malignancy (16%) and pneumonia (23%) (Sadovnick et al., 1991). In a study of outpatients with MS, suicidal intent was *not* related to gender, employment status, disease duration, physical disability, or cognitive status. The three most important variables for predicting suicidal intent were severity of major depression, living alone, and alcohol abuse, which in combination had an 85% predictive accuracy for suicidal intent. Poor social support and living alone are also associated with suicide in MS.

Depression in MS is frequently underdiagnosed and undertreated. One study found that 67% of subjects with current major depression, all suicidal, had not received antidepressant medication, whereas 31.4% of the patients with a lifetime history of suicidal intent and 35% of the patients with a lifetime diagnosis of major depression had received neither antidepressant medication nor psychotherapy.

Impact of Depression on Caregivers

The majority of individuals providing care to a person with MS report that the demands of caregiving disrupt their obligations to friends, family, and career, but that the perception of the person with MS about the degree of the caregiver's burden is less than that reported by the caregivers themselves. The well-being of the patient, however, is often vitally dependent on the continued efforts and support from the caregiver, which can best be furnished by a healthy individual.

Poor social support and living alone are both associated with significantly higher rates of suicide in MS patients (Aronson, Cleghorn, and Goldenberg, 1996). Poor social support has also been implicated as a factor in increasing the rate of MS exacerbations (Warren, Warren, and Cockerill, 1991). Conversely, social support acts to dampen the effects of depression on promoting immune activation (Mohr and Genain, 2004). This suggests that maximizing social support might buffer the effects of stress and depression on the pathogenesis of MS and be a crucial part of the treatment of patients with the disease.

Care recipient variables associated with increased caregiver burden include depression, an unstable course, increased physical disability, and pain. Because depression exacerbates all of these variables, caregivers often also benefit when a patient receives adequate treatment for the mood disorder.

Causes

As already noted, the finding that there is no correlation between the rate or severity of depression in MS and the degree of physical disability argues against psychosocial stress being a primary cause of the high prevalence of major depression in MS (Patten and Metz, 1997; Feinstein, 2002; McGuigan and Hutchinson, 2006). The extensive interactions between the immune and nervous systems raises the possibility that the immune system plays a role in the development of both MS and major depression. One link may be cytokines, messenger molecules produced by immunocompetent cells that mediate communication between cells of the immune system. Several authors have proposed that proinflammatory cytokines such as interleukin (IL)-6, tumor necrosis factor-α, and IL-1 are involved in depression. Multiple lines of evidence support this hypothesis: (1) various conditions that are associated with enhanced immune function have a high incidence of comorbid depression; (2) administration of cytokines results in the symptoms of depression; (3) cytokine production is elevated in depressed patients; (4) antidepressant drugs decrease cytokine levels and can reverse the depressive symptoms induced by cytokine administration; (5) cytokines cause alterations in brain systems that have been implicated in depression; and (6) stress, which may contribute to the development of depression, has effects on cytokines. This proposal is supported by the finding that immune abnormalities may precede the development of depression in MS.

The existing evidence suggests a role for cytokines in the pathogenesis of depression in MS, with these same mediators of inflammatory damage to the central nervous system (CNS) causing perturbations in mood regulation. Taken from this vantage point, depression can be viewed as both a pathophysiologic complication as well as a clinical symptom of MS. This would suggest that the management of depression is an integral part of the general management of MS, analogous to the treatment of other disease-related disabilities involving motor, sensory, and autonomic dysfunction, with potential prognostic implications for the overall course of the disease progression.

The high-dose corticosteroids used to treat MS exacerbations can result in depression. The U.S. Food and Drug Administration (FDA) requires that interferon-beta (IFNβ) preparations used to treat MS patients include the warning, "depression and suicide have been reported to occur with increased frequency in patients receiving IFN compounds." The evidence supporting these warnings is mixed, and there is no consensus on whether IFNβ can cause or exacerbate depression in patients with MS. While active, severe depression is a relative contraindication to IFNβ treatment, patients who are good candidates for IFN treatment should probably not be excluded based on a family or prior personal history of depression that might be kept in check by the impact of IFNβ treatment on the progression of MS and appropriate psychiatric treatment.

It has been shown that treatment for depression can have a specific effect on immune factors that are key players in the pathogenesis of the inflammation and exacerbation of MS. This has led the authors to speculate that treating depression might prove to be an important disease-modifying component in MS treatment.

Poor social support has been implicated as a factor in increasing the rate of exacerbations of MS. Conversely, social support acts to dampen the effects of depression on promoting immune activation. This suggests that maximizing social support might buffer the effects of stress and depression on the pathogenesis of MS and be a crucial part of the treatment of patients with MS.

Treatment

The correct diagnosis and management of depression in MS avoids the use of symptomatic treatments that might worsen depression. For example, modafinil, prescribed to treat fatigue, can lead to worsening insomnia; benzodiazepines, used to treat insomnia, can worsen cognition and cause falls; and donepezil, prescribed to treat cognitive impairment, can worsen appetite, lower energy, and cause fatigue.

Unlike depression in the general population that resolves spontaneously in roughly 75% of patients in an average of 6 to 12 months, depression in MS is generally unremitting and tends to worsen without therapeutic intervention. However, treatment outcomes studies are limited and largely anecdotal. One randomized double-blind placebo-controlled trial compared desipramine to placebo over 5 weeks; there was greater improvement in the desipramine-treated group, but side effects limited desipramine dosage in half of the treated patients (Schiffer and Wineman, 1990). A 3-month open label study of fluvoxamine 200 mg reported a 79% response rate and few side effects. Two separate open label 3-month trials of sertraline and moclobemide reported positive responses in 90% of subjects.

In selecting antidepressants, the side-effect profile of the medication is often tailored to alleviate the patient's depressive symptoms. For example, bupropion, fluoxetine, and venlafaxine tend to be activating and may ameliorate fatigue in some patients with MS. In contrast, desipramine, mirtazapine, and paroxetine cause sedation and stimulate appetite; these side effects can be beneficial for patients with insomnia and loss of appetite.

Antidepressant selection is also influenced by the opportunity to treat conditions comorbid with depression simultaneously. Tricyclic antidepressants (such as nortriptyline and desipramine) can help with incontinence (because they are anticholinergic) and neuropathic pain, both of which are common in patients with MS. Duloxetine also is effective in treating neuropathic pain, for which it has an FDA indication, in addition to treating depression.

Empirical studies of psychotherapy to treat MS depression have examined cognitive-behavioral, relaxation, and supportive group therapies. Psychotherapy with an emphasis on coping skills have been found more likely to be effective than insight oriented therapy in treating depression MS patients. Cognitive-behavioral therapy (CBT) has been found to be effective in treating depression in MS, and a number of small studies—some of them randomized—demonstrate the short and long-term efficacy of this form of treatment (Mohr et al,. 2001a).

There are no randomized controlled trials of exercise as an adjunctive treatment for depression in MS, but exercise has been shown to improve mood, sexual function, pain, and fatigue. The two limitations of this intervention are the difficulty of motivating depressed patients to begin a new schedule of exercise and the rapid loss of efficacy for depression if regular exercise is terminated.

The idea that psychologic states could trigger disease activity was originally described by Charcot, who speculated that grief, vexation, and adverse changes in social circumstances were related to disease onset (Butler and Bennett, 2003). Depression is a state of extreme, prolonged psychologic stress, and there has been a growing consensus in the literature that specific types of stress can cause MS exacerbations (Mohr and Pelletier, 2006). Studies have shown that chronic stress has been linked to increased risk of clinical exacerbations as well as accrual of disability.

It has been shown that treatment of depression can have a highly specific effect on immune factors that are key players in the pathogenesis of inflammation and exacerbation in MS, leading the authors to speculate that treating depression might prove to be an important disease-modifying component in treating MS (Mohr et al., 2001b). These preliminary studies suggest (1) that depression has effects on the immune system and brain, and (2) that some of these effects may be related to worsening the course of MS. Treating the depression may therefore be an integral component in managing the neurologic as well as the psychiatric manifestation of this autoimmune disease.

Bipolar Disorder

Epidemiology and Presentation

Epidemiologic studies report a lifetime prevalence of bipolar disorder of 2% in MS, twice the rate in the general population, whereas clinical studies have identified bipolar disorder in up to 13% of patients with MS (Joffe et al., 1987). This association between bipolar disorder and MS has further been supported by evidence that there may be a genetic link between bipolar disorder and MS in certain females. However, there are few studies of bipolar disorder in MS.

Causes

Steroid medications used to treat exacerbations in MS can induce an activated state characterized by increased energy, decreased sleep, and variable euphoria; this is sometimes described as a "steroid psychosis," although the term likely has a broader meaning. Risk factors for the onset of steroid-induced hypomania or mania in patients with MS include past episodes of major depression both before and after the onset of MS and a family history of depression (Minden, Orav, and Schildkraut, 1988). Hence these patients may have a predisposition to development of mood disorders. This is similar to antidepressant medication–induced mania in which a family and personal history of bipolar disorder are strong risk factors. Both show good response to treatment with lithium.

Evidence against the argument that steroid-induced affective changes are the major cause of the increased rates of bipolar disorder is the finding that mania can precede symptoms (and hence treatment) of MS. Furthermore, in some case studies, steroid treatment of acute psychosis in MS has ameliorated the symptoms of psychosis.

Numerous studies have implicated lesions in the frontal lobes as a cause of bipolar disorder and other neuropsychiatric symptoms in MS, some more specifically in the right frontal lobe. However, other studies have implicated left temporal lobe lesions as a cause.

Both bipolar depression and mania have been shown to be associated with increased plasma concentrations of the proinflammatory cytokines IL-6, IL-8, and TNF-α, raising the possibility that similar immune mechanisms may be involved in both mania and depression. TNF-α, IL-1, and IL-6 stimulate the hypothalamic-pituitary-adrenal (HPA) axis during immune activation, and this may play a homeostatic regulatory role by leading to the production of cortisol, which in turn dampens cytokine production. Hypercortisolemia has been linked to major depression, and steroid administration has been linked to affective changes as described. Raised levels of IL-6 have been found in patients with MS, and this may account for some of their increased susceptibility to the development of bipolar disorder.

Treatment

There are scant data on the treatment of bipolar mania occurring in MS. In addition to the use of standard psychotropic medications some authors have suggested that medications aimed at alleviating the demyelinating process such as corticosteroids, interferon-beta-1b (IFNß-1b) and glatiramer acetate are helpful, but supportive studies are lacking.

Euphoria

Epidemiology and Presentation

The association between euphoria and MS was originally described by Charcot in 1877 in his *Lectures on the Diseases of the Nervous System* as a "cheerful indifference without cause." It was subsequently labeled *euphoria sclerotica* by Smith and Kinnier. More recently it has been shown to have a prevalence of 9% in the population with MS (Fishman et al., 2004); it is more common in those suffering from secondary progressive MS. These patients were also found to be impatient, inconsiderate, and quarrelsome, and they have poor insight and impaired cognition. Furthermore, informants also reported distressing behaviors such as childishness, outbursts of anger, and lack of empathy, and caregivers reported it to make their relationship with the patient difficult. Charcot associated euphoria with disinhibition, impulsivity, and emotional lability.

Causes

In some patients euphoria may be due to bipolar disorder, manic phase, or steroid-induced affective changes. However, there is increasing evidence that many cases are linked to extensive underlying brain injury. In one magnetic resonance imaging (MRI) study, smaller gray matter volume was associated with greater euphoria and disinhibition, leading the authors to propose a link between loss of gray matter in the prefrontal cortex, an area responsible for inhibitory effects on the limbic system, and euphoria (although this was not found for patients with "severe" frontotemporal pathology [Diaz-Olavarrieta et al., 1999]). These findings led to a second hypothesis that the euphoria and disinhibition in MS stem from loss of gamma-aminobutyric acid neurons that ordinarily provide widespread inhibitory effects on cortical functioning. This hypothesis is supported by evidence that (unsegmented) whole brain atrophy is related to greater euphoria and disinhibition (Benedict, Carone, and Bakshi, 2004).

Treatment

In cases of euphoria due to bipolar disorder or steroid-induced affective changes, treatment is targeted to those etiologies. For cases thought to arise directly from structural and functional brain involvement by MS, treatment relies on the principles utilized in treating individuals with extensive brain injury.

Pseudobulbar Affect

Epidemiology and Presentation

A variety of terms have been used to describe this condition, including pathologic laughing and crying, emotional incontinence, emotional lability, involuntary emotional expression disorder (IEED), and pseudobulbar affect (PBA). Although there is some debate concerning the definition of the condition because of disagreement over the level of congruity with subjective mood and the level of voluntary control, PBA is defined here as an inappropriate and uncontrollable display of emotional output that is independent of experienced mood. It includes uncontrollable laughing that persists for an excessively long period of time, is out of proportion to the stimulus (eg, in response to something that is only moderately amusing), or is unrelated emotionally to the situation (eg, when the patient is angry or frustrated [mood incongruent]). Similar descriptions apply to crying, which is more common.

The prevalence of PBA in MS is approximately 10% (Feinstein et al., 1997). In this study the patients had been diagnosed with MS for a mean of 10 years and had entered the chronic phase of the illness. PBA was not associated with disease exacerbations, depression, or anxiety, but with more severe intellectual impairment. In another study, 36% of patients with cognitive impairment had PBA in contrast with 8% of patients without significant cognitive deficits (Sartori and Edan, 2006).

PBA can be extremely distressing for patients because they are often aware that their expressed emotion does not reflect their emotional state and they feel unable to control it. It can also be extremely distressing for those around the patient, particularly if they do not understand the incongruity in the expressed and subjectively experienced emotion.

Causes

PBA is more frequent in diseases with bilateral brain involvement, such as Alzheimer's disease, traumatic brain injury, and MS, and thus it is associated with degree of intellectual deterioration. A wide range of brain areas have been implicated in the pathophysiology of PBA. An association between PBA and disease in the prefrontal cortex has been suggested by studies linking PBA in MS to poorer performance on the Stroop Test, verbal fluency tests, and the Wisconsin Card Sorting Test (Feinstein et al., 1999). However, it has also been proposed that it may be due to disconnection in the cerebropontocerebellar pathway (Parvizi et al., 2001). This is based on the clinical association between PBA and pseudobulbar palsy in patients with MS (in which pontine lesions are implicated) and links between subcortical atrophy and PBA on computed tomography scan in patients with Alzheimer's disease.

Treatment

Clinical trials support the efficacy of tricyclic antidepressants and selective serotonin reuptake inhibitors (SSRIs), using amitriptyline in patients with MS (Schiffer, Herndon, and Rudick, 1985), nortriptyline in poststroke patients (Robinson et al., 1993), and fluoxetine in both post-stroke and MS patients. This efficacy in PBA is independent of the drugs' effects on depression. More recently a phase III 90-day placebo-controlled trial of dextromethorphan (DM; a sigma-1 receptor agonist that inhibits glutaminergic signaling), plus quinidine, added to increase the availability of DM, has shown both safety and efficacy in the treatment of PBA in MS (Panitch et al., 2006). Sigma-1 receptor sites are concentrated in the brainstem and cerebellum, supporting the hypothesis that disease in these areas is implicated in the pathogenesis of PBA.

Apathy

Epidemiology and Presentation

Apathy is characterized by a loss of motivation and is manifest in the affective realm as a blunted emotional response, in the cognitive realm as a lack of insight and initiative, and in the behavioral realm as social isolation and withdrawal. Therefore, differentiating apathy from depression can be challenging because they share similar symptoms. However, blunted emotional responses, indifference, low social engagement, diminished initiation, and poor persistence are most commonly symptoms of apathy, whereas dysphoria, suicidal ideation, self-criticism, guilt, pessimism, and hopelessness are symptoms of depression.

Apathy has been found to have a prevalence of 20% in MS. It has a profound impact on both patients and their caregivers. In

Alzheimer's disease, apathetic patients are more impaired in their ability to perform basic activities of daily living (ADL) than would be indicated by their cognitive level. Furthermore, caregivers may misinterpret the apathetic behavior as laziness or deliberate opposition, an interpretation that puts added strain on their relationship and leads to reports of higher levels distress.

Causes

Because the prevalence of apathy in other neurologic diseases is higher than in MS, most research has been carried out in these patient populations. Damage to the frontal lobes, and more recently the anterior cingulate, have been implicated in its pathogenesis.

Treatment

The importance of distinguishing apathy from depression is that their treatments differ. Modes efficacy for the treatment of apathy has been shown with psychostimulants (eg, methylphenidate, cholinergic therapies, or dopaminergic therapies). This has been postulated to be due to their enhancement of prefrontal cortical activity. Distinguishing these syndromes is also important, because some medication for depression can worsen apathy; for example, SSRIs may increase apathy and withdrawal from engagement with the environment.

Psychosis

Epidemiology and Presentation

Reports of psychosis, defined as the presence of hallucinations and/or delusions and formal thought disorder (a dysfunction of goal-directed verbal discourse), in MS have variably described syndromes resembling schizophrenia, delusional disorders, and affective psychoses.

Traditionally the prevalence rates of psychosis in MS have not been considered to exceed that of the general population (Joffe et al., 1987), although numerous case descriptions of psychosis and MS have been published, some of which report it as the initial symptom. A recent epidemiologic study reported a greater prevalence of psychotic disorders in MS than in the general population, an association that lessens with age (Patten, Svenson, and Metz, 2005).

The development of psychosis in MS has profound impact both on the patients and their caregivers. By definition, the patient will maintain his or her delusional beliefs despite evidence to the contrary and experience his or her hallucinations as if they were a normal percept. This can be extremely distressing to the caregiver and others close to the patient, particularly if they are incorporated into the delusion. However, this also may be extremely distressing to the patient particularly if the delusions or hallucinations are threatening.

Causes

Studies linking psychosis in MS to temporal lobe pathology include the following: (1) an association between more temporoparietal pathology on MRI in patients with flattening of affect, delusions, and thought disorder (Ron and Logsdail, 1989), (2) MRI studies correlating hallucinations and frontotemporal MRI lesions, and (3) a case report linking psychosis in MS with left temporal lobe MRI lesions.

As with depression and bipolar disorder, psychosis in the absence of known autoimmune CNS disease has been associated with alterations in the immune system. The studies have generally investigated schizophrenia and found increased plasma

IL-6 in untreated patients and that is reduced after treatment with neuroleptics and, more recently, correlations between IL-6 levels and severity of psychopathology in schizophrenia.

Treatment

The only data regarding the use of antipsychotics in MS are case reports of the successful use of clozapine, efficacy of ziprasidone following unsatisfactory results with olanzapine and quetiapine, and good tolerance and efficacy of aripiprazole following the development of akathisia with risperidone and ziprasidone.

Cognitive Dysfunction

Epidemiology and Presentation

Cognitive dysfunction in MS is frequently underrecognized, perhaps because it is characterized by the slowed rate of mental processing, forgetfulness, executive dysfunction, and apathy of a subcortical dementia. In one study, 48% of patients with MS failed four or more of the cognitive test indices in a 31-test battery when compared with 5% of healthy controls (Rao et al., 1991). Patients with MS were particularly impaired in recent memory, sustained attention, verbal fluency, conceptual reasoning, and visuospatial perception. Cognitive impairment was not associated with illness duration, disease course, or medication usage, although it was weakly associated with physical disability. A stronger association with physical disability was found in a 10-year natural history study in patients with early onset MS (Amato et al., 2001). At 10 years, 56% of the cohort demonstrated cognitive dysfunction, including 17 of the 37 patients who were cognitively normal at the start of the study. The degree of physical disability, progressive course, and increasing age predicted the extent of cognitive decline.

The importance of accurate recognition of cognitive dysfunction is underscored by the strong relationship between cognitive dysfunction and disability in MS. Patients with the disease and cognitive impairment have fewer social interactions, more sexual dysfunction, greater difficulty with household tasks, and higher unemployment than those without cognitive dysfunction.

Although cognitively intact patients with MS may remain stable over long periods of time, those who show deficits on testing generally show progressive cognitive decline over time. Improvement is uncommon except following acute cognitive deterioration during acute attacks of MS; in one study, improvement of cognitive function 6 weeks following an attack paralleled the resolution of gadolinium-enhancing lesions on MRI (Foong et al., 1998).

Causes

The extent of white matter lesions on conventional brain MRI scans correlates modestly (although statistically significantly) with performance on a wide variety of neuropsychologic tests. This correlation is higher than that found between physical disability and MRI white matter lesions. Several MRI studies have found that the patterns of white matter lesions correspond to specific patterns of MS-related cognitive deficits. For example, extent of frontal lobe involvement best predicts impairments of abstract problem solving, memory, and word fluency, and extent of left parieto-occipital involvement best predicts deficits in verbal learning and complex visual-integrative skills.

Measurements of brain atrophy with MRI have demonstrated even more robust between the extent or type of disability and T1- and T2-weighted MRI lesions (Lucchinetta, Bruck, and Noseworthy, 2001). However, many studies have found either poor or no correlation between white matter lesions and performance and have led to closer examination of what has been termed "normal appearing brain tissue" (NABT) (Lucchinetta, Bruck, and Noseworthy 2001). Abnormalities detected in NABT by novel imaging modalities, such as magnetic resonance spectroscopy (MRS), correlate better with disability and cognitive impairment than do T1 or T2 lesions by MRI. MRS provides a noninvasive method for examining regional changes in brain neurochemistry. This allows for a safe means of ascertaining direct information about the function of the brain, whereas MRI provides only structural details. Diffusion tensor imaging abnormalities also correlate with the degree of cognitive impairment, though further research is needed.

Treatment

Although it has been suggested that disease-modifying drugs such as interferon beta-1a (IFNβ-1a), IFNβ-1b, and glatiramer acetate (GA) should prevent or reduce the progression of cognitive dysfunction by preventing the development or progression of cerebral lesions or brain atrophy, evidence is modest except for IFNβ-1a (Fischer et al., 2000). IFNβ-1b may also improve cognitive performance in MS patients, although larger studies are required. Evidence for an effect of GA on cognitive function in MS is poor, but it has also not been extensively studied.

Acetylcholinesterase inhibitors, currently FDA approved for use in Alzheimer's disease, have been tested in MS. Donepezil has shown efficacy for improved verbal learning and memory but not other cognitive tasks or overall cognition score) in a randomized controlled trial (Krupp et al., 2004).

The results of the few studies that have assessed the efficacy of cognitive rehabilitation in MS have been disappointing. One single-blind randomized controlled trial of cognitive rehabilitation that targeted specific deficits showed no significant benefits on mood, quality of life, subjective cognitive impairment, or independence (Lincoln et al., 2002). However, compensation— the use of residual or undisturbed functions as a basis for compensatory strategies—and adaptation (the use of external aids) have been shown to be beneficial. For example, "positively reframing" a memory problem as an organizational problem and using a written notes or a "to do" list is associated with better adaptation.

Conclusion

That there are devastating neuropsychiatric manifestations of MS has been known since its original neurologic description and characterization. It has taken a century, however, for systematic investigations to be undertaken. Although studies of the diagnosis and treatment of psychiatric comorbidities of MS are still in their infancy, evidence has been mounting that clinically addressing these issues can have profound impact on patient's function, quality of life, longevity, and comfort. Scientific inquiry into the nature of the insults in MS that result in specific psychiatric syndromes promises to shed much needed neuroscientific light onto how the brain elaborates higher cortical functions related to the mind, such as mood regulation, cognition, and the maintenance of coherent thought processes.

References

Amato, M.P., Ponziani, G., Siracusa, G., Sorbi, S. (2001). Cognitive dysfunction in early-onset multiple sclerosis: a reappraisal after 10 years. *Archives of Neurology* 58: 1602–6.

Anderson, D.W., Ellenberg, J.H., Leventhal, C.M., Reingold, S.C., Rodriguez, M., Silberberg, D.H. (1992). Revised estimate of the prevalence of multiple sclerosis in the United States. *Annals of Neurology* 31: 333–6.

Aronson, K.J., Cleghorn, G., Goldenberg, E. (1996). Assistance arrangements and use of services among persons with multiple sclerosis and their caregivers. *Disability and Rehabilitation* 18: 354–61.

Benedict, R.H., Carone, D.A., Bakshi, R. (2004). Correlating brain atrophy with cognitive dysfunction, mood disturbances, and personality disorder in multiple sclerosis. *Journal of Neuroimaging* 14: 36S-45S.

Benedict, R.H., Wahlig, E., Bakshi, R., Fishman, I., Munschauer, F., Zivadinov, R., Weinstock-Guttman, B. (2005). Predicting quality of life in multiple sclerosis: accounting for physical disability, fatigue, cognition, mood disorder, personality, and behavior change. *Journal of Neurological Sciences* 231: 29–34.

Butler, M.A., Bennett, T.L. (2003). In search of a conceptualization of multiple sclerosis: a historical perspective. *Neuropsychology Review* 13: 93–112.

Caine, E.D., Schwid, S.R. (2002). Multiple sclerosis, depression, and the risk of suicide. *Neurology* 59: 662–3.

Diaz-Olavarrieta, C., Cummings, J.L., Velazquez, J., Garcia de la Cadena, C. (1999). Neuropsychiatric manifestations of multiple sclerosis. *Journal of Neuropsychiatry and Clinical Neurosciences* 11: 51–7.

Feinstein, A. (2002). An examination of suicidal intent in patients with multiple sclerosis. *Neurology* 59: 674–8.

Feinstein, A., Feinstein, K., Gray, T., O'Connor, P. (1997). Prevalence and neurobehavioral correlates of pathological laughing and crying in multiple sclerosis. *Archives of Neurology* 54: 1116–21.

Feinstein, A., O'Connor, P., Gray, T., Feinstein, K. (1999). Pathological laughing and crying in multiple sclerosis: a preliminary report suggesting a role for the prefrontal cortex. *Multiple Sclerosis* 5: 69–73.

Fischer, J.S., Priore, R.L., Jacobs, L.D., Cookfair, D.L., Rudick, R.A., Herndon, R.M., Richert, J.R., Salazar, A.M., Goodkin, D.E., Granger, C.V., Simon, J.H., Grafman, J.H., Lezak, M.D., O'Reilly Hovey, K.M., Perkins, K.K., Barilla-Clark, D., Schacter, M., Shucard, D.W., Davidson, A.L., Wende, K.E., Bourdette, D.N., Kooijmans-Coutinho, M.F. (2000). Neuropsychological effects of interferon beta-1a in relapsing multiple sclerosis. Multiple Sclerosis Collaborative Research Group. *Annals of Neurology* 48: 885–92.

Fishman, I., Benedict, R.H., Bakshi, R., Priore, R., Weinstock-Guttman, B. (2004). Construct validity and frequency of euphoria sclerotica in multiple sclerosis. *Journal of Neuropsychiatry and Clinical Neurosciences* 16: 350–6.

Foong, J., Rozewicz, I.., Quaghebeur, G., Thompson, A.J., Miller, D.H., Ron, M.A. (1998). Neuropsychological deficits in multiple sclerosis after acute relapse. *Journal of Neurology, Neurosurgery, and Psychiatry* 64: 529–32.

Frank, J.D., Frank, J.B. (1991). *Persuasion and Healing: A Comparative Study of Psychotherapy.* (3rd ed.). Baltimore, MD: Johns Hopkins University Press.

Fruehwald, S., Loeffler-Stastka, H., Eher, R., Saletu, B., Baumhackl, U. (2001). Depression and quality of life in multiple sclerosis. *Acta Neurologica Scandinavica* 104: 257–61.

Joffe, R.T., Lippert, G.P., Gray, T.A., Sawa, G., Horvath, Z. (1987). Mood disorder and multiple sclerosis. *Archives of Neurology* 44: 376–8.

Krupp, L.B., Christodoulou, C., Melville, P., Scherl, W.F., MacAllister, W.S., Elkins, L.E. (2004). Donepezil improved memory in multiple sclerosis in a randomized clinical trial. *Neurology* 63: 1579–85.

Lincoln, N.B., Dent, A., Harding, J., Weyman, N., Nicholl, C., Blumhardt, L.D., Playford, E.D. (2002). Evaluation of cognitive assessment and cognitive intervention for people with multiple sclerosis. *Journal of Neurology, Neurosurgery, and Psychiatry* 72: 93–8.

Lucchinetti, C., Bruck, W., Noseworthy, J. (2001). Multiple sclerosis: recent developments in neuropathology, pathogenesis, magnetic resonance imaging studies and treatment. *Current Opinion in Neurology* 14: 259–69.

McGuigan, C., Hutchinson, M. (2006). Unrecognised symptoms of depression in a community-based population with multiple sclerosis. *Journal of Neurology* 253: 219–23.

Minden, S.L., Orav, J., Schildkraut, J.J. (1988). Hypomanic reactions to ACTH and prednisone treatment for multiple sclerosis. *Neurology* 38: 1631–4.

Mohr, D.C., Genain, C. (2004). Social support as a buffer in the relationship between treatment for depression and T-cell production of interferon gamma in patients with multiple sclerosis. *Journal of Psychosomatic Research* 57: 155–8.

Mohr, D.C., Pelletier, D. (2006). A temporal framework for understanding the effects of stressful life events on inflammation in patients with multiple sclerosis. *Brain, Behavior, and Immunity* 20: 27–36.

Mohr, D.C., Hart, S.L., Goldberg, A. (2003). Effects of treatment for depression on fatigue in multiple sclerosis. *Psychosomatic Medicine* 65: 542–7.

Mohr, D.C., Dick, L.P., Russom D., Pinn, J., Boudewyn, A.C., Likosky, W., Goodkin, D.E. (1999). The psychosocial impact of multiple sclerosis: exploring the patient's perspective. *Health Psychology* 18: 376–82.

Mohr, D.C., Boudewyn, A.C., Goodkin, D.E., Bostrom, A., Epstein, L. (2001a). Comparative outcomes for individual cognitive-behavior therapy, supportive-expressive group psychotherapy, and sertraline for the treatment of depression in multiple sclerosis. *Journal of Consulting and Clinical Psychology* 69: 942–9.

Mohr, D.C., Goodkin, D.E., Islar, J., Hauser, S.L,, Genain, C.P. (2001b). Treatment of depression is associated with suppression of nonspecific and antigen-specific T(H)1 responses in multiple sclerosis. *Archives of Neurology* 58: 1081–6.

Panitch, H.S., Thisted, R.A., Smith, R.A., Wynn, D.R., Wymer, J.P., Achiron, A., Vollmer, T.L., Mandler, R.N., Dietrich, D.W., Fletcher, M., Pope, L.E., Berg, J.E., Miller, A. (2006). Randomized, controlled trial of dextromethorphan/quinidine for pseudobulbar affect in multiple sclerosis. *Annals of Neurology* 59: 780–7.

Parvizi, J., Anderson, S.W., Martin, C.O., Damasio, H., Damasio, A.R. (2001). Pathological laughter and crying: a link to the cerebellum. *Brain* 124: 1708–19.

Patten, S.B., Metz, L.M. (1997). Depression in multiple sclerosis. *Psychotherapy and Psychosomatics* 66: 286–92.

Patten, S.B., Svenson, L.W., Metz, L.M. (2005). Psychotic disorders in MS: population-based evidence of an association. *Neurology* 65: 1123–5.

Provinciali, L., Ceravolo, M.G., Bartolini, M., Logullo, F., Danni, M. (1999). A multidimensional assessment of multiple sclerosis: relationships between disability domains. *Acta Neurologica Scandinavica* 100: 156–62.

Rabkin, J.G., Albert, S.M., Del Bene, M.L., O'Sullivan, I., Tider, T., Rowland, L.P., Mitsumoto, H. (2005). Prevalence of depressive disorders and change over time in late-stage ALS. *Neurology* 65: 62–7.

Rao, S.M., Leo, G.J., Bernardin, L., Unverzagt, F. (1991). Cognitive dysfunction in multiple sclerosis. I. Frequency, patterns, and prediction. *Neurology* 41: 685–91.

Robinson, R.G., Parikh, R.M., Lipsey, J.R., Starkstein, S.E., Price, T.R. (1993). Pathological laughing and crying following stroke: validation of a measurement scale and a double-blind treatment study. *American Journal of Psychiatry* 150: 286–93.

Ron, M.A., Logsdail, S.J. (1989). Psychiatric morbidity in multiple sclerosis: a clinical and MRI study. *Psychological Medicine* 19: 887–95.

Sadovnick, A.D., Eisen, K., Ebers, G.C., Paty, D.W. (1991). Cause of death in patients attending multiple sclerosis clinics. *Neurology* 41: 1193–6

Sartori, E., Edan, G. (2006). Assessment of cognitive dysfunction in multiple sclerosis. *Journal of Neurological Sciences* 245: 169–75.

Schiffer, R.B., Wineman, N.M. (1990). Antidepressant pharmacotherapy of depression associated with multiple sclerosis. *American Journal of Psychiatry* 147: 1493–7.

Schiffer, R.B., Herndon, R.M., Rudick, R.A. (1985). Treatment of pathologic laughing and weeping with amitriptyline. *New England Journal of Medicine* 312: 1480–2.

Smith,C.S., Kinnier,W.S.A. (1926) The affective symptomatology of disseminated sclerosis. *Journal of Neurology and Psychopathology* 1–30.

Warren, S., Warren, K.G., Cockerill, R. (1991). Emotional stress and coping in multiple sclerosis (MS) exacerbations. *Journal of Psychosomatic Research* 35: 37–47.

7

Epilepsy

LAURA MARSH

As many as 50% of patients with epilepsy have psychiatric syndromes, with mood, anxiety, and psychotic disturbances being the most common. Recognition and treatment of neuropsychiatric disturbances in individuals with epilepsy is influenced by the complexity of the epilepsies, which are a heterogeneous group of chronic conditions. Epileptic syndromes are classified according to seizure type and differ in their respective diagnostic criteria, epidemiology, etiologies, medical and surgical treatments, and associated psychiatric conditions. This chapter focuses on interictal psychiatric disturbances. Periictal and ictal psychiatric phenomena are addressed in the discussions of the differential diagnosis for the various interictal phenomena and in other reviews (Trimble, 1991; Schwartz and Marsh, 2000; Marsh and Rao, 2002).

The prevalence of epilepsy ranges from 0.4% to 1%, with variation attributed to actual differences in the frequency of epilepsy among population subgroups as well as varying definitions of seizures and of epilepsy (Hauser and Rocca, 1996). The idiopathic generalized epilepsies comprise nearly one-third of all epilepsies and are primarily genetic in origin (Jallon and Latour, 2005). Partial seizures are the most common seizure type and localization-related or focal epilepsy, especially of temporal lobe origin, is the most common epilepsy syndrome (Keranen, Sillanpaa, and Riekkinen, 1988). The incidence of epilepsy in industrialized countries is highest in the first year of life; it then remains stable until it peaks again after the age of 60 years, when epilepsy is associated with vascular and neurodegenerative conditions. In older adults, however, seizure presentations can be subtle and the diagnosis of epilepsy is frequently missed. Epilepsy is more common in men than women.

Psychiatric Assessment

Multiple factors contribute to higher rates of psychiatric illness in patients with epilepsy. Whether epilepsy itself increases the risk of psychiatric disturbance is unclear; it is important to understand the type and severity of the patient's epilepsy syndrome, the ictal and peri-ictal features of the seizure, and the relationship of these to the occurrence of the psychiatric phenomena. It is also important to identify whether the patient has any of the special vulnerabilities that influence the risk of psychiatric dysfunction such as the presence of brain injury (eg, from head injury, a congenital neurodevelopmental disorder); use of medications to treat seizures or other conditions that have the potential for adverse psychoactive effects (eg, phenobarbital, benzodiazepines); untoward environmental and psychosocial circumstances; global versus selective cognitive impairments; and temperamental (ie, personality) traits that limit adaptability (Reynolds, 1981). Although focal epilepsy, especially of temporal lobe origin, is often reported to have a higher incidence of associated psychiatric problems, this association is confounded by higher prevalence rates for temporal lobe epilepsy relative to other epilepsy syndromes. Genetic disorders, inherited syndromes, and other situations that affect seizure threshold also influence the risk of comorbid psychiatric disorders.

The risk of psychiatric pathology is also compounded by the frequent co-occurrence of other impairments (Cowan et al., 1989). Mental retardation, seen in as many as 28% of epilepsy patients, motor deficits, and hearing and visual dysfunction are the most common comorbid conditions among epilepsy patients. Among patients with mental retardation, epilepsy is associated with even greater severity of cognitive deficits as well as higher rates of comorbid developmental disturbances such as autism or cerebral palsy. Individuals with epilepsy who have more than one developmental disability in addition to intellectual disability are more likely to present with psychiatric pathology (Matson et al., 1999).

Characteristics of Psychiatric Disturbances

Psychiatric disturbances in epilepsy can be categorized according to whether they are direct expressions of the seizure (ie, ictal state), features of a peri-ictal state (ie, postictal or preictal/prodromal phase), or phenomena of the interictal period (Table 7–1). The transition from one state to the next can be ambiguous, but there is usually a consistent pattern across seizures.

Table 7.1. Psychiatric Disturbances during Ictal, Postictal, and Interictal States

Ictal	Postictal	Interictal
Anxiety	Confusion	Major depression
Intense sense of horror	Depression	Adjustment disorders
Panic attacks	Agitation	Dysthymia
Dysphoria	Paranoia	Atypical depressive syndromes
Tearfulness (dacrystic seizures)	Hallucinations	Affective lability
Laughter (gelastic seizures)	Mania	Medication-induced mood changes
Sexual excitement	Aggression/ violence	Mania
Paranoia		Panic disorder
Hallucinations		Generalized anxiety
Illusions		Obsessive-compulsive disorder
Forced thoughts (resembling obsessions)		Phobias
Déjà vu, other memory experiences		Psychogenic nonepileptic seizures
Confusion		Adverse medication-induced cognitive effects
Aggression/violence		Psychotic syndromes
		Aggression/violence

Therefore, the patient's history should include a description of the patient's seizure semiology (ie, the sequence of clinical manifestations of the seizure), the patient's behavior and mental state relative to the actual seizure, and plausible precipitating factors such as emotional events. Because most patients experience amnesia or are confused during or after their seizures, interviews with a family member or other suitable informant are critical to obtain accurate information, determine when a psychiatric disturbance occurs relative to epileptic events, and assess whether more than one psychiatric disturbance is present across the different seizure phases. In some cases, video-electroencephalogram (EEG) monitoring is needed to clarify the relationship between the epileptic seizure and the psychiatric disturbance.

Ictal psychiatric disturbances are characterized by the typical features of epileptic seizures. The events are stereotyped, have a sudden onset, and are brief, lasting from less than 1 to up to 3 minutes. Consciousness is altered with complex partial seizures, although impairment or confusion may be subtle. Some ictal phenomena such as staring, motor or oral automatisms, nonsensical speech or simple phrases, and undirected pacing or other semipurposeful activities can be identified as behavioral or neuropsychiatric. Nonconvulsive partial status epilepticus can be manifest as prolonged states of fear, mood changes, or psychosis and resemble an acute schizophrenic or manic state. Epilepsy can be misdiagnosed in the setting of intermittent emotional or aggressive episodes or other states that include changes in responsiveness such as catatonia, severe depression, or delirium.

Peri-ictal psychiatric disturbances can be postictal or preictal. One epilepsy monitoring unit reported an annual incidence of postictal disturbances of 7.8%, but an average prevalence is unknown (Kanner et al., 1996). Postictal disturbances may present in the context of a delirium or in clear consciousness.

Compared with interictal disturbances, postictal states usually have a shorter duration and may follow a lucid interval. Psychotic symptoms are most common, but diverse motor, somatosensory, autonomic, and cognitive deficits can occur. Duration varies from full recovery to baseline immediately or shortly after a seizure to states lasting up to several weeks. Although many disturbances remit spontaneously, medication may be needed, especially when there is distressing or disruptive psychosis. For some patients, postictal mental phenomena such as paranoia are so intense and disturbing that the prospect of repeatedly experiencing the postictal disturbance becomes a focus of anxiety during the interictal phase. One series showed higher rates of interictal psychiatric disturbances in patients with postictal psychiatric events (Kanner et al., 1996).

Preictal disturbances, also called prodromal phenomena, can develop and last for several minutes, hours, or days before a seizure. Irritability, mood lability, apprehension, depression, and, in some cases, directed aggression are common. They may begin suddenly or represent an aggravation of an interictal disturbance, often with fluctuations in their intensity, ending only with the seizure. Preictal disturbances should be distinguished from emotional distress that precipitates a seizure. For example, one patient described that the distress associated with arguments with her mother was associated with a greater likelihood of having a seizure shortly after the argument.

Cognitive Disturbances

Cognitive dysfunction is frequent in patients with epilepsy, but its impact is often overlooked. Mental slowness, memory dysfunction, and attentional deficits are common cognitive complaints in adults (van Rijckevorsel, 2006), whereas generalized impairments, learning disabilities, and language deficits are frequently evident when epilepsy begins early in life. Memory deficits are most prevalent in focal epilepsy syndromes. Short-term memory is especially affected and most pronounced in patients whose seizures originate in the medial temporal lobe. The severity of the memory deficit varies and is influenced by the extent of structural pathology in the hippocampus and surrounding structures (Hermann et al., 1997). Language disturbances include word-finding difficulties, anomia, and lexical knowledge, and tend to be a greater problem in children.

Cognitive decline is also observed in a subset of patients with epilepsy (Vingerhoets, 2006). As many as 25% of children experience significant deterioration in cognitive abilities; this is associated with greater seizure frequency, an earlier age onset of epilepsy, antiepileptic medications, psychosocial factors, and symptomatic generalized epilepsies. Presumably, these deficits persist into adulthood and represent the impact of epilepsy on the developing brain. In adults, prospective studies show mild cognitive declines in patients with treatment-refractory epilepsy, with memory affected more than general intelligence (Vingerhoets, 2006). Improved seizure control, including after successful resective surgery, can stabilize progressive deficits, although there is considerable individual variation in performance patterns (Engman et al., 2006).

A number of factors contribute to cognitive dysfunction, often in an additive and interactive fashion. In routine clinical practice, it is important to identify the various causes, because targeted interventions can reduce cognitive difficulties, improve overall function, and reduce the risk of additional psychopathology. Poor seizure control, including subclinical seizures, and interictal epileptiform activity interfere with learning and memory (Holmes and Lenck-Santini, 2006). Mood disturbances, which are treatable, also have a negative effect on cognition. Inattention can be related to subclinical seizures, undiagnosed learning disabilities, disrupted sleep resulting from anti-epileptic drugs (AEDs), side effects, or an attention deficit disorder. Adverse effects of AEDs, especially polytherapy, are a major cause of cognitive complaints and frequently aggravate baseline memory deficits, even in patients with well-controlled epilepsy (Uijl et al., 2006). Among the "older" AEDs, phenobarbital results in the most significant adverse effects, including intelligence quotient (IQ) decline in children. Phenytoin and benzodiazepines are also common offenders. Carbamazepine and valproate also cause modest cognitive side effects. Newer AEDs such as topiramate, lamotrigine, oxcarbazepine, and levetiracetam appear to have fewer adverse cognitive effects at therapeutic doses, although topiramate and gabapentin cause dose-related cognitive difficulties, including inattention.

Affective Disturbances

Depression

Depressive disturbances are the most common psychiatric disturbance in epilepsy, but they tend to be underdetected and undertreated (Hermann, Seidenberg, and Bell, 2000). Reported rates of depression vary according to how "depressive disorders" is defined and what population is studied. Among patients admitted to tertiary epilepsy centers, as many as 50% have clinically significant depression, but population-based studies report lifetime prevalence estimates between 6% and 30% (Kanner, 2003b). Rates of depression are higher in patients who are surgical candidates for epilepsy and depression is common after surgery as well, even when the surgery is effective at controlling seizures (Hermann et al., 1997). For this reason, psychiatric assessment should be an integral part of the comprehensive care of patients with treatment-refractory epilepsy.

The clinical presentation of interictal depressive disturbances is often similar to that of nonepileptic patients, but one-third of affected patients present with atypical features. Several investigations of interictal depressive disturbances describe intermittent recurrent affective syndromes that resemble dysthymia and can last for several hours to several weeks (Hermann et al., 1991). Another presentation involves a chronic dysthymic-like presentation with anhedonia, fatigue, anxiety, irritability, low frustration tolerance, and mood lability with tearfulness (Kanner, 2003b). A final presentation, referred to as interictal dysphoric disorder (Blumer, Montouris, and Hermann, 1995), is characterized by a changeable mood with intermittent dysthymic-like episodes mixed with brief bouts of euphoria, extreme irritability, explosiveness, anxiety, paranoia, neurovegetative symptoms (reduced energy and sleep disturbance), self-injurious behavior, and distress.

The rate of suicide is four times greater in patients with epilepsy and 25 times more common in patients with temporal lobe epilepsy than in the general population (Harris and Barraclough, 1997). The highest suicide rates are in surgically treated patients with epilepsy. Other risk factors for suicidality in epilepsy include a prior history of attempts, a family or personal history of psychiatric illness, and stressful life events (Robertson, 1997). This underscores the importance of recognizing and treating psychopathology.

The course and prognosis of depression in epilepsy has not been studied, but multiple risk factors for developing interictal depression have been reported. Important psychosocial variables include problems with perceived stigma, a pessimistic attributional style, low social supports, and learned helplessness (Hermann, Seidenberg, and Bell, 2000). Temporal lobe epilepsy, male gender, left-sided seizure foci, and frontal lobe cognitive deficits are risk factors, whereas no consistent associations are

reported for age, education, IQ, and seizure-related characteristics (eg, age at epilepsy onset, duration of epilepsy, or laterality
of seizure focus) (Hermann et al., 1997).

The differential diagnosis for interictal depressive syndromes is broad. It includes peri-ictal depression or sadness, in
which case the treatment should focus on improved seizure
control. Preictal affective changes include increased irritability,
mood lability,and depression for several minutes, hours, or even
days before a seizure; this may represent an aggravation of
an interictal psychiatric disturbance (Blanchet and Frommer,
1986). Pre-ictal mood changes should be distinguished from
reactive mood changes that can precipitate a seizure. Ictal depression sometimes presents as marked dysphoria with severe
guilt, sadness, and hopelessness, and it can lead to suicide. This
underscores the importance of careful history-taking to determine the relationship of the mood changes to other features of a
discrete seizure.

The diagnosis of epilepsy can be especially difficult to establish when partial seizures manifest as emotional phenomena.
For example, ictal crying (dacrystic seizures) is rare, but it may
appear to be a primary affective disturbance when other typical
ictal phenomena (such as staring, changes in consciousness,
motor automatisms, or convulsions) are not obvious or present.
Ictal events should be considered when events are brief (about
90 seconds) and accompanied by recurrent and stereotyped
phenomena. Postictal depression and anxiety are also common.
They frequently have associated psychotic symptoms and may
accompany a postictal delirium. Suicide attempts can also occur
during this phase.

AEDs frequently induce mood changes. Phenobarbital is a
well-established cause of depression, as are primidone, tiagabine, vigabatrin, and felbamate. Treatment with AEDs that have
mood-stabilizing properties such as carbamazepine, valproate,

and lamotrigine can also be associated with depressive episodes, especially when the dose is lowered in patients with a history of depression.

Mania and Bipolar Disorder

Few studies have investigated manic phenomena in patients with epilepsy, and the prevalence of manic disturbances or of classic bipolar disorder in epilepsy is unclear. Prevalence was reported as less than 5% in one early study (Gibbs, Gibbs, and Furster, 1948). Manic symptoms are typically associated with ictal or postictal states or are transient phenomena after temporal lobectomy (Schmitz, 2005). A predominance of right-sided hemispheric lesions or seizure foci has been noted (Robertson, 1998). Classic bipolar disorder, with defined interictal episodes of depression and mania, is not more prevalent in epilepsy patients relative to the general population (Lyketsos et al., 1993).

For any patient, it is important to establish whether the manic phenomena are interictal or related to manifestations of the patient's seizures or postictal state because this determines the focus of treatment. The occurrence of peri-ictal mania, especially in patients with established interictal depression, should raise suspicions of uncontrolled epilepsy as a cause of manic symptoms. For example, one patient with an established diagnosis of epilepsy involving partial seizures manifest as macropsia or micropsia, orgasmic sensations, and the idea that "something great might happen" was later admitted to an epilepsy monitoring unit in nonconvulsive status epilepticus with sustained grandiose delusions. Without knowledge of his seizure semiology, his diminished awareness and ictal automatisms consisting of purposeless stereotyped hand movements and pacing as well as his grandiosity might have been interpreted as a primary manic state.

No distinct clinical features of interictal mania have been reported. In my clinical experience, patients with epilepsy and interictal bipolar disorder present with mood symptoms that resemble those seen in idiopathic conditions (eg, elevated mood, increased goal-directed activity, irritability, and decreased need for sleep). Although certain AEDs can be used to treat epilepsy and provide mood stabilization, it is important to determine whether each disturbance is being adequately treated pharmacologically because mood stabilization may be achieved at doses of an AED that are ineffective for seizure control. Occasionally, convulsive seizures relieve depression or precipitate mania.

The concurrent use of AEDs to treat epilepsy and bipolar disorder can also confound diagnosis. This point was demonstrated by a patient who was being treated with sodium valproate monotherapy for the diagnoses of bipolar disorder and primary generalized epilepsy. Although his interictal depressive episodes were clearly established, detailed inquiry revealed that the patient's epilepsy syndrome involved complex partial seizures that intermittently secondarily generalized. The postictal state after a partial seizure was stereotypically followed by several days of increased mood and self-attitude and irritability as well as mild confusion. In this case, the confusion and stereotyped sequence of events suggested the diagnosis of peri-ictal mania.

Anxiety

Anxiety symptoms occur at a higher rate in patients with epilepsy than in the general population (Mittan and Locke, 1982), with prevalence rates between 10% and 30% in surgical candidates. They are the second most common affective disturbance in epilepsy and frequently are present with comorbid depressive disorders (Mendez, Cummings, and Benson, 1986). Anxiety is often attributed to the unpredictability of seizures, social stigma, and psychosocial difficulties. Although many patients are fearful of having seizures, frank seizure phobias are rare (Newsom Davis, Goldstein, and Fitzpatrick, 1998). Panic disorder affects about 21% of epilepsy patients (Pariente, Lepine, and Lellouch, 1991). The episodes resemble idiopathic panic disorder with recurrent episodes of apprehension lasting 5 to 30 minutes; they are accompanied by physical and emotional symptoms such as dyspnea, palpitations, gastrointestinal upset, dizziness, and fears of losing control or dying. These episodes should be readily distinguishable from panic associated with seizures, which are typically brief (<2 minutes) and stereotyped. Obsessive-compulsive disorder or symptoms is uncommon in patients with epilepsy (Kanner et al., 1993). Postoperative anxiety is associated with persistent seizures, preoperative psychiatric complaints (including anxiety), and new cognitive complaints.

AEDs can be associated with increases or decreases in anxiety. AEDs are generally mood stabilizing and anxiolytic, which may lead to emergence of anxiety when an AED is stopped or tapered.

The course of anxiety in patients with epilepsy has not been studied. Careful inquiry, and sometimes video-EEG monitoring, may be necessary to distinguish interictal anxiety from ictal panic or other anxiety states. Fear and apprehension is a component of the typical aura in up to one-third of patients with partial seizures (Engel. 1989). This diagnosis is challenging because such patients are also more likely to have interictal anxiety disturbances. Panic attack–like phenomena, including depersonalization or derealization, can occur during simple or complex partial seizures. Ictal fear refers to an extreme feeling of unprovoked terror that is also a manifestation of the seizure and may be accompanied by ictal paranoia, hallucinations, or autonomic symptoms. Postictal anxiety is less common than postictal depression but should be distinguishable from an emotional reaction in response to seizures (Kanner et al., 1996).

Psychosis

The prevalence of interictal psychosis, defined as hallucinations or delusions, is estimated to be about 7% (Umbricht et al., 1995). Interictal psychotic disturbances most often involve chronic schizophrenia-like states, but psychotic affective syndromes, brief psychotic states, and delirium also occur. The most common symptoms are paranoid or religious delusions as well as visual and auditory hallucinations. Other symptoms seen in idiopathic schizophrenia, such as negative symptoms (amotivation, apathy, flattened affect), disorganized behavior, or thought disorder may be seen (Mace, 1993). Cognitive impairment is more severe in epilepsy patients with psychosis than those without; there are higher rates of mental retardation (Matsuura et al., 2005) as well as greater impairment of executive and memory tasks (Nathaniel-James et al., 2004). Some reports have emphasized the specific association of temporal lobe pathology and seizure foci with interictal schizophrenia-like psychosis. However, signs of more extensive brain injury such as bilateral temporal foci on EEG, seizure clustering, an absence of past febrile convulsions, temporal and extratemporal pathology (Bruton, Stevens, and Frith, 1994), structural imaging abnormalities (Marsh et al., 2001), and dopaminergic abnormalities (Reith et al., 1994) are also associated with interictal psychosis.

The course and prognosis of patients with interictal psychosis has not been specifically studied. but some patients with recurrent episodes of postictal psychosis develop chronic interictal psychosis (Kanner et al., 1996). In clinical experience, patients tend to have chronic symptoms that require medication management. However, medication compliance with psychosis and epilepsy treatments seems to be associated with functional stability, which improves prognosis from a psychosocial standpoint. It is not known whether interictal psychosis is associated with a decline in intellectual abilities.

As with the other psychiatric disturbances in epilepsy, the differential diagnosis of interictal psychosis includes peri-ictal phenomena. A variety of phenomena present as ictal psychosis. Olfactory and gustatory hallucinations are more commonly associated with ictal than interictal disturbances. Ictal visual and auditory hallucinations can consist of complex scenes or speech but usually are vague shapes or sounds. Paranoid or grandiose ideas can also occur and can be frightening. The prevalence of post-ictal psychosis is about 10% (Lancman, 1999). It usually develops within hours to a few days after a seizure or cluster of seizures that may or may not involve secondary generalization. The symptoms can emerge from a delirium or a period of lucidity and include delusions or mood changes with mood-congruent psychotic phenomena. Prompt recognition and treatment is important, because the combination of confusion and the psychotic experiences can lead to self-destructive or aggressive behavior.

Behavioral Disturbances

Psychogenic Nonepileptic Seizures

A number of terms have been used to describe time-limited paroxysmal behaviors that mimic epileptic seizures but are not associated with abnormal electrical discharges in the brain. Nonepileptic seizures (NES) is a general term that includes physiologic NES, which are caused by some physical disturbance such as a cardiac arrhythmia, and psychogenic NES, in which the event is related to a psychiatric disturbance. Like an epileptic seizure, the NES can manifest as a disturbance in any form of mental experience, including motor, sensory, autonomic, cognitive, and emotional functions, or some combination of these. Most commonly, psychogenic nonepileptic seizures (PNES), also called behavioral seizures or pseudoseizures, are associated with somatoform disorders, but factitious disorders or malingering are also a cause of PNES.

The use of video-EEG has allowed for better identification of PNES and revealed that they are more common than had been realized. Among patients previously regarded as having true epilepsy, PNES were diagnosed in 5% of patients in a primary care practice, 10% of patients with medication-refractory seizures in an epilepsy clinic, and 30% of patients referred to extensive video-EEG monitoring in an epilepsy center (Reuber et al., 2005). PNES are frequently accompanied by additional psychopathology, especially depressive disorders and anxiety. Suicidality is also reported, sometimes after resolution of PNES behavior (Ettinger et al., 1999).

Violence

Several studies report increased rates of aggressive or violent behaviors, but valid prevalence rates for violence in epilepsy are not established (Marsh and Krauss, 2000). Interictal violence is rarely associated with epilepsy-specific variables such as EEG findings, although it has been suggested that interictal epileptiform discharges may be predisposing.

A key feature of interictal aggression is that it is purposeful and significantly related to the social context in which it occurs. The behaviors are directed, coordinated, and not stereotyped, and they are often precipitated by emotionally salient circumstances. Memory may be impaired during the outbursts, but that is not evidence for an epileptic seizure. At its offset, the patient recovers quickly, and there may or may not be remorse.

A number of factors are associated with higher rates of interictal aggression. Brain injury is a major influence, with damage to frontal, left hemisphere, and limbic regions conferring greater risk. Other risk factors are the presence of cognitive impairment, which often accompanies brain injury, low innate intelligence, low educational level, unemployment, lower socioeconomic status, and a prior history of behavioral problems. Concurrent psychosis can lead to violence, particularly in the setting of paranoid delusions and low intelligence.

The differential diagnosis of aggression in patients with epilepsy includes several conditions. Episodic dyscontrol syndrome refers to uncontrollable rage attacks usually stimulated by limited provocation. The attacks are not epileptic, but similarities such as premonitory auras with visual illusions or hyperacusis, amnesia for the event, and headache or drowsiness afterward are noted. Extreme remorse is common afterward, and the behavior is viewed negatively by the perpetrator. Ictal violence is extremely rare (Delgado-Escueta et al., 1981), although epileptic automatisms have been used as an explanation for violent crimes. Ictal violence usually consists of nondirected, spontaneous, stereotyped aggressive movements accompanied by the usual features of the seizure with impaired consciousness, brief duration, and sudden onset and offset. Property can be damaged, and there may be shouting or spitting. There may be resistive violence during the ictus that becomes more aggressive with continued confusion and resistive aggression during the postictal state. Resistive violence refers to aggression toward others that is unintended and occurs when someone attempts to restrain or assist the person during a seizure.

With postictal violence, there may be confusion, delirium, depressive symptoms, or psychosis that influence symptoms. The duration of the aggression varies, just as all postictal states vary, but the behavior remains out of character for the individual, and there is usually amnesia for the event.

Impact of Neuropsychiatric Disturbances in Epilepsy

Cognitive Dysfunction

Cognitive problems range from mild difficulties with academic achievement, to mental retardation, or progressive intellectual decline. The impact of cognitive deficits varies according to developmental stage and psychosocial status. Many aspects of daily life are affected, such as the ability to live independently, maintain employment, adhere to medication regimens, and sustain interpersonal relations. Attentional difficulties can be marked and have a greater influence on academic failure than memory deficits and socioeconomic status (van Rijckevorsel, 2006). Greater severity of cognitive deficits increases the risk of other psychiatric difficulties and the complexity of psychiatric assessment and treatment. For example, patients with mental retardation often experience multiple seizure types refractory to medication management; behavioral disturbances include aggression, self-injury, or temper tantrums; and other psychopathology, including depressive, and anxiety, and schizophrenia-like conditions. Poor seizure control further increases the likelihood of psychiatric comorbidities. Intellectual limitations that affect communication can make it difficult to distinguish behavioral nonepileptic events from epileptic seizures or other abnormal movements and behaviors that occur in this population (eg, myoclonus or staring), some of which may be a complication of anti-epileptic therapy itself.

Mood Disorders

Depressive disorders have a substantial adverse impact in individuals with epilepsy, affecting general functioning, quality of life, health care costs, mortality, and adherence to medical treatment. In patients with refractory epilepsy, depression has a stronger influence on quality of life than epilepsy variables such as seizure frequency, number or anti-epileptic drugs, and other variables (Gilliam, Hecimovic, and Sheline, 2003). The impact of mania in epilepsy has not been specifically studied.

Higher rates of anxiety are associated with lower health–related quality of life, with a greater influence than seizure or demographic variables (Beyenburg et al., 2005). Patients with anxiety appear more likely to be disabled by anticipatory anxiety about having a seizure in unfamiliar situation, which can lead to maladaptive avoidant behaviors and isolation (Newsom Davis, Goldstein, and Fitzpatrick, 1998).

Psychosis

Psychosis in epilepsy is associated with increased risk of cognitive impairment and brain injury. Many such patients are unable to live independently and require supervision to live safely. The long-term prognosis of psychosis in epilepsy has not been studied, but patients function better when their psychiatric symptoms and seizures are both well-controlled.

Behavioral Disorders

The risks of PNES include injury, admissions to intensive care settings, and iatrogenic harm, including death that can result from inappropriate medication administration. Many patients continue to report problems with anxiety and depression and fail to resume their prior occupational status, even with remission of PNES (Walczak et al., 1995).

Violent interictal behavior can have legal consequences. Because many patients with violent behavior also have intellectual limitations and other psychiatric comorbidities, they are at high risk for institutional placement.

Treatment

General Principles

Psychiatric treatments must target symptoms and syndromes according to their relationship to seizures. Decisions about treatment are significantly influenced by the extent to which the clinical picture is due to the primary neurologic condition (epilepsy), an interictal psychiatric disturbance, and medication effects. When the disturbance has a peri-ictal basis, the focus of treatment is improved seizure control, whereas the treatment of interictal disturbances is generally similar to the treatment of comparable idiopathic conditions. The presence of cognitive impairment, the proconvulsant effects of psychiatric medications, and the potential for interactions between psychiatric medications and AEDs influence decisions as well.

Pharmacologic and nonpharmacologic strategies are necessary components of treatment. Patients and families benefit from education about the psychiatric disturbance and how it relates to epilepsy and seizures. Comanagement by the neurologist and psychiatrist or psychologist is often optimal. For example, cognitive-behavior therapy can help with depression and anxiety and may reduce seizure frequency (Spector et al., 1999).

In patients with intellectual and developmental disabilities, high rates of mixed and generalized seizures usually warrant treatment with drugs that are effective for both partial and generalized seizures, including valproate, lamotrigine, topiramate, and zonisamide. Because patients frequently present with more than one neuropsychiatric disturbance (eg, major depression and cognitive difficulties), management requires recognition of the relative contributions of seizures, inherent brain injury, AEDs, cognitive, and psychiatric status to the clinical picture as well as how each of these realms interacts. Coordination among practitioners is often needed to ensure that the simplest, most effective, and safest medication regimen is used.

Psychiatric consultation should be obtained whenever there are concerns about suicidality or other forms of danger to self or others and if initial attempts at treatment with pharmacologic or nonpharmacologic strategies are unsuccessful. Inpatient psychiatric hospitalization is necessary for suicidality, severe depression, anxiety, or agitation that cannot be managed with usual outpatient care. It can also be useful for clarifying the diagnosis(es) or initiating therapies safely in patients when poor seizure control, cognitive impairment, or lack of psychosocial supports contributes to poor adherence to treatment.

Pharmacologic Treatment

A detailed review on the use of psychiatric medications in patients with epilepsy is available (McConnell and Duncan, 1998).

Cognitive abnormalities. Because all AEDs can have detrimental effects on the central nervous system, clinicians must balance the need for maximal seizure control with avoidance of neuropsychiatric side effects. Some AEDs (eg, lamotrigine, oxcarbazepine) may have beneficial effects on cognition. Effective and early seizure control using AEDs, resective surgery, or vagal nerve stimulation can limit the impact of epilepsy on cognitive status.

Donepezil has been evaluated in randomized, double-blind, placebo-controlled trial in patients with epilepsy (Hamberger et al., 2007). It did not show any benefits on memory, other cognitive functions, mood, social functioning, or quality of life. Donepezil was not associated with increased seizure severity or frequency. Memantine has not been studied as a treatment for cognitive dysfunction in patients with epilepsy. Stimulants other than bupropion appear to be safe and effective for attentional deficits, including attention deficit disorder, but controlled data are lacking. Atomoxetine has not been shown to have adverse effects in individuals with epilepsy.

Depression. The treatment of depression in epilepsy has been studied in one randomized, double-blind trial comparing nomifensine to amitriptyline, showing greater improvement in patients on nomifensine at 12 weeks (Robertson and Trimble, 1985). The recommendations are based on general consensus and clinical experience.

The primary concern in using antidepressants, especially tricyclic antidepressants (TCAs), is that many lower seizure threshold. However, this concern may be more theoretical than actual, because the proconvulsant effects of these medications are based on studies in animal models or on the effects of overdoses of antidepressants. Although patients with treated depression often have improved seizure control, possibly because of improved medication adherence, maprotiline, bupropion, amoxapine, and clomipramine should probably be avoided in patients with epilepsy because they lower seizure threshold the most (Curran and de Pauw, 1998).

Selective serotonin reuptake inhibitors (SSRIs) are generally used as initial treatment for depressive disorders and appear to be well tolerated and effective in patients with epilepsy and a low seizure propensity (Kanner, Kozak, and Frey, 2000). Venlafaxine, the selective noradrenergic and serotonergic antidepressant, also appears effective and safe in open-label use (Kanner, 2003a). TCAs alone and in combination with SSRIs are reported to be well-tolerated (Blumer and Zielinski, 1988). However, risks associated with TCA overdose make use of this class less desirable. Monoamine oxidase inhibitors also appear well-tolerated but are less likely to be used because of dietary restrictions. To minimize the risk of inducing or worsening seizures, it is prudent to start at low doses of antidepressants (eg, sertraline 25 mg/day or venlafaxine 37.5 mg/day), with smaller incremental increases until a satisfactory clinical effect is achieved.

Pharmacokinetic interactions between AEDs and antidepressant medications are another important concern (McConnell and Duncan, 1998). Phenytoin, carbamazepine, phenobarbital, primidone, oxcarbazepine, and topiramate have enzyme-inducing properties that affect antidepressant metabolism, an effect not seen with lamotrigine, gabapentin, tiagabine, levetiracetam, and zonisamide. Conversely, fluoxetine, paroxetine, fluvoxamine, and sertraline inhibit cytochrome p450 enzymes that can affect AED levels. Sertraline can also increase phenytoin levels via competitive protein binding. Monoamine oxidase inhibitors administered with carbamazepine can result in a hypertensive crisis. Simultaneous use of fluoxetine and carbamazepine can result in a serotonin syndrome (Dursun, Mathew, and Reveley, 1993).

Electroconvulsive therapy (ECT) can be used to treat major depression that fails to respond to antidepressant medications or when there is a need for more rapid treatment. ECT may improve seizure control, but it is rarely a cause of status epilepticus or increased seizure frequency (Keller and Bernstein, 1993).

Mania and bipolar disorder. Several AEDs are used to treat both seizures and bipolar disorder. Although lithium is a first-line agent for bipolar disorder, it may not be tolerated in patients with epilepsy because of neurotoxicity and proconvulsant effects, especially when used with antipsychotic medications. Antipsychotic medications may need to be added for agitated or manic states. Use of antipsychotics is described below.

Anxiety. There are no controlled trials regarding the medical treatment of interictal anxiety disorders. The usual approaches include a combination of pharmacotherapy and psychotherapy.

Antidepressants, namely SSRIs, are commonly used. Benzodiazepines (eg, clonazepam 0.5 mg /day) are indicated for short-term treatment only because of the risk of dependence, withdrawal-related anxiety, or lowering of the seizure threshold. Benzodiazepines also have the potential to cause confusion, impaired memory, and a predisposition to falls or paradoxical disinhibition. Buspirone lowers seizure threshold in animal experiments and should be used with caution. AEDs with anxiolytic effects include GABAergic drugs such as gabapentin and pregabalin. Vigabatrin, tiagabine, and valproate also have anxiolytic properties.

Psychosis. Overall, antipsychotic agents are associated with a 1% risk of seizures (Lancman, 1999). High-potency antipsychotics have a lower risk than low-potency agents. Clozapine, an atypical agent, is associated with a dose-related increased risk of seizures as well as epileptiform EEG abnormalities. Atypical agents such as risperidone, olanzapine, aripiprazole, and quetiapine are less likely to lower the seizure threshold.

In clinical experiences, patients with epilepsy may be more vulnerable to extrapyramidal side effects of antipsychotics, even with atypical agents. Low starting doses (eg, quetiapine 25 mg nightly, risperidone 0.5 mg twice daily, olanzapine 2.5 mg nightly) are recommended to allow monitoring for such effects.

Psychogenic nonepileptic seizures. There are no standard treatment approaches for PNES. The key element of treatment is accurate diagnosis. Psychotherapy is a major component of treatment, and approaches should be individualized to the patient's needs and circumstances. Discontinuation of AED treatment in patients with PNES is controversial.

Violence. Treatment of interictal violence depends largely on the specific circumstances. Lowering and elimination of medications that might be aggravating behaviors is sometimes beneficial. Adjunctive AED therapy, in addition to the AED therapy for epilepsy, may be useful if the patient is not using a mood-stabilizing antipsychotic. "Serenic" medications that may be used include lithium, propranolol, and SSRIs.

References

Beyenburg, S., Mitchell, A.J., Schmidt, D., Elger, c.e., Reuber, M. (2005). Anxiety in patients with epilepsy: systematic review and suggestions for clinical management. *Epilepsy & Behavior* 7: 161–71.

Blanchet, P, Frommer, G.P. (1986). Mood change preceding epileptic seizures. *Journal of Nervous and Mental Disease* 174: 471–76.

Blumer, D., Zielinski, J. (1988). Pharmacologic management of psychiatric disorders associated with epilepsy. *Journal of Epilepsy* 1: 135–50.

Blumer, D., Montouris, G., Hermann, B. (1995). Psychiatric morbidity in seizure patients on a neurodiagnostic monitoring unit. *Journal of Neuropsychiatry and Clinical Neurosciences* 7: 445–56.

Bruton, C.J., Stevens, J.R., Frith, C.D. (1994). Epilepsy, psychosis, and schizophrenia: clinical and neuropathologic correlations. *Neurology* 44: 34–42.

Cowan, L.D., Bodensteiner, J.B., Leviton, A., Doherty, L. (1989). Prevalence of the epilepsies in children and adolescents. *Epilepsia* 30: 94–106.

Curran, S., de Pauw, K. (1998). Selecting an antidepressant for use in a patient with epilepsy. Safety considerations. *Drug Safety* 18: 125–33.

Delgado-Escueta, A.V., Mattson, R.H., King, L., Goldensohn, E.S., Spiegel, H., Madsen, J., Crandall, P., Dreifuss, F., Porter, R.J. (1981). The nature of aggression during epileptic seizures. *New England Journal of Medicine* 305: 711–16.

Dursun, S.M., Mathew, V.M., Reveley, M.A. (1993). Toxic serotonin syndrome after fluoxetine plus carbamazepine [letter]. *Lancet* 342: 442–43.

Engel, J. (1989). *Seizures and Epilepsy*. Philadelphia, PA: F.A. Davis Co.

Engman, E., Andersson-Roswall, L., Samuelsson, H., Malmgren, K. (2006). Serial cognitive change patterns across time after temporal lobe resection for epilepsy. *Epilepsy & Behavior* 8: 765–72.

Ettinger, A.B., Devinsky, O., Weisbrot, D.M, Ramakrishna, R.K., Goyal, A. (1999). A comprehensive profile of clinical, psychiatric, and psychosocial characteristics of patients with psychogenic nonepileptic seizures. *Epilepsia* 40: 1292–98.

Gibbs, F.A., Gibbs, E.L., Furster, B. (1948). Psychomotor epilepsy. *Archives of Neurology and Psychiatry* 60: 331–39.

Gilliam, F., Hecimovic, H., Sheline, Y. (2003). Psychiatric comorbidity, health, and function in epilepsy. *Epilepsy & Behavior* 4: S26–S30.

Hamberger MJ, Palmese CA, Scarmeas N, Weintraub D, Choi H, Hirsch LJ (2007). A randomized, double-blind, placebo-controlled trial of donepezil to improve memory in epilepsy. *Epilepsia* 48:1283–91.

Harris, E.C., Barraclough, B. (1997). Suicide as an outcome for mental disorders. A meta-analysis. *British Journal of Psychiatry* 170: 205–28.

Hauser, W.A., Rocca, W.A. (1996). Descriptive epidemiology of epilepsy: contributions of population-based studies from Rochester, Minnesota. *Mayo Clinic Proceedings* 71: 576–86.

Hermann, B.P., Seidenberg, M., Bell, B. (2000). Psychiatric comorbidity in chronic epilepsy: identification, consequences, and treatment of major depression. *Epilepsia* 41: S31–S41.

Hermann, B.P., Seidenberg, M., Haltiner, A., Wyler, A.R. (1991). Mood state in unilateral temporal lobe epilepsy. *Biological Psychiatry* 30: 1205–18.

Hermann, B.P., Seidenberg, M., Schoenfeld, J., Davies, K. (1997). Neuropsychological characteristics of the syndrome of mesial temporal lobe epilepsy. *Archives of Neurology* 54: 369–76.

Holmes, G.L., Lenck-Santini, P.P. (2006). Role of interictal epileptiform abnormalities in cognitive impairment. *Epilepsy & Behavior* 8: 504–15.

Jallon, P., Latour, P. (2005). Epidemiology of idiopathic generalized epilepsies. *Epilepsia* 46: 10–14.

Kanner, A.M. (2003a). Depression in epilepsy: a frequently neglected multifaceted disorder. *Epilepsy & Behavior* 4: 11–19.

Kanner, A.M. (2003b). Depression in epilepsy: prevalence, clinical semiology, pathogenic mechanisms, and treatment. *Biological Psychiatry* 54: 388–98.

Kanner, A.M., Kozak, A.M., Frey, M. (2000). The use of sertraline in patients with epilepsy: is it safe? *Epilepsy & Behavior* 1: 100–5.

Kanner, A.M., Morris, H.H., Stagno, S., Chelune, G., Luders, H. (1993). Remission of an obsessive-compulsive disorder following a right temporal lobectomy. *Neuropsychiatry, Neuropsychology, and Behavioral Neurology* 6: 126–9.

Kanner, A.M., Stagno, S., Kotagal, P., Morris, H.H. (1996). Postictal psychiatric events during prolonged video-electroencephalographic monitoring studies. *Archives of Neurology* 53: 258–63.

Keller, C.H., Bernstein, H.J. (1993). ECT as a treatment for neurologic illness. In C.E. Coffey (Ed.), *The Clinical Science of Electroconvulsive Therapy*. Washington, DC: American Psychiatric Press. pp. 183–210.

Keranen, T., Sillanpaa, M., Riekkinen, P.J. (1988). Distribution of seizure types in an epileptic population. *Epilepsia* 29: 1–7.

Lancman, M. (1999). Psychosis and peri-ictal confusional states. *Neurology* 53: S33–8.

Lyketsos, C.G., Stoline, A.M., Longstreet, P., Lesser, R., Fisher, R., Folstein, M.F. (1993). Mania in temporal lobe epilepsy. *Neuropsychiatry, Neuropsychology, and Behavioral Neurology* 6: 19–25.

Mace, C.J. (1993). Epilepsy and schizophrenia. *British Journal of Psychiatry* 163: 439–45.

Marsh. L., Rao, V. (2002). Psychiatric complications in patients with epilepsy: a review. *Epilepsy Research* 49: 11–33.

Marsh, L., Krauss, G.L. (2000). Aggression and violence in patients with epilepsy. *Epilepsy & Behavior* 1: 160–8.

Marsh, L., Sullivan, E.V., Morrell, M., Lim, K.O., Pfefferbaum, A. (2001). Structural brain abnormalities in patients with schizophrenia, epilepsy, and epilepsy with chronic interictal psychosis. *Psychiatry Research* 108: 1–15.

Matson, J.L., Bamburg, J.W., Mayville, E.A., Kahn, I. (1999). Seizure disorders in people with intellectual disability: an analysis of differences in social functioning, adaptive functioning, and maladaptive behaviors. *Journal of Intellectual Disability Research* 43: 531–39.

Matsuura, M., Adachi, N., Muramatsu, R., Kato, M., Onuma, T., Okubo, Y., Oana, Y., Hara, T. (2005). Intellectual disability and psychotic disorders of adult epilepsy. *Epilepsia* 46: 11–14.

McConnell, H., Duncan, D. (1998). Treatment of psychiatric comorbidity in epilepsy. In H.W. McConnell, P.J. Snyder (Eds.), *Psychiatric Comorbidity in Epilepsy: Basic Mechanisms, Diagnosis, and Treatment*. Washington, DC: American Psychiatric Press. pp. 245–361.

Mendez, M.F., Cummings, J.L., Benson D.F. (1986). Depression in epilepsy. *Archives of Neurology* 43: 766–70.

Mittan, R.J., Locke, G.E. (1982). Fear of seizures: epilepsy's forgotten problem. *Urban Health* Jan/Feb: 40–1.

Nathaniel-James, D.A., Brown, R.G., Maier, M., Mellers, J., Toone, B., Ron, M.A. (2004). Cognitive abnormalities in schizophrenia and schizophrenia-like psychosis of epilepsy. *Journal of Neuropsychiatry and Clinical Neurosciences* 16: 472–9.

Newsom Davis, I., Goldstein L.H., Fitzpatrick, D. (1998). Fear of seizures: an investigation and treatment. *Seizure* 7: 101–6.

Pariente, P.D., Lepine, J.P., Lellouch, J. (1991). Lifetime history of panic attacks and epilepsy: an association from a general population survey [letter]. *Journal of Clinical Psychiatry* 52: 88–9.

Reith, J., Benkelfat, C., Sherwin, A., Yasuhara, Y., Kuwabara, H., Andermann, F., Bachneff, S., Cumming, P., Diksic, M., Dyve, S.E., Etienne, P., Evans, A.C., Lal, S., Shevell, M., Savard, G., Wong, D.F., Chouinard, G., Gjedde, A. (1994). Elevated dopa decarboxylase activity in living brain of patients with psychosis. *Proceedings of the National Academy of Sciences of the United States of America*. 91: 11651–4.

Reuber, M., Mitchell, A.J., Howlett, S., Elger, C.E. (2005). Measuring outcome in psychogenic nonepileptic seizures: how relevant is seizure remission? *Epilepsia* 46: 1788–95.

Reynolds, E. (1981). Biological factors in psychological disorders associated with epilepsy. In E.H. Reynolds (Ed)., *Epilepsy and Psychiatry*. Edinburgh, Scotland: Churchill Livingstone. pp 264–90.

Robertson, M.M. (1997). Suicide, parasuicide, and epilepsy. In J. Engel, Jr., T.A. Pedley, (Eds.), *Epilepsy: A Comprehensive Textbook*. Philadelphia, PA: Lippincott-Raven.

Robertson, M. (1998). Mood disorders associated with epilepsy. In H.W. McConnell, P.J. Snyder (Eds.), *Psychiatric Comorbidity in Epilepsy: Basic Mechanisms, Diagnosis, and Treatment*. Washington, DC: American Psychiatric Press. pp. 133–67.

Robertson, M.M., Trimble, M.R. (1985). The treatment of depression in patients with epilepsy. A double-blind trial. *Journal of Affective Disorders* 9: 127–36.

Schmitz, B. (2005). Depression and mania in patients with epilepsy. *Epilepsia* 46: 45–9.

Schwartz, J.M., Marsh, L. (2000).The psychiatric perspectives of epilepsy. *Psychosomatics* 41: 31–8.

Spector, S., Tranah, A., Cull, C., Goldstein, L.H. (1999). Reduction in seizure frequency following a short-term group intervention for adults with epilepsy. *Seizure* 8: 297–303.

Trimble, M.R. (1991). *The Psychoses of Epilepsy*. New York, NY: Raven Press.

Uijl, S.G., Uiterwaal, C.S., Aldenkamp, A.P., Carpay, J.A., Doelman, J.C., Keizer, K., Vecht, C.J., de Krom, M.C., van Donselaar, C.A. (2006). A cross-sectional study of subjective complaints in patients with epilepsy who seem to be well-controlled with anti-epileptic drugs. *Seizure* 15: 242–8.

Umbricht, D., Degreef, G., Barr, W.B., Lieberman, J.A., Pollack, S., Schaul, N. (1995). Postictal and chronic psychoses in patients with temporal lobe epilepsy. *American Journal of Psychiatry* 152: 224–31.

van Rijckevorsel, K. (2006). Cognitive problems related to epilepsy syndromes, especially malignant epilepsies. *Seizure* 15: 227–34.

Vingerhoets, G. (2006). Cognitive effects of seizures. *Seizure* 15: 221–26.

Walczak, T.S., Papacostas, S., Williams, D.T., Scheuer, M.L., Lebowitz, N., Notarfrancesco, A. (1995). Outcome after diagnosis of psychogenic nonepileptic seizures. *Epilepsia* 36: 1131–7.

8

Parkinson's Disease

LAURA MARSH

Parkinson's disease (PD), the second most common neurodegenerative disorder after Alzheimer's disease (AD), causes a progressive neurologic syndrome characterized by bradykinesia, tremor, rigidity, and, in its later stages, postural instability. The motor signs of PD correspond to loss of dopaminergic neurons in the substantia nigra pars compacta within the ventral midbrain. Neuronal inclusions, called Lewy bodies, are also present in the same region, but they can also be present in limbic and cortical regions and, along with other neurotransmitter deficits, are associated with nonmotor aspects of the disease. PD is to be distinguished from parkinsonism, a general term that refers to clinical conditions with the same motor phenomena, but without reference to a specific etiology.

Prevalence rates of PD vary. Epidemiologic studies show age-adjusted prevalence rates (per 100,000 individuals) range from 104.7 in Japan, 114.6 in the United States, 168.8 in Taiwan, and 258.8 in Sicily (Korell and Tanner, 2005). The disease affects about 1 million individuals in North America—approximately 0.5% to 1% of the population older than age 65 years of age. The average age of onset is about 60 years, but 5% to 10% of patients have young-onset PD, beginning before age 40 (Tanner and Ben-Shlomo, 1999). The disease affects all races, and there is a slightly higher prevalence of PD among men.

The diagnosis of PD relies on the clinical history and motor examination, which usually distinguish it from other parkinsonian disorders. However, because there is no biological marker that verifies the diagnosis of PD, neuropathologic findings remain the gold standard for confirmation of the clinical diagnosis. Even at specialized movement disorder centers, autopsy studies reveal that 10% to 20% of patients with clinical diagnoses of PD have other neuropathologic diagnoses (Hughes, Daniel, and Lees, 2001).

Two of the three cardinal motor signs (tremor, akinesia/ bradykinesia, and rigidity) are required to establish the diagnosis of PD, but these motor features overlap with other parkinsonian disorders. However, in patients without an overt tremor, early signs of PD such as decreased arm swing, limb stiffness, and diminished facial expression can be subtle, and the diagnosis of PD maybe delayed for several years. For example, the diagnosis of PD is not uncommonly missed in geriatric patients who present for evaluation of physical complaints or depressed mood. When distinguishing PD from other conditions, it is always important to remember that motor signs in PD begin unilaterally and remain asymmetric as the disease progresses, usually with the initially affected side showing more severe deficits. In addition, motor symptoms in PD typically respond to levodopa therapy, in contrast to most other parkinsonian conditions. About 70% to 80% of patients with PD experience a tremor that most commonly occurs at rest, but postural and kinetic tremors can also be present. Postural instability occurs later in the course of typical PD.

Because there are many causes of parkinsonism, evaluation and treatment of psychiatric complications in PD first requires confirmation of the clinical diagnosis of PD, as discussed above, and consideration of other parkinsonian conditions. Often, psychiatric disturbances are similar across conditions, but differences in their etiologies and course have implications for treatment. Drug-induced parkinsonism is associated with a number of agents. In psychiatric settings, neuroleptics are a common cause, but antiepileptic, antidepressant, anti-emetic, and antihypertensive agents also cause parkinsonism, as do a variety of toxins and chemicals. A number of neurodegenerative disorders involve parkinsonian features. Progressive supranuclear palsy is frequently misdiagnosed as PD early in its course. Other neurodegenerative disorders sometimes mistaken for PD include multiple system atrophy and corticobasal ganglionic degeneration. Parkinsonism often accompanies dementia. Dementia with Lewy bodies, in which the dementia syndrome is evident before or within the first year after onset of parkinsonism, is an important example of a condition that overlaps clinically with late-stage PD. Other dementing disorders that can share clinical phenomena with PD include AD, frontal-temporal dementia, and vascular dementia. Hereditary disorders with parkinsonism include Wilson's disease, Huntington's disease, dentatorubral-pallido luysian atrophy, and certain spinocerebellar ataxia syndromes.

Characteristics of Psychiatric Disturbances

A summary of psychiatric disturbances in PD is presented in Table 8–1.

Table 8.1.   Psychiatric Disturbances in Parkinson's Disease

Cognitive Impairments	Affective	Psychotic Phenomena	Behavioral
Executive dysfunction	Depression	Hallucinations	Impulse control disorders
Explicit memory deficits	Emotional Incontinence	Delusions	Hypersexuality
Slowed intellectual processing	Anxiety disorders Panic Disorder		Gambling Excessive
Attentional deficits	Phobias Generalized		Spending L-Dopa abuse
Visuospatial dysfunction	Anxiety Situational anxiety		Repetitive behaviors
Dementia	"Wearing-off"		Punding
Delirium	Anxiety Apathy Mania/hypomania		Compulsions

Cognitive Disturbances

Most patients with PD experience some degree of cognitive impairment, ranging from mild selective disturbances to global dementia (Dubois and Pillon, 1997). The extent to which these deficits contribute to the clinical picture and dysfunction is frequently underappreciated, in part, because screening tests for dementia such as the Mini-Mental State Examination are often in the "normal" range, even in patients with dementia. Early in the course of PD, selective impairments especially affect executive functions, memory, attention, and visuospatial dysfunction. In terms of daily life, this can be manifest by disorganization, trouble setting priorities, forgetfulness, and distractibility. Other affected domains involve information processing (eg, slowed thinking) and verbal fluency. The memory deficit in PD primarily affects explicit recall, with relative sparing of recognition memory and the absence of "rapid forgetting" seen in AD. Thus, for example, a patient with PD can learn the specifics of their medication regimen but might have difficulty retrieving these details when asked about them unless given a cue or reminder.

Dementia syndromes in PD generally develop later in the disease course and involve global impairments that preclude independent living (Tröster and Kaufer, 2005). The prevalence of dementia in PD is 25% to 40%, and its incidence increases with disease progression: at the end stages of PD, about 70% of patients have a severe dementia syndrome (Aarsland et al., 2003). In general, dementia syndromes in PD fall into three subgroups. The first involves intensification of selective deficits, especially in memory and information processing. The second shows increased involvement of cortical functions, including aphasia, apraxia, and memory, although the course and presentation is distinct from AD. The third has features of both PD and AD, with especially pronounced language deficits. Dementia with Lewy bodies (DLB) has many clinical features that overlap with dementia in PD, except that the cognitive disturbance either precedes the onset of parkinsonism or develops within the first year of onset of motor signs (Marsh and Aarsland, 2005).

Delirium is another cause of global cognitive impairment in patients with PD. Similar to delirium in patients without PD, it often develops in the setting of dementia, so that patients present with greater cognitive impairments, especially confusion and disorientation, than is their usual baseline. There are also fluctuations in the mental state over the course of the day; a patient may be relatively lucid and calm in the morning and confused and agitated in the evening. Because PD often involves fluctuating motor and mental states related to antiparkinsonian medications (Racette et al., 2002), it can be difficult to determine whether some patients, especially those with advanced PD and dementia, have a delirium. However, because delirium is a treatable condition, the possibility of its presence should always be considered. Delirium is usually the result of acute comorbid medical conditions (eg, urinary tract infections, pneumonia) or psychoactive medications used to treat PD or other conditions such as opiates, corticosteroids, benzodiazepines, and anticholinergics. More than one cause may be contributing to the delirium. Once the cause of the delirium is addressed, the cognitive status of the patient generally improves back to baseline, but some patients sustain a permanent diminution in their function after acute medical events.

Affective Disturbances

Depression. Depressive disturbances are common in PD. Although rates tend to be higher among patients in tertiary care centers, the prevalence of depression is about 40% to 50% (Slaughter et al., 2001). Slightly less than half of those affected have major depression, but a majority of patients have milder forms of depression (eg, dysthymia, minor, and subsyndromal depression). Unfortunately, depression in PD is undetected by clinicians in over half of affected patients—a phenomenon that may be due to overlap of physical and cognitive disturbances between PD itself and the syndrome of major depression (Shulman et al., 2002) (Table 8–2). Without direct inquiry about mood symptoms, a nondepressed patient can appear very similar to someone with severe depression. However, because most patients with PD are not followed by psychiatrists, clinicians may not be consistently attentive to psychiatric disturbances. Advanced age of patients or the presence of PD can also lead patients and clinicians to conclude that depressive phenomena are "understandable" in light of the patients' physical disabilities.

Similar to major depression in patients without neurologic disease, the core features of major depression in patients with PD are the presence of a persistent and pervasive low mood, a

Table 8.2. Overlapping Features of Major Depression and Parkinson's Disease

	Major Depression	Parkinson's Disease
Motor disturbances	Psychomotor Retardation	Bradykinesia
	Stooped posture	Stooped posture
	Restricted/depressed affect	Masked face/hypomimia
	Agitation	Tremor
Other physical disturbances	Decreased energy	
	Fatigue	
	Muscle tension	
	Sleep/appetite changes	
	Decreased libido	
Cognitive disturbances	Poor concentration	
	Decreased memory	
	Impaired problem-solving	

diminished ability to enjoy activities that would otherwise be enjoyable (anhedonia), or a decline in interest level from ones' usual baseline (Marsh et al., 2005). In nondepressed PD patients, motor symptoms can limit the ability to pursue previous interests (eg, detailed woodworking), but depressed PD patients fail to find alternative activities to enjoy that are within their physical capacities. Anxiety symptoms and comorbid anxiety disorders such as panic disorder are common in PD-related major depression and may precede onset of the depressive syndrome, in some cases even before the onset of PD (Menza, Robertson-Hoffman, and Bonapace, 1993). Some studies suggest that self-blame, negative self-attitude, delusions, and suicidality are less common in PD patients with major depression than they are in depressed patients without PD, but it is important to keep in mind that these phenomena can still be present. Similar phenomena are present in the nonmajor forms of depression in PD, but symptoms are more mild and fewer in number.

The course and prognosis of PD-related major depression has not been studied extensively (Weintraub et al., 2004). There are no consistent relationships among the age of onset or duration of PD, motor severity, or PD stage or subtype, and the timing of depression onset. Commonly, patients with very mild PD symptoms can be profoundly disabled by depressive symptoms that are more problematic than the actual movement disorder. Diagnosis of a depressive disorder should be considered when self-reported disability exceeds what is present on examination.

The differential diagnosis of PD-related depression includes other affective conditions as well as medical conditions. Unique to PD is the occurrence of drug-induced or fluctuating mood states that correspond to "on-off" periods induced by anti-parkinsonian medications (Racette et al., 2002). Patients may have pronounced sadness, agitation, or anxiety, usually in the "off" state when dopaminergic effects on motor function have subsided. Conversely, but less frequently, there may be hypomanic phenomena in the "on" state. There are also patients who develop a severe psychologic dependence on dopaminergic therapy that is associated with excessive use of antiparkinsonian medications and frequently severe mood swings, with dysphoria in the "off" state and enhanced well-being, if not hypomania or mania, in the "on" state. As indicated in Chapter 2, a sad mood in PD may represent demoralization rather than a major depressive disorder. Pathologic tearfulness (also called emotional incontinence), in which there is excessive and involuntary crying in response to a sad or poignant stimulus, can be a feature of a depressive disturbance, but it may also be present in the absence of a mood disorder. Other disturbances in which features overlap with depression include apathy, dementia and milder forms of cognitive impairment, or delirium. Medical conditions, including delirium from any number of causes, hypothyroidism, and testosterone deficiency can also mimic PD-related depressive disorders.

Anxiety. Anxiety disturbances are very common in PD but have not received as much attention as depressive disorders. Clinical series indicate that as many as 40% of PD patients have anxiety disorders, with men and women affected equally (Marsh, 2000). Panic disorder is especially common, with prevalence rates of 25% in some series (Stein et al., 1990). Similar to patients without PD, panic disorder in patients with PD includes the spontaneous and usually sudden onset of severe apprehension and anxiety, often with fears that one is having a heart attack, dying, or losing control of oneself. There are a number of accompanying physical symptoms, including shortness of breath, chest discomfort, indigestion, nausea, lightheadedness, paresthesias, and various autonomic symptoms (eg, tachycardia, facial flushing). Generalized anxiety, social phobias, claustrophobia, and other phobias are also seen, but many patients have persistent or recurrent anxiety phenomena that do not meet specific diagnostic criteria for specific anxiety disorders in the *Diagnostic and Statistical Manual of Mental Disorders* (APA, 1994). Comorbid depressive disorders are common in PD patients with anxiety disorders. Fluctuations in levodopa levels and "on-off" states can also be associated with anxiety. Such "nonmotor fluctuations" frequently involve severe panicky states that persist even after motor function improves in the "on" state. Some patients have severe situational anxiety that aggravates motor symptoms. For example, one patient was so anxious about being able to answer the phone on time in light of his PD symptoms that he became akinetic whenever the phone rang, even at times when his motor symptoms were minimal. Unlike catastrophic reactions seen in patients with dementia, these anxious episodes tend to be stereotypical and somewhat predictable, and the patient is not confused or disoriented.

The course of anxiety disorders in PD has not been studied. Epidemiologic studies show that anxiety disturbances in the general population confer a higher relative risk of developing PD (Gonera et al., 1997; Shiba et al., 2000; Weisskopf et al., 2003). In clinical practice, anxiety disturbances often develop during a prodromal period before onset of motor symptoms, or as much as 20 years before the onset of motor signs. Pathologic anxiety may therefore represent either a risk factor for PD or an early nonmotor sign of the disease. After onset of PD, anxiety disturbances can occur at any time. Like depression, pathologic anxiety may be underrecognized because its manifestations are often episodic or situational and regarded as a reasonable reaction to the difficulties related to PD motor symptoms. In fact, PD patients with anxiety disturbances frequently describe their anxiety as excessive for their circumstances.

Mania/hypomania. The prevalence of manic or hypomanic disturbances in PD is not established, and these phenomena have not been well-characterized in studies of PD. In the majority of cases, manic phenomena appear to develop in the context of a treatment-induced state. There have been reports of manic phenomena developing with levodopa use, especially when it first became available to treat PD and higher doses were used (Goodwin, 1971). Mania can also develop in response to other dopaminergic agents or after neurosurgical treatments for PD (eg, deep brain stimulation or pallidotomy) (Anderson and Mullins, 2003). As noted above, some patients fluctuate between manic states when "on" and depressive states when "off" (Racette et al., 2002). Another way in which mania can appear in PD is in patients with a history of bipolar disorder before the onset of PD. Such patients are more likely to present with sustained manic states that resemble prior episodes. Finally, there are patients with PD and a history of unipolar depression who develop hypomanic or manic phenomena in the setting of combined use of antidepressants and antiparkinsonian medications.

Aside from the fluctuating nature of the mental state in some patients, the features of mania and hypomania resemble those in patients without PD and include an elevated mood; grandiosity; irritability; hyperactivity; and increased goal-directed behavior, including risk-taking behaviors. One patient who developed hypomania after unilateral pallidotomy wanted to redecorate the clinic and start a support group for patients considering a second pallidotomy. Another patient with advanced PD started sky-diving and spending money excessively. Mood-congruent psychotic phenomena can be present. For example, one patient with extreme motor fluctuations had grandiose delusions in "on" states.

Psychotic Phenomena

Psychotic phenomena in PD include hallucinations and delusions. Over the course of the disease, about 50% of patients experience hallucinations, and cross-sectional prevalence is 25% to 40% (Fénelon et al., 2000) Delusions occur in as many as 30% of patients (Marsh et al., 2004). Development of psychotic phenomena in PD is associated with concurrent dopaminergic therapy, but the dose of dopaminergic therapy is not correlated with the presence of hallucinations and delusions. Underlying cognitive impairment, especially dementia, is also an important risk factor, as is sleep deprivation. Delirium should be considered in the differential diagnosis of psychotic phenomena, but typical PD-related psychotic phenomena are not a component of a delirious state or medication toxicity related to nondopaminergic drugs.

Visual hallucinations are the most common hallucinatory phenomenon, experienced by 15% to 40% of patients cross-sectionally and by nearly 50% of patients over the course of PD (Fénelon et al., 2000). These may be fleeting simple images (eg, shadows) or complex scenes with well-formed people that are usually stereotyped each time they occur. Minor hallucinations, reported by about 25% of patients (Fénelon et al., 2000), include a sensation of a presence (eg, a person), a brief vision of something (usually a person or animal) passing sideways in the peripheral visual field, or illusions. Patients in earlier stages of PD often have insight into the "nonreal" nature of the hallucinations. In the absence of insight, patients can develop suspiciousness, become agitated about intruders, or try to feed unwanted houseguests.

Up to half of patients with visual hallucinations experience other types of hallucinations (Fénelon et al., 2000; Marsh et al., 2004). About 10% of patients with PD who have hallucinations have auditory hallucinations; other types of hallucinations are less prevalent (Marsh et al., 2004). Psychotic affective syndromes can be associated with either depression or mania in PD. Most often, however, hallucinations and delusions present as phenomena independent of mood disorders.

Hallucinations and delusions are usually present at the same time in a patient, but the content of each may be unrelated. Delusions most often have paranoid themes and focus on a single subject or theme. Common examples are spousal infidelity, fears of being poisoned or injured, or elaborate conspiracies (Factor et al., 1995). Occasionally, there are bizarre delusions, such as beliefs that one's motor symptoms are controlled by an outside force. Nonmotor "on-off" fluctuations can also involve psychotic phenomena. The diagnosis of DLB should be considered when hallucinations, especially visual hallucinations, occur in the absence of dopaminergic treatment. Psychotic phenomena in PD can be distinguished from those of Charles Bonnet syndrome, in which there are also complex visual hallucinations in the setting of visual impairment, but patients are otherwise neurologically normal and not taking dopaminergic medications.

Behavioral Disturbances

Impulse control disorders. The core feature of impulse control disorders (ICDs) is the inability to resist the drive to behave in a way that is ultimately harmful to oneself or others. Such behavioral disturbances in patients with PD include hypersexuality, pathologic gambling, excessive spending, and overeating behaviors, and some patients demonstrate more than one such behavior. The hypersexuality can range from an increased desire for sexual activity with one's usual partner to involvement in multiple sexual relationships to the onset of paraphilic behaviors. In general, the behaviors in ICDs appear to be induced by dopaminergic medications or neurosurgical treatment for PD (Anderson and Mullins, 2003), but the underlying factors that render some patients vulnerable to ICDs are not known. The behaviors are not occurring in the context of a manic state, and most patients describe them as alien to their usual selves. The exact prevalence of ICDs in PD is unknown because the behaviors are frequently covert and the association with PD is not appreciated.

Repetitive behaviors. "Punding" is a phenomenon first described in amphetamine addicts that involves the repetitive handling of objects, frequently taking them apart and attempting to reassemble them (Fernandez and Friedman, 1999). Examples involve dissembling and reassembling mechanical items in the home such as flashlights and other appliances, shelving and reshelving books, and repetitive entering of sums on a calculator. The prevalence of such behaviors in PD may be as high as 14% (Kurlan, 2003). Unlike ICDs, which are driven by the prospect of a reward, punding is obsessive-compulsive–like in that the behaviors are repetitive and stereotypical, and they are often conducted with the goal of feeling more relaxed. Obsessive-compulsive behaviors as such occur rarely and appear to be less common than the other behavioral and anxiety disturbances.

Apathy. Apathy, a state of diminished motivation and goal-directed behavior, is present as an independent syndrome in at least 10% of patients (Pluck and Brown, 2002). About 25% of patients have apathy and a concurrent depressive disorder (Starkstein et al., 1992). Apathy is also a common feature of dementia, delirium, and demoralization. As an independent disturbance, apathy is often overlooked or misdiagnosed as depression, but its recognition is important to guiding treatment. In apathy independent of other syndromes, patients typically show poor motivation as well as indifference to their circumstances, including a lack of concern over their health. The patient experiences pleasure and participates in structured activities if they are organized by others but is otherwise inactive. It is important to distinguish apathy from neurologic phenomena such as akinesia, hypomimia, hypophonia, cognitive dysfunction, and bradyphrenia. Predictors of apathy or its effects on the course of PD are not known.

Impact of Psychiatric Disturbances in Parkinson's Disease

Even in the absence of psychiatric pathology, PD is already a complex disorder with its heterogeneous and progressive motor and nonmotor physical features. Fluctuating medication effects on motor function add to its complexity, i.e."on-off" phenomena and hyperkinetic "on" state choreiform movements referred to as dyskinesias and dystonias. There is substantial interplay among the motor, cognitive, affective, and behavioral disturbances such that the impact of each on functional abilities is at least additive. Fortunately, successful treatment of psychiatric disturbances reduces excess disability.

Cognitive Disturbances

Early in the course of PD, cognitive dysfunction can be relatively subtle, so the extent to which deficits cause dysfunction often relates to a patient's circumstances. Individuals attempting to remain in the workforce or live independently can be profoundly disabled and demoralized by executive dysfunction, but this is less of a problem for individuals who are retired. However, untreated psychiatric disturbances such as mood disorders aggravate selective impairments, especially executive dysfunction. Dementia is devastating for individuals who live alone, as independent living becomes unsafe and compliance with the complicated antiparkinsonian dosing regimens is largely impossible. Dementia appears to be associated with an increased risk of many additional psychiatric disturbances, including depression, psychotic phenomena, punding, and apathy. For family members, individual cognitive impairments such as executive dysfunction are challenging because the patient's performance can be erratic. With the global cognitive impairments of dementia, caregiver burden can be substantial and nursing home admission may be necessary.

Mood Disturbances

The impact of untreated affective disorders is substantial (McDonald, Richard, and DeLong, 2003). Major depression is associated with greater motor and cognitive deficits, excessive and accelerated progression of disability, worsened quality of life, and greater caregiver burden and depression. The patient's negativism and reduced activity strains daily interactions with caregivers and others. Patients often think that their depression is the result of deficient coping skills, but the opposite is actually true. With PD (or any chronic illness), successful coping and adaptation is nearly impossible when there is an untreated mood disorder. Treatment of the depressive disorder enables the person to better compensate and face the challenges associated with the underlying disease. Motor symptoms are often aggravated by anxiety symptoms, which can lead to overmedication with antiparkinsonian drugs if the anxiety disturbance is not addressed. Anxiety disorders are especially challenging for caregivers because patients in states of acute anxiety frequently seek reassurance but can be difficult to reassure and redirect.

Psychotic Phenomena

Hallucinations and delusions tend to occur in patients with more severe cognitive deficits (especially dementia) and with depressive disorders. Psychotic phenomena in patients with PD produce increased caregiver burden, a greater risk of nursing home placement, and an overall worse prognosis with greater mortality (Fernandez and Lapane, 2002). Fortunately, the effectiveness of certain atypical neuroleptics has improved outcomes for patients with PD-related hallucinations and delusions (see below).

Behavioral Disturbances

Behavioral disturbances in PD frequently have profound social effects (Marsh, 2005). With gambling, sexual indiscretion, or excessive spending, the trust of others is often betrayed, and the financial consequences can be devastating. Patients with punding often do not recognize their time-consuming behaviors as abnormal. Often, patients with behavioral disturbances become distressed or irritable when redirected and they neglect medication adherence and sleep, which results in motor deterioration and greater caregiver burden and frustration. By definition, apathetic states are not distressing to the affected patient. The patients' inactivity and indifference over their health can accelerate physical debility, and families and caregivers are frequently more frustrated by the patients' inertia and lack of spontaneous effort.

Treatment

General Steps in Treatment of Psychiatric Disturbances in Parkinson's Disease

Pharmacologic and nonpharmacologic strategies are both necessary components in the treatment of psychiatric conditions in PD. Because patients frequently present with more than one psychiatric disturbance (eg, major depression, dementia, drug-induced mood changes), treatment is complex. The following guidelines are recommended:

• The relative contributions of motor, cognitive, affective, and other psychiatric phenomena to the clinical picture should be recognized, as well as how each of these realms interacts with and is affected by antiparkinsonian, psychiatric, and other medications.
• Comorbid medical conditions, including delirium, should be addressed.
• Careful attention should be paid to the role of the antiparkinsonian regimen on the mental state and to the possibility of adverse effects of all other psychoactive drugs taken by the patient. Importantly, "nonmotor fluctuations" in mood states require modification of the PD regimen rather than psychiatric medications.
• Given the risk of adverse drug effects, including drug-drug interactions, starting doses of psychiatric medications should be low in order to evaluate tolerability. All psychoactive medications should also be monitored for aggravating parkinsonism or cognitive dysfunction.
• To assess treatment response, patients started on psychiatric medications should be evaluated more frequently in follow-up than is customary for treatment of motor symptoms. Unfortunately, many PD patients with psychiatric disturbances are undertreated and remain symptomatic (Weintraub et al., 2003). Therefore, after initiating medication therapy, subsequent dosage adjustments should be aimed at remission of the psychiatric symptoms.

Nonpharmacologic treatments include a variety of strategies. Because motor features generally receive the most emphasis in PD, many patients and families benefit from additional education about the psychiatric aspects of PD, their impact on other aspects of PD and quality of life, and the importance of adequate treatment. Caregivers are vulnerable to depressive disturbances and may need referral for treatment. Caring for patients with combined motor and psychiatric dysfunction poses substantial burdens, especially as the disease progresses. Respite care, day programs, and nursing home placement can be integral adjuncts to the overall treatment plan.

Psychiatric consultation should be obtained when initial attempts at treatment with pharmacologic or nonpharmacologic strategies are unsuccessful and whenever there are concerns about suicidality or other forms of danger to self or others. Inpatient psychiatric hospitalization is necessary for suicidality, severe depression, anxiety, or agitation that cannot be managed with usual outpatient care. It can also be useful for clarifying the diagnosis, initiating therapies safely in patients with advanced disease and complex medical regimens, and providing a structured situation that can assess triggers of problem behaviors, ranging from punding to anxiety disorders, while ensuring that there is compliance with medical treatment.

Cognitive Dysfunction

Studies on treatment of cognitive dysfunction in PD have mainly focused on dementia. Several double-blind placebo-controlled studies have demonstrated the effectiveness and relative safety of all of the available cholinesterase inhibitors for treatment of dementia in PD (Leroi, Collins, and Marsh, 2006). Common side effects of cholinesterase inhibitors include nausea and other gastrointestinal side effects, as well as worsened tremor. To limit such side effects and increase the overall tolerability of the cholinesterase inhibitors, it is often best to begin treatment with doses that are lower than the recommended starting doses (eg, 2.5 mg of donepezil daily or 4 mg of galantamine daily). Whether cholinesterase inhibitors are useful for early-stage cognitive impairment in PD has not been studied. Medications that have potential use for treatment of executive dysfunction and other selective deficits in PD include modafinil (starting at 200 mg in the morning) and atomoxetine (starting at 25 mg daily) (Bassett, 2005). Other cognition-enhancing medications indicated for AD and vascular dementias such as memantine can be helpful in some patients with PD and dementia, and controlled studies are underway.

Delirium is treated by decreasing or stopping the offending medication or medications (if possible) and addressing other nonmedication causes of delirium. Treating agitation, delusions, or hallucinations from delirium in patients with PD is challenging. When delirium is caused by one or more of the PD medications, these must be reduced or eliminated. Amantadine, anticholinergic agents, and dopamine agonists often contribute to delirium, but abrupt elimination or reduction of these medications can also cause agitation or aggravate parkinsonism. Although it occurs rarely, a clinical state resembling neuroleptic malignant syndrome can be associated with discontinuation or reduction of antiparkinsonian medications (Ueda et al., 1999). Therefore, the medications should be tapered expeditiously and with careful monitoring of motor and mental status in response to dosage adjustments. Because most patients with PD, even when delirious, require ongoing dopaminergic therapy, immediate-release levodopa preparations are usually best tolerated from the psychiatric standpoint and are generally associated with a more predictable motor response than other antiparkinsonian agents.

In acute settings, when the patient is agitated and has dangerous behaviors that might lead to self-harm or harm to others or property, benzodiazepines (eg. starting doses of oral or intramuscular lorazepam, 0.25–1.0 mg every 6 hours, with repeat doses as needed) are recommended for the treatment of delirium in PD. Because benzodiazepines are a common cause of delirium in vulnerable patients, their use may seem counter-intuitive. However, in PD, medication options for treatment of delirium are limited because of the need to balance treatment of both motor and psychiatric phenomena without adverse side effects that aggravate either. Neuroleptics such as quetiapine (starting dose range, 6.25–25 mg/day, with smaller doses used to initiate therapy in frail patients) may not be as readily effective as benzodiazepines. Typical neuroleptics (eg, haloperidol), which are often used to control symptoms in non-PD patients with delirium, are contraindicated in patients with PD because they block dopamine receptors and cause severe parkinsonism. This can result in medical complications such as fractures, aspiration pneumonia, deep venous thrombosis, or decubiti. Ondansetron (starting dose of 4 mg/day), and related serotonin-blockers (usually used to combat chemotherapy-related nausea) can be given intravenously, intramuscularly, or orally, but they are very expensive and their use is probably most appropriate in settings of postoperative delirium. When agitation is not an issue or behaviors can be controlled by redirection or environmental manipulations (eg, moving the patient to a place that is less stimulating, providing adequate lighting, having someone stay with the patient for reassurance), the best approach for treatment of delirium is to address the cause and to not add additional medications.

Cognitive rehabilitation for selective impairments in PD and behavioral interventions to maximize functioning and reduce disruptive behaviors in other dementias may also be useful in PD, but they have not been specifically studied. It is often helpful to advise families about behavioral strategies that can enhance function (eg, memory aides, structured environment, assistance from others to reduce the impact of executive dysfunction, avoidance of tasks that exceed the patient's abilities). Occupational and speech therapies can individualize strategies to maximum daily functioning and address communication deficits.

Mood Disturbances

Depression. There is little more than anecdotal evidence and case series reports on which to base advice regarding treatment of mood disturbances in PD (Weintraub et al., 2005). For non-major forms of depression, it is often appropriate to monitor symptoms (ie, watchful waiting) and provide a referral to rehabilitative therapies that can assist with problem-solving and help maximize function, thereby overcoming demoralization.

If symptoms persist, are prolonged, or are at least moderately disruptive, use of antidepressant medications should be considered. Selective serotonin reuptake inhibitors (SSRIs) are frequently used for treatment of depression (Richard, Kurlan, and Parkinson Study Group, 1997), but clinical trials have been limited; there is no evidence that one antidepressant is more effective than another. Dosing strategies are similar to what is recommended in geriatric psychiatry. For example, it is common to use low starting doses (eg, sertraline 25 mg daily, escitalopram 5 mg daily, venlafaxine 37.5 mg daily, bupropion 50 mg daily, nortriptyline 10 mg daily) in order to assess tolerance. If symptoms persist, it is important to increase the dose to the usual target doses for antidepressants or switch antidepressants if there has been an inadequate response after 12 weeks at a maximum dose. Electroconvulsive therapy (ECT) is indicated when patients are severely depressed and have not responded to antidepressant medication or in danger of death from inanition or suicide. Interestingly, ECT is also beneficial for motor symptoms of PD in the absence of a concurrent mood disturbance (Faber and Trimble, 1991).

There are no data on the duration of antidepressant treatment for major depression. In many cases, patients require chronic maintenance therapy because depressive symptoms return when the antidepressant medicines are reduced or discontinued.

Anxiety. There are no published studies on treatment of anxiety disorders, but SSRIs appear to be helpful. A "serotonin syndrome" has the potential to occur when there is coadministration of selegiline, a monoamine oxidase-B inhibitor, and SSRIs or tricyclic antidepressants, but clinical experience suggests that such combinations are usually well-tolerated depression (Richard et al., 1997). Patients on selegiline and an antidepressant should, however, be assessed frequently; many of the symptoms associated with the serotonin syndrome (eg, agitation, confusion, hyperreflexia, myoclonus, restlessness, rigidity, tremor, tachycardia) overlap with the motor phenomena of PD and its psychiatric complications. In addition, because SSRIs and other antidepressants have the potential to aggravate anxiety when doses are first initiated, it is best to start treatment of anxiety disturbances with low doses of antidepressants (eg, escitalopram 5 mg daily) and to warn patients and their caregivers of this possibility. Similarly, when discontinuing an antidepressant, it is important to taper the drug and monitor for withdrawal-emergent symptoms, which often involve anxiety phenomena.

Psychotic phenomena. In contrast to other psychiatric disturbances in PD, a number of studies have addressed the treatment of psychotic phenomena (Friedman and Fernandez, 2002). When psychotic phenomena are mild or have no functional impact (eg benign visual hallucinations), educating patients and families about the occurrence of psychotic phenomena in PD may be sufficient. Cholinesterase inhibitors can be added to enhance cognition, but they have also been shown to reduce hallucinations (Leroi, Collins, and Marsh, 2006). Improving nocturnal sleep with trazodone or neuroleptics (see below) is often very helpful. The typical dose range for trazodone, when used as a hypnotic in patients with PD, ranges from 25 to 150 mg nightly. As noted above, except in states of extreme agitation

(Factor and Molho, 2000), it is best to avoid benzodiazepines for agitation or as hypnotics because they can contribute to delirium.

Neuroleptics should be used for disruptive hallucinations and delusions. The only available neuroleptics that are recommended are quetiapine and clozapine. Both are generally well tolerated and effective, but clozapine appears to be the most effective and does not aggravate parkinsonism—something that is still possible but less common with quetiapine. However, quetiapine is the first-line agent because it does not require hematologic monitoring for agranulocytosis. Starting doses for both quetiapine and clozapine are 6.25–12.5 mg at night, and maintenance doses range from 6.25 mg every other night to as high as 200 mg nightly. Sometimes, symptom control is better when several small doses (eg, 12.5 mg) are given during the day and a larger dose is given at bedtime. This strategy also helps patients with insomnia to sleep and settles patients with increased agitation at nighttime.

Behavioral disturbances. ICDs can be challenging to treat because the behaviors are often covert. The first step is to educate patients and families about the potential for impulsive behaviors in PD before medications are started. When such behaviors do occur, the next step is to adjust the PD medications and taper or eliminate the offending agents—often dopamine agonists. Quetiapine or clozapine can be used for symptom control acutely and if symptoms persist after medication adjustments. Some patients require inpatient hospitalization to control symptoms, especially when there are concurrent psychotic phenomena. To prevent devastating financial losses, families often have to control the patient's access to money until the symptoms are well-controlled. Agents for impulse control and lability (eg, lithium, oxcarbazepine) can be considered, especially when there are hypomanic phenomena, but there are little data regarding this strategy. It should also be noted that mood-stabilizing agents such as lithium and valproate can aggravate parkinsonism, and monitoring for this side effect is warranted. Psychiatric referral is recommended for such treatment.

When punding is a problem, the PD regimen should be adjusted to see if the symptoms become less intense. Day programs and other structured daytime activities can decrease opportunities for repetitive behaviors and often enhance nocturnal sleep. Trazodone or quetiapine are often used to facilitate nocturnal sleep. SSRIs can be considered as they may target the obsessive-compulsive nature of these symptoms.

Treatment of apathy, when it is not part of a depressive disturbance, first involves adjusting the patient's daily schedule so as to maximize functioning and activity level. Structured day programs are often helpful in this regard. Cognition-enhancing medications (eg, galantamine, 4 mg daily starting dose; memantine, 5 mg daily starting dose) and amphetamines (D-amphetamine, 5 mg in the morning) can also be helpful, but there are no studies on such use of these medications in PD.

References

Aarsland, D., Andersen, K., Larsen, J.P., Lolk, A., Kragh-Sørensen, P. (2003). Prevalence and characteristics of dementia in Parkinson disease. *Archives of Neurology* 60: 387–92.

[APA] American Psychiatric Association (1994). *Diagnostic and Statistical Manual of Mental Disorders* (3rd ed.). Washington, DC: American Psychiatric Association.

Anderson, K.E., Mullins, J. (2003). Behavioral changes associated with deep brain stimulation surgery for Parkinson's disease. *Current Neurology and Neuroscience Reports* 3: 306–13.

Bassett, S.S. (2005). Cognitive impairment. In M. Menza and L.Marsh (Eds.) *Psychiatric Issues in Parkinson's Disease—A Practical Guide*. London, England: Taylor & Francis. pp. 63–75.

Dubois, B., Pillon, B. (1997). Cognitive deficits in Parkinson's disease. *Journal of Neurology* 244: 2–8.

Faber, R., Trimble, M.R. (1991). Electroconvulsive therapy in Parkinson's disease and other movement disorders. *Movement Disorders* 6: 293–303.

Factor, S.A., Molho, E.S. (2000). Emergency department presentations of patients with Parkinson's disease. *American Journal of Emergency Medicine* 18: 209–15.

Factor, S.A., Molho, E.S., Podskalny, G.D., Brown, D. (1995). Parkinson's disease: drug-induced psychiatric states. *Advances in Neurology* 65: 115–38.

Fénelon, G., Mahieux, F., Huon, R., Ziégler, M.(2000). Hallucinations in Parkinson's disease. Prevalence, phenomenology, and risk factors. *Brain* 123: 733–45.

Fernandez, H.H., Friedman, J.H. (1999). Punding on L-dopa. *Movement Disorders* 14: 835–8.

Fernandez, H.H., Lapane, K.L. (2002). Predictors of mortality among nursing home residents with a diagnosis of Parkinson's disease. *Medical Science Monitor* 8: 241–6.

Friedman, J.H., Fernandez, H.H. (2002). Atypical antipsychotics in Parkinson-sensitive populations. *Journal of Geriatric Psychiatry and Neurology* 15: 156–70.

Gonera, E.G., van't Hof, M., Berger, J.C., van Weel, C., Horstink, M.W. (1997). Symptoms and duration of the prodromal phase in Parkinson's disease. *Movement Disorders* 12: 871–6.

Goodwin, F.K. (1971). Psychiatric side effects of levodopa in man. *Journal of the American Medical Association* 218: 1915–20.

Hughes, A.J., Daniel, S.E., Lees, A.J. (2001). Improved accuracy of clinical diagnosis of Lewy body Parkinson's disease. *Neurology* 57: 1497–99.

Korell, M., Tanner, C.M. (2005). Epidemiology of Parkinson's disease: an overview. In M.P.R. Ebadi (Ed.), *Parkinson's Disease*. Boca Raton, FL: CRC Press. pp. 39–50.

Kurlan, R. (2003). Disabling repetitive behaviors in Parkinson's disease. *Movement Disorders* 19: 433–69.

Leroi, I., Collins, D., Marsh, L. (2006). Non-dopaminergic treatment of cognitive impairment and dementia in Parkinson's disease: a review. *Journal of Neurological Sciences* 248:104–14.

Marsh, L. (2000). Anxiety disorders in Parkinson's disease. *International Review of Psychiatry* 12: 307–18.

Marsh, L. (2005). Behavioral disturbances. In M.A. Menza and L. Marsh (Eds.), *Psychiatric Aspects of Parkinson's Disease: A Practical Guide*. London, England: Taylor & Francis. pp. 193–218.

Marsh, L., Aarsland, D. (2005). Dementia secondary to Parkinson's disease versus dementia with Lewy bodies. In M. Menza and L. Marsh (Eds.), *Psychiatric Issues in Parkinson's Disease—A Practical Guide.* London, England: Taylor & Francis. pp. 97–117.

Marsh, L., Williams, J.R., Rocco, M., Grill, S., Munro, C., Dawson, T.M. (2004). Psychiatric comorbidities associated with psychosis in patients with Parkinson's disease. *Neurology* 63: 293–300.

Marsh, L., McDonald, W.M., Cummings, J., Ravina, B. (2005). Provisional diagnostic criteria for depression in Parkinson's disease: report of an NINDS/NIMH Work Group. *Movement Disorders* 21: 148–58.

McDonald, W.M., Richard, I.H., DeLong, M.R. (2003). Prevalence, etiology, and treatment of depression in Parkinson's disease. *Biological Psychiatry* 54: 363–75.

Menza, M.A., Robertson-Hoffman, D.E., Bonapace, A.S. (1993). Parkinson's disease and anxiety: comorbidity with depression. *Biological Psychiatry* 34: 465–70.

Pluck, G.C., Brown, R.G. (2002). Apathy in Parkinson's disease. *Journal of Neurology, Neurosurgery, and Psychiatry* 73: 636–42.

Racette, B.A., Hartlein, J.M., Hershey, T., Mink, J.W., Perlmutter, J.S., Black, K.J. (2002). Clinical features and comorbidity of mood fluctuations in Parkinson's disease. *Journal of Neuropsychiatry and Clinical Neurosciences* 14: 438–42.

Richard, I.H., Kurlan, R., Parkinson Study Group (1997). A survey of antidepressant usage in Parkinson's disease. *Neurology* 49: 1168–70.

Richard, I.H., Kurlan, R., Tanner, C., Factor, S. Hubble, J., Suchowersky, O., Waters, C. (1997). Serotonin syndrome and the combined use of deprenyl and an antidepressant in Parkinson's disease. Parkinson Study Group. *Neurology* 48: 1070–7.

Shiba, M., Bower, J.H., Maraganore, D.M., McDonnell, S.K., Peterson, B.J., Ahlskog, J.E. Schaid, D.J., Rocca, W.A. (2000). Anxiety disorders and depressive disorders preceding Parkinson's disease: a case-control study. *Movement Disorders* 15: 669–77.

Shulman, L.M., Taback, R.L., Rabinstein, A.A., Weiner, W.J. (2002). Nonrecognition of depression and other non-motor symptoms in Parkinson's disease. *Parkinsonism and Related Disorders* 8: 193–7.

Slaughter, J.R., Slaughter, K.A., Nichols, D., Holmes, S.E., Martens, M.P. (2001). Prevalence, clinical manifestations, etiology, and treatment of depression in Parkinson's disease. *Journal of Neuropsychiatry and Clinical Neurosciences* 13: 187–96.

216 PSYCHIATRIC ASPECTS OF NEUROLOGIC DISEASES

Starkstein, S.E., Mayberg, H.S., Preziosi, T.J., Andrezejewski, P., Leiguarda, R., Robinson, R.G. (1992). Reliability, validity, and clinical correlates of apathy in Parkinson's disease. *Journal of Neuropsychiatry and Clinical Neurosciences* 4: 134–9

Stein, M.B., Heuser, I.J., Juncos, J.L., Uhde, T.W. (1990). Anxiety disorders in patients with Parkinson's disease. *American Journal of Psychiatry* 147: 217–20.

Tanner, C., Ben-Shlomo, Y. (1999). Epidemiology of Parkinson's disease. *Parkinson's Disease: Advances in Neurology* 80: 153–9.

Tröster A.I., Kaufer, D.I. (2005). Dementia. In M. Menza and L. Marsh (Eds.), *Psychiatric Issues in Parkinson's Disease—A Practical Guide*. London, England: Taylor & Francis. pp. 77–95.

Ueda M., Hamamoto, M., Nagayama, H., Otsubo, K., Nito, C., Miyazaki, T. Terashi, A., Katayama, Y. (1999). Susceptibility to neuroleptic malignant syndrome in Parkinson's disease. *Neurology* 52: 777–81.

Weintraub D., Moberg, P.J., Duda, J.E., Katz, I.R., Stern, M.B. (2004). Effect of psychiatric and other nonmotor symptoms on disability in Parkinson's disease. *Journal of the American Geriatrics Society* 52: 784–8.

Weintraub D., Moberg, P.J., Duda, J.E., Katz, I.R., Stern, M.B. (2003). Recognition and treatment of depression in Parkinson's disease. *Journal of Geriatric Psychiatry and Neurology* 16: 178–83.

Weintraub, D., Morales, K.H., Moberg, P.J., Bilker, W.B., Balderston, C., Duda, J.E., Katz, I.R., Stern, M.B. (2005). Antidepressant studies in Parkinson's disease: a review and meta-analysis. *Movement Disorders* 20: 1161–69.

Weisskopf, M.G., Chen, H., Schwarzschild, M.A., Kawachi, I., Ascherio, A. (2003). Prospective study of phobic anxiety and risk of Parkinson's disease. *Movement Disorders* 18: 646–51.

9

Alzheimer's Disease

MARTIN STEINBERG

Alzheimer's disease (AD), a progressive degenerative dementia, causes suffering for millions of patients as well as their caregivers. Among the elderly, the prevalence of AD increases dramatically with age: it is about 5% to 7% in people 65 years of age and older and rises to 40% to 50% in those older than 90 years of age (Rabins, Lyketsos, and Steele, 1999). AD typically affects short-term memory first; over time, impairment in language, praxis, recognition, and executive function occur. In the late stages, patients become completely dependent on others.

In addition to this cognitive and physical burden, psychiatric signs and symptoms are nearly universal. These psychiatric phenomena, which include depression, delusions, hallucinations, apathy, and aggression, affect as many as 90% of patients with dementia over the course of their illness (Steinberg et al., 2003). Psychiatric phenomena often present differently in patients with AD than in the population without dementia. Uncertainty remains regarding how to best classify many of these phenomena. For example, delusions can be described as occurring in isolation, or as part of a psychotic syndrome, with associated features such as irritability and agitation. Delusions can also occur as part of a depressive syndrome or delirium. Little research is currently available to guide treatment. Nevertheless, many syndromes can be accurately diagnosed and can respond to a variety of pharmacologic and nonpharmacologic treatments.

Depression

Depressive phenomena are common in AD. Estimates for the prevalence of major depression in patients with AD are 20% to 25%, (Lyketsos et al., 2003). Due to their dementia, patients with AD are often poor historians. They may not be aware of depressive phenomena or able to recall them, and their aphasia may make describing symptoms difficult. Therefore, information from a reliable caregiver is crucial for making a proper diagnosis.

Depressive disorders in AD are often somewhat different from those occurring in the absence of dementia. In particular, patients with AD may not endorse hopelessness, suicidal thoughts, or worthlessness (Zubenko et al., 2003). Patients with AD, however, express symptoms such as anxiety, anhedonia, irritability, lack of motivation, and agitation (Rosenberg et al., 2005). Anxiety is often the most prominent symptom, and delusions, often of a paranoid nature, are also common. Because major depression in AD has a somewhat atypical presentation, relying on the *Diagnostic and Statistical Manual*, fourth edition (DSM-IV), diagnostic criteria may result in an underdiagnosis of depression, with resulting undertreatment.

Use of a rating instrument is often helpful in diagnosis. One of the best validated instruments for this purpose is the Cornell Scale of Depression in Dementia (Alexopoulos et al., 1988). This is a 19-item scale administered by a clinician. The clinician interviews both the patient and a caregiver and, taking data from both informants into account, rates each item on a scale from 0 (absent) to 2 (severe). A score of 8 or greater is commonly considered indicative of significant depression; a score of 12 or greater of severe depression.

Differentiating major depression from other psychiatric phenomena that occur in AD is sometimes difficult. Because major depression in this population may involve delusions, and (less commonly) auditory or visual hallucinations, and because psychotic phenomena can occur in AD without depression, the depression may be missed. In depressive disorders, the delusions and hallucinations always occur in the setting of other depression symptoms.

Apathy can also be mistaken for major depression. This syndrome, which is likely distinct from affective disorders, is discussed in more detail below.

Demoralization is common in patients with AD and often occurs when they learn of their diagnosis or are faced with a new limitation (eg, are no longer able to drive, need assisted living). Demoralization does not involve irritability, agitation, delusions, or hallucinations, and it often improves as patients adjust to their new situation.

Finally, medical comorbidity needs to be considered in the differential diagnosis. This can be of relevance in two ways: (1) depressive syndromes can be associated with a variety of medical conditions (eg, hypothyroidism, cancer) as well as certain medications (eg, prednisone), and (2) depression can be mistakenly diagnosed when the symptoms are actually due to another medical condition (eg, poor appetite and fatigue due to cancer; irritability and sleep disruption due to a delirium). Psychiatric consultation can be useful when such diagnostic problems arise.

Delusions and Hallucinations

Delusions and hallucinations often occur in AD. Delusions tend to be more common than hallucinations. In population-based studies (Lyketsos et al., 2000; Aalten et al., 2005), the prevalence of delusions in dementia is approximately 25%; for hallucinations, it is 10% to 15%.

Patients with AD rarely experience the systematized delusions characteristic of schizophrenia. They often report isolated paranoid beliefs. Common examples of such beliefs include that their home is not their home and that others (often their spouses) are not who they say they are. When patients have misplaced something due to their memory impairment, they may become convinced the item was stolen and persist in this belief despite being presented with evidence to the contrary. Grandiose delusions are rare. Visual hallucinations are more common than auditory ones in AD. This is in contrast to many psychotic disorders separate from AD, in which auditory hallucinations are more common. Hallucinations in AD commonly involve seeing people, including those who are dead. Unlike the hallucinations of many psychotic disorders, those occurring in AD tend not to distress patients; they may even find the experiences pleasurable.

A physician assessing a patient with AD and delusions or hallucinations should perform a comprehensive history and mental state examination to rule out other medical and psychiatric etiologies before concluding that a nondepressive psychotic disorder due to AD is present. As discussed above, major depression in AD can be associated with delusions and (less commonly) hallucinations. In fact, when delusions occur in AD, they may be more likely to be part of a depressive syndrome than a nondepressive one. In the major depression of AD, symptoms such as low mood, anxiety, irritability, and sleep and appetite disturbance are present and tend to be more prominent than hallucinations and delusions. Because the recommended treatment of major depression in AD is different from that of a psychotic syndrome, psychiatry consultation is wise when this differential diagnosis is in question.

Delirium such as from an infection (eg, urinary tract infection) or medication (eg, anticholinergic) side effect also needs to be considered in the differential diagnosis of cognitive dysfunction associated with delusions or hallucinations. The presence of a clouded sensorium, attentional disturbance, and sleep-wake disruption should raise concerns for delirium. A thorough medical history and medication review is thus indicated in all cases of new-onset delusions or hallucinations in AD.

Executive Dysfunction Syndrome

A variety of mood, personality, and behavioral phenomena can result from damage to frontal-subcortical neuronal circuits in dementias. These phenomena are most common in the late stages of the disease and can include disinhibition, stimulus-bound behaviors, perseverative speech (eg, near-constant repetition of a phrase), pacing, and psychomotor restlessness (Lyketsos, Rosenblatt, and Rabins, 2004). This syndrome occurs more commonly in frontotemporal dementias such as Pick's disease, and if prominent, especially early in the dementia, may warrant re-evaluation of the AD diagnosis. Studies suggest a prevalence of 6% to 9% for disinhibition in dementia and 15% to 25% for aberrant motor behavior (eg, pacing, repetitive behaviors) (Lyketsos et al., 2000; Aalten et al., 2005).

The executive dysfunction syndrome typically distresses caregivers more than patients. For example, a spouse may find a patient's repetitive comments irritating, and disinhibition (eg flirtatiousness) can make taking the patient out in public difficult, which then increases the caregiver's sense of isolation. Although relatively uncommon, pacing with exit-seeking and sexually inappropriate touching require immediate attention. Such phenomena are more common in later stages of AD and thus tend to be seen more often in the nursing home setting.

Apathy

Likely the most common psychiatric phenomenon in AD, the prevalence of apathy is estimated at 27% to 40% (Lyketsos et al., 2000; Aalten et al., 2005). Apathetic patients with AD typically show diminished volition, low self-motivation, low vitality, diminished emotions, and decreased goal-directed behavior. Although apathy can be a symptom of depression, it is also likely a distinct phenomenon. Depressed patients with AD typically present with associated symptoms such as anxiety, sadness, sleep or appetite changes, and delusions; these are not characteristic of apathy. Unlike depressed patients, apathetic patients usually are not distressed, and they often appear contented.

Agitation and Aggression

Agitated behaviors such as irritability, yelling, restlessness, and physical aggression (especially striking out at caregivers) are common in AD, with an estimated prevalence of 20% to 25% (Lyketsos et al., 2000; Aalten et al., 2005). Physicians are frequently contacted because a patient is "agitated"; this is often accompanied by a plea to "give him something."

Physicians should keep in mind that agitation is a nonspecific phenomenon with a broad differential diagnosis. Evaluation should start with a clear description of what the behavior entails (eg, "he strikes at staff when they attempt to shower him" or "she is anxious, tearful and screams 'help' from early afternoon until dinnertime"). This history, combined with a thorough examination, allows the physician to develop a differential diagnosis. The common causes to consider are a psychiatric syndrome (eg, major depression, nondepressive psychosis), a medical problem (eg, pain, delirium), a caregiver's behavior (eg, rushing the patient when helping him or her dress), and an environmental problem (eg, too much or too little stimulation). Of the above, pain is probably the most overlooked and undertreated contributor. This situation can be most unfortunate when a demented patient with agitation from unrecognized pain is given neuroleptic medication that not only fails to treat the underlying problem but also can place the patient at risk for falls with injury and increased pain.

Catastrophic Reactions

A catastrophic reaction can be defined as a sudden expression of negative emotion (eg, sadness, anxiety, anger) that is precipitated by an environmental event or task failure (Rabins, Lyketsos, and Steele, 1999). An example would be a woman with AD becoming tearful and throwing objects when frustrated because she cannot figure out how to use a familiar kitchen appliance. Such reactions can occur with little warning in a patient who otherwise has appeared calm and content, and they are typically time-limited. They can, however, be frightening for the patient as well as the caregiver and can sometimes be associated with physical aggression.

Impact of Neuropsychiatric Symptoms on Patients and Caregivers

The cognitive impairment and functional decline caused by AD produce suffering for patients as well as their loved ones and caregivers. This distress is further exacerbated when patients have any of the psychiatric phenomena described above. Many studies have linked psychiatric symptoms in AD to poorer quality of life, excess disability, more rapid cognitive decline, and earlier institutionalization for patients, as well as to distress for caregivers (Rabins, Lyketsos, and Steele, 1999). When phenomena such as depression, agitation, delusions, and disinhibition are severe, caregivers often find these symptoms more distressing than the cognitive and functional ones. This is especially true when caregivers do not fully understand or accept that their loved one's behavior is a manifestation of AD. Thus a wife, for example, may be stung by her husband's accusation of infidelity, or an inadequately trained nursing assistant in a comprehensive care setting may scold a resident for being "difficult." In the most severe cases, a family member or paid caregiver may become physically aggressive toward a patient in response to agitated or combative behavior. Patient and caregiver distress can often be ameliorated by compassionate education and support. Explaining the nature of these behaviors as symptoms of the disease can provide comfort to loved ones. Such explanations also help caregivers to respond in ways that are less likely to provoke further behaviors. Similarly, when institutional care providers receive dementia-specific education and training (preferably hands-on), their caregiving skills and tolerance for patients' distressing behaviors can markedly improve. Effective treatment of psychiatric phenomena also lessens distress for all.

Treatment of Psychiatric Phenomena in Alzheimer's Disease

Depression

Both nonpharamacologic and pharmacologic treatments for depression are available. For mild major depression, interventions such as providing increased structure and pleasurable activities (eg, a dementia-specific day activity program), may be sufficient. In most cases of major depression, however, a trial of antidepressant medication is warranted. Limited evidence is yet available to guide physicians in this regard. Many earlier studies showed either inconsistent benefits from antidepressant treatment, or a high response rate with either placebo or antidepressant. Some of these studies were probably limited by inadequate selection criteria (eg, DSM criteria, which often do not fit dementia patients well), insufficient dosing, or insufficient treatment length. In one recent 12-week study (Lyketsos et al., 2003), patients with AD and depression not only experienced improved mood on sertraline versus placebo, but also had less functional decline with antidepressant treatment.

Physicians commonly start with a serotonin-specific re-uptake inhibitor (SSRI) as the treatment of choice, given that these are among the most-studied antidepressants in AD and are well tolerated overall in people with AD. Mirtazapine (starting at 7.5 mg before bed), bupropion (starting at 100 mg daily of the extended-release preparation), and serotonin-norepinephrine reuptake inhibitors (eg, venlafaxine starting at 37.5 mg of the extended-release preparation) are also reasonable first or second choices. Tricyclic antidepressants (eg, nortriptyline) can be effective in this population. However, because of potential side effects such as orthostatic hypotension, constipation, blurry vision, and anticholinergic-induced delirium, these drugs require close monitoring and are rarely first choices. As in other frail populations, it is important to begin at a low antidepressant dose (eg, 25 mg of sertraline) and increase slowly as tolerated, with close monitoring for side effects. At the same time, it is important not to undertreat, recognizing that some patients with AD have optimal responses in the higher dose ranges (eg, 100 mg of sertraline).

In severe or treatment-refractory cases, electroconvulsive treatment (ECT) may be indicated. Clinical experience suggests that patients with AD tolerate ECT well and experience high response rates, similar to those of depressed patients without dementia. However, patients with AD are more susceptible to delirium during the treatment course. If this occurs, decreasing treatment frequency (eg, to twice instead of three times weekly) can be helpful. In one case series study of ECT in depressed patients with dementia, most individuals had improvement in depression and (to a slight extent) in cognitive function (Rao and Lyketsos, 2000).

Due to the impairments in memory and complex thought processes that occur in AD, psychotherapy is contraindicated in all but the most mildly impaired patients. A supportive relationship with a compassionate care provider, as in all patient care, remains essential.

Delusions and Hallucinations

The treatment of hallucinations and delusions depends on their cause. In the case of hallucinations and delusions due to the process of AD, options include behavioral interventions and neuroleptic treatment. When hallucinations and delusions are not severe, behavioral interventions such as distraction and avoiding arguments (described in Table 9–1) are often sufficient. These interventions are implemented by the caregiver who, in confronting the patient about his or her delusions or hallucinations, may have unintentionally increased the patient's distress. For example, when patients are delusional that they need to "go home" when already home and their caregivers try to persuade them otherwise, this can escalate the patients' distress and paranoia (eg, "Why are you lying? What are you trying to do to me?"). Sometimes acknowledging the distress while distracting the patient with reassuring comments can be helpful (eg, "I understand how upset you must feel. Come have a cup of tea and tell me about your home."). There are no "fail-safe" responses suitable for all patients. Physicians, nurses, and social workers experienced in AD care can assist when needed in educating caregivers and helping them formulate the best method of response for a given patient.

When hallucinations or delusions are severe, very distressing, and/or pose a safety risk (eg, patients threatening spouses they believe are imposters), pharmacotherapy is indicated. Neuroleptics are the treatment of choice. Unfortunately, their efficacy has not been well demonstrated, and recent safety concerns have arisen regarding use of atypical neuroleptics in dementia. These medications are associated with a small increased stroke and transient ischemic episode risk in dementia patients

Table 9.1. Nonpharmacologic Interventions for Common Behavioral Problems in Alzheimer's Disease

Behavioral Problem	Avoid	Try
"In the evening, she asks where her mother is. When I remind her she passed away twenty years ago, she accuses me of lying."	1. Arguing or rationalizing (eg, "You're mother passed away. Don't you remember?") 2. Expressing own frustration or exasperation (eg, "I've told you ten times, and you keep …")	1. Responding with calm reassuring tone of voice. 2. Addressing the underlying emotion (ie, misses mother). Examples: "What was your mother like?" "What did you enjoy doing with her?" 3. Using distraction (eg, snack, short walk, or TV show) Attempting transition to another topic (eg. "I remember your mother loved figure skating. Did you know a girl from our neighborhood just won …")
"He strikes out at me when I attempt to dress him."	1. Rushing patient 2. Using multistep directions (eg, "Put your shirt on and button it") 3. Persisting when behavioral interventions not successful or if agitation escalating.	1. Having all items ready before starting task 2. Assessing whether pain or another medical problem may be contributing 3. Using single-step instructions (eg, "Put your arm into this")

Situation	Don't	Do
"He just sits and watches TV all day. Any activity I suggest, he refuses."	1. Exhorting patient (eg, "You just sit there all day. You've got to get up and do things.") 2. Asking if patient wishes to do something using "yes-or-no" format (eg, "Would you like to take a walk?") 3. Offering multiple options (eg, "We could play cards or you can help me set the table")	1. Using gentle leading commands instead of requests (eg, "Come to the table for our card game. I've set everything up") 2. Offering a single option instead of a multiple ones (eg, "It's time for our walk")
"She refuses to go to her doctor's appointments" (or day activity program, or other activity important for the patient's care)	1. Arguing or rationalizing (eg, "Don't you realize what can happen if your blood pressure gets too high?") 2. Engaging in advance discussions about the unwanted activity (eg, "This day program is a good idea. I'd like you to give it 2 weeks ...")	1. Deferring informing patient of the appointment until as late as possible (eg, on the drive over) 2. Planning a pleasurable activity to follow the one the patient resists (eg, "After your doctor's appointment, we'll go out for lunch")
"He's awake several hours every night pacing."	1. Requesting sleeping medication before nonpharmacologic interventions are tried	1. Increasing daytime stimulation, minimizing napping, or engaging in light exercise in the early evening 2. Ensuring comfortable sleeping environment (eg, reducing noise). Instituting safety measures for the home (eg, locks or alarms on doors, no throw rugs) to minimize wandering and fall risk

(Schneider, Dagerman, and Insel, 2005) and in April 2005, the U.S. Food and Drug Administration (FDA) added a "black box" warning for use in dementia because of a 1.7-fold increased mortality rate compared with placebo found in patients with dementia (Schneider, Dagerman, and Insel, 2005). This risk is in addition to other neuroleptic side effects such as sedation, parkinsonism, and orthostatic hypotension, to which the frail elderly are particularly susceptible. Nevertheless, some patients do improve on these medicines and tolerate them well, especially at low doses (eg, 0.25–1 mg of risperidone daily, 2.5–5 mg of olanzapine daily, 12.5–50 mg of quetiapine daily). Although recent safety reports focus on the newer "atypical" neuroleptics, some evidence suggests similar concerns exist for older neuroleptics (eg, haloperidol) as well (Schneider, Dagerman, and Insel, 2005). The decision to initiate neuroleptic treatment involves careful consideration of the risks involved in possible treatment of hallucinations or delusions and an open discussion of these with the patient and family. Close monitoring for response and medication side effects, as well as frequent re-evaluation of the need for continued treatment, is indicated.

If the hallucinations or delusions are part of a depressive disorder, both the mood changes and the psychotic phenomena may respond to antidepressant treatment alone; addition of neuroleptic can be considered in certain severe cases. In the case of hallucinations or delusions from delirium, treating the underlying medical cause (eg, urinary tract infection) and/or removing the offending medication (eg, diphenhydramine) typically result in symptom resolution.

Executive Dysfunction Syndrome

As with major depression and psychotic phenomena, severity of symptoms influences the nature of treatment indicated. Milder symptoms (eg, embarrassing comments, restless pacing) can be managed by educating caregivers, who may not realize that the behavior in question is not under the patient's voluntary control. Techniques such as distraction and reassurance, instead of confrontation, should be encouraged (Table 9–1). Environmental interventions should be instituted as needed. Examples of such interventions include locking hazardous items out of reach of a pacing, stimulus-bound patient and using a one-piece coverall in patients with a propensity to expose themselves. Treatment of more severe disinhibited and inappropriate behavior frequently involves trials of pharmacotherapy; very little evidence-based guidance exists in this matter. Depending on the clinical presentation, trials of SSRIs, mood stabilizers (eg, valproic acid), neuroleptics, and amantadine may be helpful. Given the complexities involved, pharmacotherapeutic intervention for these disorders is best carried out with consultation from a specialist.

Apathy

Mild apathy is common in AD, and in many cases no specific treatment is needed. Caregivers often benefit from learning that decreased motivation and interests can be expected as part of the disease. Gently encouraging pleasant activities and enrolling the patient in a dementia-specific day activity program can help maximize stimulation (Table 9–1). In severe cases, it may be difficult to motivate the patient to engage in any activity, including getting dressed or even out of bed. Such inactivity can place the patient at risk for medical complications (eg, deep vein thrombosis). Little is known about pharmacotherapy for apathy in dementia, but in small case studies, psychostimulants (eg, methylphenidate), bupropion, and amantadine have shown benefit. A physician may begin with a trial of methylphenidate (5–20 mg daily), and if no improvement occurs, consider switching to bupropion (75–150 mg daily) or amantadine (100–300 mg daily). Studies also suggest that cholinesterase inhibitors (eg, donepezil 5–10 mg daily) may be beneficial (Lyketsos, Rosenblatt, and Rabins, 2004).

Agitation and Aggression

Treatment depends on the underlying cause of the behavior (eg, depression, delirium, pain). When the agitation or aggression is severe and no clear underlying psychiatric or medical etiology is identified, empiric use of a neuroleptic can be considered (eg, 0.25–1 mg of risperidone daily, 2.5–5 mg of olanzapine daily, 12.5–50 mg of quetiapine daily). Whether or not pharmacotherapy is indicated, caregiving and environmental factors can be modified, with consultation, as needed, from a physician, nurse, or social worker with expertise in dementia care. Several common management problems with suggestions for behavioral interventions are presented in Table 9–1.

Catastrophic Reactions

Catastrophic reactions are typically time-limited, and it is important that the caregiver maintain a calm and reassuring demeanor. If these episodes are severe, a low dose of an as-needed medication may be helpful during the acute crises. Examples of potential pharmacotherapy interventions include lorazepam (0.25–0.5 mg), risperidone (0.25–0.5 mg), and trazodone (25–50 mg). Precipitants should be explored and interventions devised to modify the environmental or situational trigger. Guidance from a dementia-care professional can be beneficial in this regard.

References

Aalten, P., de Vugt, M.E., Jaspers, N., Jolles, J., Verhey, F.R.J. (2005). The course of neuropsychiatric symptoms in dementia, Part I: findings from the two-year long Maasbed study. *International Journal of Geriatric Psychiatry* 20: 523–30.

Alexopoulos, G.S., Abrams, R.C., Young, R.C., Shamoian, C.A. (1988). Cornell scale for depression in dementia. *Biological Psychiatry* 23: 271–84.

Lyketsos, C.G., Rosenblatt, A., Rabins, P. (2004). Forgotten frontal lobe syndrome or "executive dysfunction syndrome." *Psychosomatics* 3: 247–55.

Lyketsos, C., Steinberg, M., Tschanz, J.T., Norton, M.C., Steffens, D.C., Breitner, J.C.S. (2000). Mental and behavioral disturbances in dementia: findings from the Cache County Study on memory in aging. *American Journal of Psychiatry* 157: 708–14.

Lyketsos, C.G., DelCampo, L., Steinberg, M., Miles, Q., Steele, C.D., Munro, C., Baker, A.S., Sheppard, J.M., Frangakis, C., Brandt, J., Rabins, P.V. (2003). Treating depression in Alzheimer disease: efficacy and safety of sertraline therapy, and the benefits of depression reduction: the DIADS. *Archives of General Psychiatry* 60:737–46.

Rabins, P.V., Lyketsos, C.G., Steele, C.D. (1999). *Practical Dementia Care*. New York, NY: Oxford University Press.

Rao, V., Lyketsos, C.G. (2000). The benefits and risks of ECT for patients with primary dementia who also suffer from depression. *International Journal of Geriatric Psychiatry* 15: 729–35.

Rosenberg, P.B., Onyike, C.U., Katz, I.R., Porsteinsson, A.P., Mintzer, J.E., Schneider, L.S., Rabins, P.V., Meinert, C.L., Martin, B.K., Lyketsos, C.G. (2005). Clinical application of operationalized criteria for 'Depression of Alzheimer's Disease.' *International Journal of Geriatric Psychiatry* 20: 119–27.

Schneider, L.S., Dagerman, K.S., Insel, P. (2005). Risk of death with atypical antipsychotic drug treatment for dementia: meta-analysis of randomized placebo-controlled trials. *Journal of the American Medical Association* 294: 1934–43.

Steinberg, M., Sheppard, J.M.E., Tschanz, J.T., Norton, M.C., Steffens, D.C., Breitner, J.C.S., Lyketsos, C.G. (2003). The incidence of mental and behavioral disturbances in dementia: the Cache County Study. *Journal of Neuropsychiatry and Clinical Neurosciences* 15: 340–5.

Zubenko, G.S., Zubenko, W.N., McPherson, S., Spoor, E., Marin, D.B., Farlow, M.R., Smith, G.E., Geda, Y., Cummings, J.L., Petersen, R.C., Sunderland, T. (2003). A collaborative study of the emergence and clinical features of the major depressive syndrome of Alzheimer's disease. *American Journal of Psychiatry* 160: 857–66.

10

Frontotemporal Dementia

DAVID M. BLASS

Frontotemporal dementia (FTD) is a family of neurodegenerative diseases and syndromes that most commonly involve the frontal and temporal lobes, producing dramatic alterations of personality, behavior, language, and other cognitive abilities (McKhann et al., 2001). Age of onset tends to be younger than in Alzheimer's disease (AD), with most patients becoming symptomatic in the sixth decade of life. Although population-based epidemiologic studies of FTD have found a prevalence of approximately 5–10 per 100,000 in patients 50 years of age and older, autopsy-based case series have found that approximately 5% to15% of people with dementia have FTD, a discrepancy suggesting that many cases go undiagnosed during life (Rosso et al., 2003). Recent advances in clinicopathologic correlation have revealed that a number of neurologic conditions previously conceived of as independent disease entities such as progressive supranuclear palsy (PSP), corticobasilar degeneration (CBD), and hippocampal sclerosis dementia are in many cases better classified in the FTD family (McKhann et al., 2001; Blass et al., 2004). Many patients with FTD develop other neurologic syndromes as well, including parkinsonism and amyotrophic lateral sclerosis (ALS).

Major Clinical Variants

FTD is actually a group of clinical syndromes with overlapping neuropathologies. The clinical expression of the disease relates primarily to the anatomic location of disease involvement rather than the neuropathologic subtype; there are many such subtypes.

Clinical variants are most distinct early in the disease course, when the degree of anatomic involvement may be limited to discrete regions. As the disease spreads through the brain, many patients have symptoms that become complex and take on characteristics of other variants. The first clinical FTD variant is one in which behavioral abnormalities and personality changes dominate the clinical presentation. This syndrome is usually associated with disease involvement of the frontal and anterior temporal lobes. In addition, there are two language presentations: primary progressive aphasia and semantic dementia (McKhann et al., 2001). The neurologic syndromes of PSP, CBD, and ALS with dementia are familiar to the neurologist because of their neurologic symptoms; it is noteworthy that patients with any of the previously mentioned syndromes routinely develop the psychiatric symptoms reviewed below. The term Pick complex is increasingly used to describe the group of FTD clinical syndromes and neuropathologies as a whole (Kertesz and Munoz, 1998).

Psychiatric Manifestations

Patients with any of the FTD clinical variants typically exhibit a wide array of psychiatric phenomena that often require treatment (Bozeat et al., 2000). Much of the treatment of patients with FTD focuses on such phenomena and on educating patients' families about them as well as providing support to families.

Behavioral Dysregulation

Behavioral dysregulation is common in FTD and causes significant distress to those around the patient (Table 10–1). There are a number of common symptom clusters. The first consists of repetitive, stereotyped behaviors, both motor and verbal. Examples of complex motor stereotypies are washing, touching, tapping, folding-unfolding, checking, attempts at defecation, and hitting. Verbal stereotypies are common and include repetition of catch phrases or even paragraphs, counting, singing, and cursing. More simple repetitive behaviors are also seen and can include grimacing, blinking, grunting, and humming.

Table 10.1. Behavior Disturbances in Fronto Temporal Dementia

Disturbance	Description
Repetitive behaviors	Repetitive/stereotyped actions, verbal stereotypy (catch phrases), counting, singing, checking
Hyperorality	Increased food intake, alcoholism, increased/new smoking, eating others' food, eating from serving dish or garbage
Disinhibition/impulsivity	Inappropriate comments/jokes, touching, reckless spending, public urination
Apathy	Reduced engagement in work, recreation, socialization
Neglect of personal hygiene	Refusal to shower, shave, change clothing
Sleep disturbance	Difficulty falling asleep, multiple nighttime awakenings, daytime sleeping
Aggression	

Dysregulation of appetite is common, and many patients eat voraciously and indiscriminately with significant weight gain. Indeed, patients may eat from others' plates and serving bowls, or even the garbage. Specific food cravings often develop, particularly for sweets, and some patients may attempt to eat inedible objects. Increased alcohol or cigarette use may also occur.

Many patients become disinhibited and impulsive in their speech or social behavior, making inappropriate comments or gestures. Patients may urinate in public, expose themselves, or make racially or sexually inappropriate jokes. Money may be spent or given away indiscriminately. Patients may touch or hug young children who they do not know, which sometimes leads to attention from the police.

Loss of motivation and drive is another manifestation of behavioral dysregulation. Patients fail to initiate activities they previously performed at home or in the workplace and may no longer engage in housework or hobbies. Many patients with FTD lose interest in personal grooming and hygiene, often refusing to change clothes, brush their teeth, or shower. These changes are not due to forgetting to perform these tasks but to a loss of interest in them. Some patients speak more about sexual matters but actually become less interested in conducting sexual relations.

Restlessness is a common and problematic phenomenon. Patients may be unable to sit or lay still and may appear to be in constant motion, leading to pacing and wandering. They often have disturbed sleep with difficulty falling asleep and multiple awakenings during the night, all of which may be related to restlessness. Finally, the ability to sustain attention, already impaired in FTD, is also exacerbated by restlessness.

Aggression can be a significant problem in a minority of patients. Aggression may be related to agnosia in some patients, but in others it is not. Agnosia can precipitate aggression when patients are unable to recognize individuals in their environment or appreciate the meaning of what is being done for them, such as dressing, bathing, or toileting. Aggression may be unpredictable or may occur in specific circumstances. Early in the disease course, some patients develop criminal behavior, including shoplifting, indecent exposure, and flagrant violations of driving norms. The combination of mental rigidity, irritability, and lack of insight makes interactions with the police or other security officials (such as in airports) potentially explosive.

Patients with all forms of dementia, including FTD, can experience episodes of severe emotional distress, often involving frustration, crying, yelling, restlessness, agitation, and occasionally even aggression, known as *catastrophic reactions*. These reactions often occur in the context of being unable to perform a cognitive or functional task that the patient perceives that he or she should be able to perform, or when presented with stimuli that confuse or frustrate the patient such as loud noise, over-stimulation, or complicated instructions. Alternatively, they may occur in the setting of significant confusion, either about where they are, who they are with, or what is occurring in the environment. Although these reactions by definition resolve with the passage of time (usually about half an hour), they reflect great distress on the part of the patient and cause significant distress to those around the patient.

Personality Changes

Personality change is one of the hallmarks of FTD and is often among the earliest manifestations. In some cases, changes in personality may cause the changes in behavior listed above. Many patients become cold and uninterested in others, even close family, and are often described as self-centered and sarcastic. Patients may lose much of their social awareness and grace and appear blind to the social expectations and demands of a given situation. Excessive jocularity may develop, with the patient appearing silly and with an inappropriately happy and superficial expression of emotion.

Many patients become rigid, inflexible, and unwilling to negotiate. This rigidity is exacerbated by their lack of insight into the social demands of most situations. They may become preoccupied with schedules and routine to the exclusion of other concerns. Previously easygoing individuals may become contentious, difficult, and irritable.

As mentioned earlier, many patients become apathetic, uninterested, and unmotivated. They do not have anhedonia per se, but they no longer initiate contact with others or appear interested in their environment. As a rule, patients have no (or at most minimal) insight into these changes.

Mood Changes

Abnormalities of mood are common in FTD. A variety of depressive syndromes may occur (Blass, 2007). Some patients develop a full syndrome of major depression, with sadness, diminished self-attitude, anhedonia, anergia, anorexia, and impaired sleep. Pseudobulbar affect with spontaneous, rapidly developing and short-lived crying and sadness is not uncommon. Patients' moods may have a labile and stimulus-bound quality to them, rapidly changing in response to the environment. Thus, for example, patients may have significant symptoms of depression only intermittently while in the presence of a specific individual or while in a particular place.

Patients with early FTD are often misdiagnosed as suffering primarily from major depression. Many symptoms of FTD such as apathy, diminished motivation, changes in sleep and appetite, social withdrawal, and inattention to personal hygiene are all commonly seen in depression as well. A number of features may be helpful in distinguishing between the two disorders. Patients with FTD who are not depressed usually do not have significant sadness, self-deprecation, or guilt, and although they may not seek out pleasurable activities, when they do engage in them, they are not actually anhedonic. Many patients with depression who are apathetic and inattentive to hygiene retain some insight into these phenomena and can identify them as being a change from their baseline and from community norms. In contrast, patients with FTD usually have quite limited insight into such matters.

Other mood abnormalities may be seen. Although frank mania is uncommon, patients may have mood symptoms resembling mania such as an inappropriately jocular mood. Patients often are anxious, and the anxiety may revolve around a somatic preoccupation, often focusing on a trivial lesion or a mild symptom that would previously not have been distressing.

Patients with FTD, particularly early in the disease course, are often demoralized, frustrated, and confused by their circumstances. For those patients who have some insight into their deficits, the loss of cognitive and functional ability at such a young age is demoralizing, leading to worry about their future and the welfare of their family. For patients without such insight (the majority of patients), the misunderstood restrictions placed upon them, such as loss of driving privileges or permission to manage their finances independently, lead to significant sadness, frustration, and anger.

Hallucinations and Delusions

Hallucinations in any sensory modality are quite uncommon in FTD. Delusions are somewhat more common, and when they occur, they often have a paranoid theme. As with mood abnormalities, the delusions may be present only intermittently, in certain settings, or with certain individuals.

Treatment

Consultation with a psychiatrist (especially one experienced in the treatment of patients with dementia) should be considered when psychiatric disturbances are severe or have not responded to treatment, or when the differential diagnosis and medication side effects are unclear.

Safety

Safety issues must be addressed for all patients and include driving, medication administration, access to handguns and other dangerous household items, kitchen appliance use and cooking, wandering, and access to finances (Talerico and Evans, 2001).

Psychiatric hospitalization (preferably on a unit expert in the care of dementia patients) may need to be pursued, often on an involuntary basis.

Although most of these safety issues are common to the care of patients with any form of dementia, some features are unique to patients with FTD. First, in contrast to AD, safety concerns are not proportional to the degree of impairment in specific cognitive domains such as visual-spatial perception, apraxia, or agnosia but relate more to the impairment in judgment, impulsivity, and distractibility. Safety issues are therefore common early in the course of care for patients with FTD, even when traditional cognitive screens such as the Mini-Mental State Examination are normal (Folstein, Folstein, and McHugh, 1975). Also, because some patients with FTD have personality changes that make them insensitive to others, cold, and prone to confabulate, they may take measures to actively elude detection of the unsafe behavior. Finally, because FTD has an earlier age of onset compared with AD, many patients are in excellent physical health early in the disease course and therefore more capable of getting into an unsafe environment than older, more frail, patients.

Behavior

Behavioral disturbances are treated with a combination of pharmacologic (Table 10–2) and environmental interventions. One easy-to-use method is the "4-D" method, in which the clinician *d*escribes and *d*ecodes the behavior, *d*evises an intervention, and *d*etermines if the intervention has succeeded (Rabins, Lyketsos, and Steele, 1999). *Description* of the behavior should be as detailed as possible and include what the patient is doing: the setting of the behavior, including the time, location, circumstances (eg mealtime, bathing, dressing); the people who were near the patient when the behavior occurred; and the consequences of

Table 10.2. Medications to Treat Mood and Behavior Disturbances

Disturbance	Medication	Starting Dose (mg/day)	Dosing Increments (mg)
Repetitive behaviors	Sertraline	12.5–25	12.5–25
	Paroxetine	5–10	5–10
	Citalopram	5–10	5–10
	Escitalopram	5	5
Disinhibited/ impulsive behaviors	Sertraline	12.5–25	12.5–25
	Paroxetine	5–10	5–10
	Citalopram	5–10	5–10
	Escitalopram	5	5
	Amantadine	50 BID	50
Sleep disturbance	Trazodone	25–50 QHS	25
Restlessness/ agitation	Trazodone	25 BID–QID	25
	Valproic acid	125–250 QHS–BID	125–150
	Carbamazepine	50 bid	50
Depression	Sertraline	12.5–25	12.5–25
	Paroxetine	5–10	5–10
	Citalopram	5–10	5–10
	Escitalopram	5	5
	Venlafaxine XR	37.5	37.5
	Mirtazapine	7.5–15 QHS	7.5
	Bupropion SR	100	100

the behavior. Once this has been done, a pattern often emerges that allows the behavior to be explained or *decoded*. Examples include a patient becoming agitated 2 to 3 hours after the last meal, suggestive of hunger-induced agitation, or agitation on being left alone for a period of time. Interventions, including environmental modifications or use of medication are logically *devised* from the results of the preceding two steps. Once the intervention is implemented, clinical follow-up helps the clinician *determine* whether the intervention has succeeded. Use of this or similar algorithms helps establish when pharmacotherapy is needed and when environmental interventions alone may suffice.

Selective serotonin reuptake inhibitors (SSRIs), even at low doses, are often very helpful in treating repetitive behaviors or speech. Over time the dose may need to be gradually increased. SSRIs may also help rigidity, negativity, and inflexibility, and disinhibition and impulsivity often improve with SSRI treatment as well. Dopamine-augmenting agents such as amantadine may also be helpful, although such medications should be used cautiously because of the risk of central nervous system toxicity such as ataxia or delirium (Merrilees and Miller, 2003).

Overeating can be a difficult problem to treat. Limiting the amount of food (and alcohol, if necessary) available and controlling the caloric content of food accessible to the patient are the cornerstones of treatment. Use of weight-reducing agents is not generally recommended, although a trial of topiramate (with a starting dose of 25 g QHS) may be considered in cases of profound weight gain. SSRIs may also reduce appetite and overeating in some patients.

Patients with difficulty settling into a bedtime ritual can be given medications such as low-dose (ie, 25–50 mg) trazodone to calm them a few hours prior to bedtime. Patients with difficulty falling asleep can also be treated with trazodone at bedtime, beginning with a low dose and increasing it slowly as needed. If patients do not sleep through the night, the bedtime dose may be increased or an extra dose may be given when the patient awakens in the middle of the night. Caution should be used to ensure the patient is not oversedated in the morning. Nonpharmacologic approaches to the treatment of sleep disturbances are listed in Table 10–3.

Restlessness, agitation, and severe aggression may improve with trazodone given an hour before the time of worst restlessness or throughout the day in divided doses if the symptom is continuous. SSRIs may also be helpful in doses similar to those

Table 10.3. Nonpharmacologic Approaches to the Treatment of Sleep Disturbances

Avoid caffeinated foods or beverages from the
  afternoon and onward
Minimize daytime napping
Minimize evening fluid consumption
Ensure the patient uses the bathroom prior
  to getting into bed
Maintain regular bedtimes and awakening times
Avoid television 30–60 minutes prior to bedtime
Review medications to identify afternoon/evening
  medications likely to interfere with sleep induction
Maintain quiet sleep environment

used for repetitive behaviors. Valproic acid and carbamazepine may prove useful for agitation and should be titrated to effect rather than to a target serum concentration. Starting doses should be low (125 mg daily or bid of valproic acid and 50 mg daily or bid for carbamazepine), and doses should not be increased more frequently than every 1 to 2 weeks in the outpatient setting. Restlessness or agitation can also be treated with very low doses of atypical neuroleptics (eg, daily or bid doses of 1.25–2.5 mg of olanzapine, 0.125–0.25 mg of risperidone, or 12.5–25 mg of quetiapine), although these agents may worsen agitation in some patients. In some cases of aggressive behavior, low doses of beta-blockers (eg, propranolol 10–20 mg qid) may be helpful.

Apathy, loss of initiation, and inattention to hygiene may be helped by using a structured schedule to help the patient get through the day. A memorandum from the physician laying out a necessary interval of bathing, teeth brushing, and clothing change may be helpful for some patients.

Catastrophic reactions can be dealt with in a number of ways. In some cases the triggers for such reactions are predictable, and the most important intervention is the elimination or avoidance of these triggers. Triggers may include being told to do something that is beyond the patient's current abilities, being told a number of things at the same time, being in a noisy environment or one with many people or other stimuli, or having to do something while tired or hungry. Once the catastrophic reaction has occurred, the patient should be gently guided to a quiet room if possible, calmed by being spoken to gently, and distracted with a different topic, if possible. Attempts to argue or reason with the patient about what occurred before or during the catastrophic reaction are usually futile and may even worsen the patient's state of mind.

Other Phenomena

Mood abnormalities can be treated with the same agents used in patients without FTD, in doses similar to those used in patients with other forms of dementia, namely the lowest possible, as outlined in Table 10–2. In patients with FTD, SSRIs, venlafaxine, mirtazapine, or bupropion may all be used to treat major depression. SSRIs or venlafaxine may be the preferred agents, because they tend to make patients easier to treat at home by reducing mental inflexibility and diminishing repetitive speech and behavior. Trying to maintain a schedule of activities for the patient, thereby keeping them active and stimulated, may combat demoralization. Pseudobulbar crying may respond to SSRIs in doses similar to those used to treat major depression. Hallucinations and delusions should be treated with atypical neuroleptics at very low starting doses (eg, QD or BID doses of 1.25–2.5 mg of olanzapine, 0.125–0.25 mg of risperidone, or 12.5–25 mg of quetiapine). Treatment of hallucinations and delusions should be instituted only when the severity of the symptoms is significant, such as if they occur frequently; cause distress or risk to the patient or those around the patient;

interfere with basic personal care, nutrition, or medical care; or jeopardize the patient's living arrangement.

Family Support

Support of the family is a critical component of FTD care. Families are at high risk for becoming socially isolated, overwhelmed, and demoralized. Caregiver burden is extremely high for FTD and may be correlated with severity of behavior symptoms, personality change, and depression.

Family support actually begins with accurate diagnosis. Dementia is often not initially suspected because of the young age of onset; the high frequency of marital discord; the relative early sparing of cognitive functions such as memory, orientation, visual-spatial orientation, and language; and the preponderance of behavioral symptoms, impaired judgment, and disturbed interpersonal functioning. As a result, patients may remain undiagnosed until symptoms have been present for a number of years. Prior to the diagnosis of FTD, patients may be diagnosed as having atypical mood disorders, mania, marital conflict, mid-life crises, personality disorders, covert substance abuse, or no disorder at all. Making the diagnosis of FTD typically is the reason for the several years of chaos in the family and provides the proper paradigm for moving forward in the care of the patient. Although the diagnosis of FTD is not "good news" per se, families are often relieved to know that there is an explanation for what has been occurring.

Educating families about the symptoms and natural history of FTD is important, as is provision of educational materials or links to informational Web sites (eg, http://www.ftd-picks.org/ or http://www.pdsg.org.uk/). Teaching strategies for managing problem behaviors is critical and families may benefit from caregiving seminars and from advice such as that provided in Table 9–1. Referral to support groups, particularly if FTD-specific, is beneficial for some families. Having an open communication with the physician is valued by most families and in and of itself provides support.

Caregiver burden should be addressed explicitly when meeting with families, and concrete suggestions should be provided to lessen that burden. Examples of such support include respite services; support groups; day care options; provision of additional help in the home; mobilizing family, friends, and community; and referrals to appropriate social service agencies.

References

Blass, D.M., Hatanpaa, K.J., Brandt, J., Rao, V., Steinberg, M., Troncoso, J.C., Rabins, P.V. (2004). Dementia in hippocampal sclerosis resembles frontotemporal dementia more than Alzheimer disease. *Neurology* 63: 492–7.

Blass, D.M., Rabins P.V. (2007). Depression in frontotemporal dementia. *Psychosomatics*. **In Press.**

Bozeat, S., Gregory, C.A., Ralph, M.A., Hodges, J.R. (2000). Which neuropsychiatric and behavioural features distinguish frontal and temporal variants of frontotemporal dementia from Alzheimer's disease? *Journal of Neurology, Neurosurgery, and Psychiatry* 69: 178–86.

Folstein, M.F., Folstein, S.E., McHugh, P.R. (1975). "Mini-mental state": a practical method for grading the cognitive state of patients for the clinician. *Journal of Psychiatric Research* 12: 189–98.

Kertesz, A., Munoz, D. (1998). Pick's disease, frontotemporal dementia, and Pick complex: emerging concepts. *Archives of Neurology* 55: 302–4.

McKhann, G.M., Albert, M.S., Grossman, M., Miller, B., Dickson, D., Trojanowski, J.Q. (2001). Clinical and pathological diagnosis of frontotemporal dementia. Report of the Work Group on frontotemporal dementia and Pick's disease. *Archives of Neurology* 58: 1803–9.

Merrilees, J.J., Miller, B.L. (2003). Long-term care of patients with frontotemporal dementia. *Journal of the American Medical Directors Association* 4: S162–4.

Rabins, P.V., Lyketsos, C.G., Steele, C.D. (1999). *Practical Dementia Care*. New York, NY: Oxford University Press.

Rosso, S.M., Donker Kaat, L., Baks, T., Joosse, M., de Koning, I., Pijnenburg, Y., de Jong, D., Dooijes, D., Kamphorst, W., Ravid, R., Niermeijer, M.F., Verheij, F., Kremer, H.P., Scheltens, P., van Duijn, C.M., Heutink, P., van Swieten, J.C. (2003). Frontotemporal dementia in The Netherlands: patient characteristics and prevalence estimates from a population-based study. *Brain* 126: 2016–22.

Talerico K.A., Evans, L.K. (2001). Responding to safety issues in frontotemporal dementias. *Neurology*;56: S52–S55.

11

Huntington's Disease

ADAM ROSENBLATT

Huntington's disease (HD) is a hereditary neurodegenerative disorder characterized by the triad of a movement disorder, dementia, and various psychiatric disturbances. HD is caused by the abnormal expansion of a trinucleotide (CAG) repeat in the *huntingtin* gene of chromosome 4—a mutation that is inherited as an autosomal dominant. When the number of CAG repeats exceeds 39, the individual harboring it goes on to develop HD. The most common time of onset is in the fourth or fifth decade, but the age of onset is inversely correlated with the size of the triplet repeat expansion. In rare instances, persons with very large expansions may have onset in childhood, and those with expansions only just into the abnormal range may have onset late in life. Children of affected fathers, if they receive the abnormal allele, tend to inherit an allele that is even further expanded, and thus usually experience the onset of symptoms at a younger age than their fathers; this phenomenon is known as *paternal anticipation.*

The progression of HD is inexorable and usually leads to death within 15 to 20 years of symptom onset; patients in the final stages have severe dementia and are unable to speak, eat, or purposefully move. Death typically results from the consequences of immobility such as pneumonia or malnutrition.

Movement Disorder in Huntington's Disease

The movement disorder of HD has two major manifestations: involuntary movements (eg, chorea, dystonia) and impairments of voluntary movement (eg, clumsiness, dysarthria, swallowing difficulties, falls, bradykinesia, rigidity). Chorea generally predominates early in the course and is gradually eclipsed by motor impairment as the disease becomes more advanced. In the end stages, patients are rigid and immobile. A variety of medications are used to suppress chorea in HD, including neuroleptics, benzodiazepines, and dopamine-depleting agents such as tetrabenazine, but it remains controversial whether these agents convey functional, as opposed to cosmetic, benefits.

Psychiatric Syndromes in Huntington's Disease

HD, like many other neurodegenerative disorders, is associated with a variety of psychiatric problems (Table 11–1). Some of these problems such as insomnia or demoralization may be thought of as nonspecific. They have a variety of causes and are associated with many different medical conditions. Other problems represent widely recognized psychiatric disorders also found in the general population such as dementia, major depression, and obsessive-compulsive disorder (OCD), for which HD is a particular risk factor. Finally, there exists a set of personality changes and altered behaviors—the executive dysfunction syndrome—which is more specific to HD and other disorders affecting the frontal and subcortical circuitry of the brain.

Table 11.1. Common Psychiatric Syndromes in Huntington's Disease

Condition	Frequency in Huntington's Disease	Typical Pharmacotherapy
Dementia	Universal in later stages	No accepted pharmacotherapy
Executive dysfunction syndrome	Very common	Various agents
Major depression	Common	Antidepressants, neuroleptics
Mania	Uncommon	Mood stabilizers, neuroleptics
Obsessive-compulsive disorder	Common	Serotonergic antidepressants
Schizophrenia-like syndromes	Uncommon	Neuroleptics

The psychiatric manifestations of HD are among the most treatable aspects of the disease. Most of the acute syndromes from which patients with HD suffer, such a major depression, can be cured, as they can in the general population. The more chronic changes are often responsive to medication and can be further improved and coped with if the family is educated about the disease and given strategies for behavioral management.

Dementia

The dementia caused by HD is often described as a subcortical dementia. In a typical cortical dementia such as that associated with Alzheimer's disease (AD), patients have disorientation, amnesia, apraxia, and aphasia, but their personalities are relatively preserved. In subcortical dementias, such as those found in HD, normal pressure hydrocephalus, Parkinson's disease, and human immunodeficiency virus (HIV) infection, patients show relatively preserved memory but great difficulty in executive function and tasks requiring attention and concentration. They also show, in general, a greater degree of personality erosion, with behavioral problems such as apathy and irritability.

Executive Dysfunction Syndrome

It has often been said that depression is the most common psychiatric manifestation of HD. Although it is probably true that major depression is the most common specific psychiatric diagnosis in HD, there is a constellation of behavioral and personality changes—the executive dysfunction syndrome—which appears to be almost universal in the course of the disease. It takes the form of a loss of inhibitions, difficulty prioritizing and making decisions, apathy, irritability, aggression, verbal perseveration, and impulsivity.

Major Depression

In his original description of the disease that bears his name, George Huntington, commented on the "tendency to insanity and suicide"(Huntington, 1872). The prevalence of major depression in HD and other disorders of the basal ganglia is indeed high, perhaps about 30% to 40% over the lifetime of an individual, with a suicide rate four to six times that of the general population (Shoenfield et al., 1984; Folstein et al., 1987) Severe cases may be accompanied by mood-congruent delusions, such as those of guilt or poverty, or by hallucinated voices making critical statements about the patient. Obstacles to diagnosis may include impaired communication on the part of the patient; the presence of confounding phenomena (eg, weight loss from dysphagia, apathy from the executive dysfunction syndrome); and a tendency on the part of physicians, family members, and even patients themselves to explain depression as an understandable reaction to the problems of living with HD. People with HD can and do become demoralized, but most of the overt depression seen in HD is thought to be the direct result of pathologic changes in the brain. Evidence in support of this idea comes from functional neuroimaging studies (Mayberg et al., 1992) and the observed phenomenon that depressive symptoms can appear before other obvious signs of HD such as chorea or dementia.

There is an important caveat to this last point. It has often been said that major depression can precede the movement disorder in HD, sometimes by years. Almost no prospective data support this contention, and major depression is a common condition in the general population. The presence of depressive symptoms in an otherwise-normal individual at risk for HD should not be used to make a diagnosis or serve as an indication for genetic testing, particularly if it is many years before that person's expected age of risk. A positive test result does not explain or help the patient's depression, and then, in addition to the depression itself, the patient has to live with the results of a predictive test that he or she was not seeking in the first place. A similar situation occurs when an at-risk child displays common behavior problems at school, and teachers and legal guardians wonder if the inattention or oppositional behavior could be due to HD.

Mania

Mania, or even a classical bipolar syndrome, has a lifetime prevalence of 5% to 10% in HD (Mendez, 1994). Patients may present with an elevated or irritable mood, impulsiveness, increased activity, hypersexuality, decreased need for sleep, and a grandiose self-attitude. In severe cases, patients may have delusions and hallucinations as well. As with major depression, mania may be the first indication of HD.

It is important to differentiate an episode of mania in HD from the chronic personality changes that are part of the executive dysfunction syndrome. Some patients with HD are chronically disinhibited, irritable, or jocose, but lack the increased energy, diminished need for sleep, and hypersexuality commonly associated with mania. Cavalier application of the term *mania* in such instances may lead to unnecessary pharmacotherapy for a condition better handled behaviorally.

Obsessive-Compulsive Disorder

Obsessive and compulsive symptoms are common in HD and have been reported in 22.3% of patients at their first clinic visit (Marder et al., 2000). However, the true lifetime prevalence of OCD is difficult to estimate. More commonly, persons with HD develop personality changes such as inflexibility and "stickiness" and a tendency to perseverate on topics of concern with single-minded intensity. Thus, they may become preoccupied with a particular type of food, with smoking, or with independence issues such as restoration of their driving privileges.

Schizophrenia-Like Syndromes

Psychotic syndromes have been reported to occur in 3% to 12% of patients with HD (Mendez, 1994). These syndromes resemble schizophrenia, with hallucinations and delusions, or occur as isolated delusional states. Some delusional states seem particularly incorrigible, as if in keeping with the inflexibility manifested by many people with HD. In one case, a woman with HD repeatedly ran away from her sister's home in response to the delusion and olfactory hallucination that she had a foul odor as well as auditory hallucinations of voices saying that she was about to be arrested. Another woman with HD developed delusions that a neighbor was in love with her, with hallucinations of his voice, declaring that love. In a final example of the schizophrenia-like syndromes that can occur in HD, a man had delusional parasitosis, excoriating his skin and expressing surprise that no one else could see the "buggies."

The Impact of Huntington's Disease on Patients and Families

Issues Related to Presymptomatic Testing for Huntington's Disease

Now that a direct assay exists for measuring CAG repeat length, it is possible to provide presymptomatic testing to individuals at risk for HD. People at risk may choose to undergo testing for a variety of reasons, including deciding whether to have children, planning their financial futures, making choices regarding work or housing, learning whether their own children are at risk, or simply desiring to know what the future holds. Given the current state of treatments for HD, however, there is no purely *medical* reason to have presymptomatic testing. HD is not a public health risk, and there are no interventions known to affect the outcome for a gene-positive person who has not yet developed any symptoms. Further, presymptomatic testing can be an extremely stressful experience, even if the results are negative. When the results are positive, there may be serious practical consequences, including difficulties with work and relationships (eg, being passed over for a promotion, or the breaking off of an engagement), difficulty obtaining various kinds of insurance, and emotional decompensation in vulnerable individuals.

These facts have several implications. Presymptomatic testing should be done only on a voluntary basis, and the clinician should adopt a neutral position, understanding that the decision to be tested is intensely personal. The standard of care is for presymptomatic testing to take place in the context of a program that includes pretest evaluation and counseling and the opportunity for post-test follow-up and support. The individual undergoing testing should enlist the support of a family member or sympathetic friend. Test results should be given in person, and testing is generally not conducted anonymously, so that individuals who are in distress are not lost to follow-up. Presymptomatic testing of children is considered unethical. Presymptomatic testing should be distinguished from confirmatory testing—testing in a person who is already showing signs of HD. Once a medical intervention for presymptomatic individuals is discovered, some of these recommendations, such as clinician neutrality or the prohibition on testing of children, would have to change.

Coping with Huntington's Disease

In contrast to AD and other neurodegenerative disorders of the elderly, HD typically strikes in the prime of life. Patients may be at their peak earning capacity and have young children. In addition to the loss of independence, patients may experience considerable guilt over their inability to provide for their families and to function fully as a parent and spouse. Children, particularly teenagers, may become embarrassed by their parent's odd appearance and disinhibited behavior, further damaging family relationships. Support groups for family members, such as those sponsored by local chapters of the Huntington's Disease Society of America, may help them to better understand and cope with the changes in their loved one.

Although patients are told that neurologic changes in HD are gradual, personal losses, such as having to leave work or stop driving, occur at discrete intervals that may be times of great vulnerability. Sometimes these losses precipitate psychiatric hospitalizations or even suicide attempts. Furthermore, the obsessionality that often develops in patients with HD may prolong the time it takes for the patients to adapt, because they may find it impossible to turn their attention to other topics. In dealing with these inevitable life changes and the ensuing grief, the physician and family should strive to be supportive and to help patients preserve their remaining autonomy, such as by arranging rides for those who are no longer able to drive.

In some ways, the progressive nature of HD itself may be a mitigating factor. As the cognitive and personality changes progress, the patient's world view tends to become constricted, and a simpler existence, which would have seemed intolerable a few years ago, may provide ample satisfaction and contentment. For this reason, when persons at risk for HD, or with early symptoms, state that they do not wish to live beyond a certain point in the disease, the clinician should listen sympathetically but not treat this understandable reaction as an emergency or assume that the person will actually become suicidal when that point is reached.

Treatment of Psychiatric Syndromes in Huntington's Disease

Dementia

The dementia of HD can be subtle to observers more familiar with cortical processes such as AD, for basic orientation is often preserved, yet patients may be substantially impaired in the areas of problem-solving and judgment. Physicians should anticipate cognitive changes in these areas after the earliest stages of the disease and act to prevent injuries and financial losses that might result from undetected impairment. Specialized neuropsychologic testing can help in questionable cases.

There is no established pharmacotherapy for the dementia of HD, but cholinesterase inhibitors and memantine, widely used for AD, have been tried empirically. An appropriate regimen might be donepezil, starting at 5 mg at bedtime and advancing after 30 days to 10 mg at bedtime, or memantine, starting at 5 mg a day and advancing by 5-mg increments each week, in divided doses, to 10 mg twice a day.

Executive Dysfunction Syndrome

There have been no large studies of treatment for the executive dysfunction syndrome in HD. Empirical pharmacotherapy depends largely on the symptom that is being targeted: apathy might respond to selective serotonin reuptake inhibitors (SSRIs) or amphetamines, irritability and aggressiveness to neuroleptics or anticonvulsants, and obsessionality to SSRIs or clomipramine.

In some cases, the results of pharmacotherapy can be remarkable but, for the most part, successful treatment of the executive dysfunction syndrome of HD consists of helping the family have reasonable expectations and teaching them how to avoid the patient's areas of vulnerability.

Apathy, for example, is much more distressing to the family than to the person experiencing it. Such patients are frequently brought to the physician as "depressed," but in fact they have no mood complaints and are puzzled as to why everyone is making such a fuss over their inactivity. One man was quite upset that his brother, who had HD, did not want to go fishing with him for his birthday, an activity he had previously enjoyed. He went reluctantly, caught several fish, and then once home, immediately turned on the television again. The patient was examined and found to be apathetic. It was explained to his brother that he did not appear to be suffering but that apathy was a common, even expected aspect of HD. It was suggested that at his next birthday they might enjoy watching a game together on television. Their relationship improved markedly thereafter. Apathetic persons have particular difficulty initiating behaviors but may function more normally if a routine is developed and someone else starts them off (eg, going to the mall every Wednesday at 2 o'clock).

In the case of perseveration, the family should be encouraged to "pick their battles." If a repetitive behavior such as adjusting the thermostat brings satisfaction to the patient, then it might be allowed to continue without trying to get the patient to accept that the temperature of the room as adequate. If being asked to do something unplanned such as to change into a different outfit precipitates an emotional outburst, it may be better simply to explain the patient's mismatched clothes to friends who do not know about HD. Confrontations should be saved for situations having to do with safety. This is easier to explain if the family understands that these changes in behavior are due to the

HD itself and that their loved one in not simply being unreasonable.

Major Depression

There have been no large controlled studies of antidepressant therapy for depression in HD, but clinical experience and smaller studies (Guttman et al., 2003) indicate that a wide variety of the standard agents can be effective; electroconvulsive therapy (ECT) may also be used. In choosing an agent, one should keep in mind that patients with HD, due to the effects of their brain disease, may show the sensitivity to adverse effects (particularly delirium) found in someone much older that the patient's chronological age. The physician must consider the complexity of the regimen and the side-effect profile of the drug. The SSRI family is probably a good place to start for two reasons: (1) safety, ease of use, and mild side-effect profile, and (2) possible usefulness in treating the apathy, irritability, and obsessiveness that may occur in the absence of major depression. A typical regimen might be sertraline, starting at 25 mg daily and advancing to 50–100 mg, with a maximal dose of 200 mg a day. In cases of depression accompanied by delusions and hallucinations, ECT or coadministration of a neuroleptic must be strongly considered, and a psychiatric consultation should therefore be obtained. A typical regimen might be haloperidol, starting at 0.5–2.5 mg daily and reaching a maximum of 20–30 mg daily or the newer agent quetiapine, beginning at 25–50 mg daily and reaching a maximum of 500–750 mg a day. A patient with HD who is oversedated on quetiapine may tolerate ziprasidone or olanzapine readily.

Typical high-potency neuroleptics such as haloperidol or fluphenazine are generally well tolerated and may be able to do "double duty" for the suppression of chorea, but they may not be a good choice in juvenile-onset HD or when rigidity and dystonia are problematic. If the neuroleptic is being used for purely psychiatric reasons, one of the newer atypical agents, such as risperidone, ziprasidone, or quetiapine, would be preferable, for reasons of overall tolerability.

Mania

Mania in HD is typically treated with a mood stabilizer such as divalproex sodium, beginning at 125 mg twice daily and advancing, in divided doses, to an eventual dose of 500–2000 mg daily, based on response and blood levels. Neuroleptics are also used, either just in the acute phase, or chronically. A typical regimen might be haloperidol, starting at 0.5–2.5 mg daily and reaching a maximum of 20–30 mg daily, or quetiapine, beginning at 25–50 mg daily and reaching a maximum of 500–750 mg daily. The conventional wisdom is that lithium is usually not a good choice for treating mania in HD. This may be due to the drug's rather narrow therapeutic range and the potential of patients with HD for poor compliance and dehydration, but it may also reflect difficulties in diagnosis, such as mistaking chronic personality changes in HD with a manic syndrome. Psychiatric consultation is almost always required for assessment and treatment of mania in HD.

Obsessive-Compulsive Disorder

Serotonergic agents such as SSRIs and clomipramine are the mainstay of pharmacotherapy for OCD in HD. A typical regimen might be sertraline, starting at 25 mg daily and advancing to 50–100 mg, with a maximal dose of 200 mg daily. The conventional wisdom is that higher doses may be required than for the treatment of major depression. However, as with symptoms of irritability and disinhibition discussed previously, particularly when the behaviors are not causing distress to the patients themselves, behavioral management, using techniques such as distraction and setting a routine, as well as managing the expectations of friends and family members through education about common personality and behavioral changes in HD, may be a more effective strategy. Consultation with a psychiatrist or psychologist about treatment of OCD in HD should prove useful.

Schizophrenia-like Syndromes

In using neuroleptics for treatment of delusions and hallucinations in HD, the clinician should bear in mind that although no particular neuroleptic has been demonstrated to be more effective than the others, the drugs differ considerably in side-effect profiles. The older, more anticholinergic agents, such as thioridazine, are usually too sedating and deliriogenic to be a good choice in HD. The atypical agents, such as risperidone, ziprasidone, or quetiapine, have the advantage in tolerability, but high-potency typical agents such as haloperidol or fluphenazine are less costly. The doses of haloperidol or quetiapine suggested in the treatment of mania would also be appropriate for schizophrenia-like syndromes. Nevertheless, many patients with these latter syndromes are poorly responsive to treatment, and psychiatric consultation is almost always required.

References

Folstein, S.E., Chase, G., Wahl, W., McDonnel, A.M., Folstein, M.F. (1987). Huntington's disease in Maryland: clinical aspects of racial variation. *American Journal of Human Genetics* 41: 168–79.

Guttman, M., Alpay, M., Chouinard, S., Como, P., Feinstein, A., Leroi, I., Rosenblatt, A. (2003). Clinical management of psychosis and mood disorders in Huntington's Disease. In M-A. Bedard, et al. (Eds.), *Mental and Behavioral Dysfunction in Movement Disorders*. Totowa, NJ: Humana Press. pp. 409–26.

Huntington, G. (1872). On chorea. *Medical and Surgical Reports of Philadelphia* 26: 317–21.

Marder, K., Zhao, H., Myers, R.H., Cudkowicz, M., Kayson, E., Kieburtz, K., Orme, C., Paulsen, J., Penney. J.B. Jr, Siemers. E., Shoulson, I., Huntington Study Group (2000). Rate of functional decline in Huntington's disease. *Neurology* 54: 452–8.

Mayberg, H.S., Starkstein, S.E., Peyser, C.E., Brandt, J., Dannals, R.F., Folstein, S.E. (1992). Paralimbic frontal lobe hypometabolism in depression associated with Huntington's disease. *Neurology* 42: 1791–7.

Mendez, M.F. (1994). Huntington's disease: update and review of neuropsychiatric aspects. *International Journal of Psychiatry in Medicine* 24: 189–208.

Shoenfield, M., Myers, R.H., Cupples, R.A., Berkman, B., Sax, D.S., Clark, E. (1984). Increased rate of suicide among patients with Huntington's disease. *Journal of Neurology, Neurosurgery, and Psychiatry* 47: 1283–7.

12

Cerebellar Diseases

RUSSELL L. MARGOLIS

After nearly 200 years, the concept that the cerebellum modulates only motor systems has been laid to rest. In the past two decades, evidence derived from neuroanatomical, neuroimaging, neuropsychologic, and psychiatric investigations has conclusively demonstrated that the normal cerebellum plays an important role in cognition and emotion and that diseases of the cerebellum may lead to cognitive impairment and psychiatric syndromes.

Diseases of the Cerebellum

Cerebellar damage can be a consequence of many different diseases (Table 12–1). The total prevalence of cerebellar disorders is unknown. Heavy alcohol use is probably the most common source of cerebellar abnormality. The cerebellum is affected in 1.5% to 8% of all strokes (Raco et al., 2003), so this is probably the second most common cause of cerebellar damage. In children, the incidence of primary brain tumors is about 2.8/100,000 per year; posterior fossa tumors account for about 40% of this total (Kuttesch and Ater, 2004). In adults, primary tumors of the cerebellum are less common than in children, but metastases are more frequent. The prevalence of recessive, dominant, and sporadic neurodegenerative diseases that primarily affect the cerebellum is, in aggregate, about 6/100,000 (Durr, 2002; Margolis, 2003). Other causes of cerebellar lesions are rare. A key point is that many of these disorders do not affect the cerebellum in isolation. Therefore, once disease affecting the cerebellum is established, it is critical to determine whether other brain regions are also involved. Other relevant clinical factors include the age of the patient and the duration of degenerative illness or the length of time since a stroke or a tumor resection.

Table 12.1. Diseases That Can Affect the Cerebellum

Disease Type	Examples
Autosomal dominant, degenerative	Spinocerebellar ataxia types 1–26
Autosomal recessive, degenerative	Friedreich's ataxia
Autosomal recessive, DNA repair	Ataxia-telangenctasia
X-linked	Rett syndrome
Mitochondrial	Neuropathy, ataxia, and retinitis pigmentosa
Nutritional	Vitamin E or thiamine deficiency
Toxic	Ethanol, phenytoin, lithium, organic solvents
Oncologic	Medulloblastoma
Infectious/post-infectious	Abscess, Whipple's disease
Vascular	Posterior circulation infarcts
Idiopathic	Sporadic late-onset cerebellar degeneration
Iatrogenic	Radiation

Psychiatric Disorders in Cerebellar Diseases

A neuroanatomic underpinning for the role of the cerebellum in cognition and emotion has been established over the past 25 years (Middleton and Strick, 2000; Schmahmann, 2001). The pathway from the cerebral cortex to the cerebellum originates with axons in cortical layer Vb in motor; somatosensory; association; and paralimbic regions, including prefrontal areas critical for attention, working memory, planning, motivation, decision-making, and language. After synapse in the pons, the pathway projects to the cerebellar cortex. The pathways back from the cerebellum to the cerebral cortex begin with axons projecting from cerebellar Purkinje cells to the deep cerebellar nuclei. These nuclei then project to both "motor" and "non-specific" nuclei of the thalamus. Both types of thalamic nuclei project to posterior parietal, superior temporal, and prefrontal association regions of the cerebral cortex, and the intralaminar nuclei also project to limbic regions (cingulate, parahippocampus). This corticocerebellar circuit is formed of discrete and relatively closed loops, similar to those detected in the circuitry between the basal ganglia and the cerebral cortex. Other cerebellar circuits of potential relevance for emotion and cognition include reciprocal pathways between the cerebellum and brainstem catecholaminergic (locus coeruleus) and serotoninergic nuclei (dorsal raphe), between the cerebellum and the hypothalamus, as well as between the cerebellum and the brainstem reticular formation, which may have a role in modulating overall alertness and activation.

Cognitive Disorders

Evidence that the cerebellum is involved in cognition and emotion in humans has emerged from functional neuroimaging studies of normal individuals engaged in various cognitive tasks and from neuropsychologic testing of individuals with cerebellar lesions. Language functions mediated by the cerebellum include verb generation, perception of temporal distinctions among phonemes, verbal fluency and word generation, and verbal working memory. Learning, especially associative motor tasks, sensory discrimination, and executive function may also be under the influence of the cerebellum. Executive tasks modulated by the cerebellum appear to include set shifting, the performance of multiple simultaneous tasks, and attention. The extent of cerebellar involvement in executive function may depend on the motor demands, automaticity, and fluency demanded by a given task.

The frequency of cognitive manifestations observed following cerebellar lesions (predominantly infarcts or hemorrhages in adults and tumors in children) is generally high. Cognitive deficits have been reported in 35% to 100% of patients after cerebellar strokes, with the lowest estimate derived from the most systematic study (Hoffmann and Schmitt, 2004). The nature of the deficits caused by these lesions varies and may include executive, language, praxic, memory, or visual-spatial dysfunction. In many cases, the abnormalities are relatively mild, and many patients improve over time. More global lesions are associated with broader cognitive deficits, and deficits associated with infarction of the posterior inferior cerebellar artery are generally milder than those associated with superior cerebellar artery or anterior inferior cerebellar artery infarction.

Resection of midline posterior fossa tumors in children leads to the "posterior fossa syndrome" in 13% of cases. This syndrome is characterized by mutism, oropharyngeal dyspraxia, impaired initiation of voluntary movements, oculomotor apraxia, incontinence, emotional liability, and personality changes that have been reported to include onset of an autistic-like syndrome (Pollack, 2001). Although most children substantially improve, longitudinal follow-up suggests that some of these deficits may not resolve completely. Resection of right hemisphere cerebellar tumors may result in deficits in language processing and auditory sequential memory, whereas resections of left hemisphere cerebellar tumors may result in impaired spatial and visual sequential memory.

Most, but not all, evidence suggests that patients with moderate degenerative disease of the cerebellum develop a mild subcortical dementia, with executive dysfunction and mild memory deficits (White, Lalonde, and Botez-Marquard, 2000; Zawacki et al., 2002). In general, impairment of executive function appears to be greater than memory impairment, which is the reverse of the pattern observed in patients with Huntington's disease (Brandt et al., 2004). Among the common hereditary spinocerebellar ataxias (SCAs), SCA1 produces the most global and severe cognitive deficits (Burk et al., 2003). The cognitive deficits in SCA6, in which pathology is largely limited to cerebellar Purkinje cells, are quite mild. The extent of cognitive impairment in Friedreich's ataxia varies from minimal to substantial impairment in multiple cognitive modalities. An important point is that executive function may be impaired in degenerative diseases affecting the cerebellum, even in the setting of overall normal intelligence and a normal bedside cognitive examination.

Noncognitive Disorders

Studies in nonhuman primates have shown that the cerebellar vermis modulates emotional arousal and fear conditioning. Similarly, in humans, stimuli with either negative or positive emotional valence activate specific cerebellar regions, and pathologic laughing and crying have been tentatively linked to cerebellar-mediated circuitry. The relationship between cerebellar topography and nonmotor function has not been fully established. The posterior lobe of the cerebellum may be associated with affect and cognition, whereas midline lesions may be associated with affective changes, potentially through pathways linking the vermis, via the fastigial nucleus, with limbic cortex (Schmahmann, 2004).

Strokes involving the cerebellum or brainstem appear to lead to mild and relatively short-lived depression, which is less severe and less prolonged than depression arising from strokes in the basal ganglia or left frontal cortex (Starkstein et al., 1988). Nonetheless, the reported depression does appear to reflect an affective disorder rather than demoralization.

Numerous case reports have suggested the presence of psychiatric disorders in patients with focal lesions, inflammatory or infectious processes, or degenerative diseases affecting the cerebellum. The syndromes described include personality changes, delusional disorders and other disorders resembling schizophrenia, and affective disorders resembling major depression or bipolar disorder. A record review of patients with degenerative cerebellar disease seen by tertiary care neurologists suggested that at least 40% of patients had readily detectable psychiatric symptoms; symptoms were more common in patients with involvement of brain regions in addition to the cerebellum (Liszewski et al., 2004). In a study based on detailed psychiatric evaluations by experienced neuropsychiatrists, the frequency of psychiatric syndromes in patients with degenerative diseases affecting the cerebellum was 80%, with 67% of patients suffering from at least one episode of major or mild depression, and 10% from a psychotic disorder (Leroi et al., 2002). Irritability and apathy were also relatively common.

Schmahmann has proposed that patients with cerebellar lesions from different etiologies tend to develop a unified set of signs and symptoms; he has termed this the "cerebellar cognitive affective syndrome" (Schmahmann, 2004). This syndrome consists of abnormalities in executive, visual-spatial, linguistic, and affective function. In the latter category he includes emotional blunting, clinically significant depression, disinhibition, and psychotic phenomena such as hallucinations and delusions. Although the concept of a single cerebellar affective cognitive syndrome has spurred considerable interest in the nonmotor dysfunction of patients with cerebellar disease, the available data suggest that cerebellar disease does not result in a unified syndrome. Rather, as with other cognitive and psychiatric manifestations of brain disease, patients may develop a number of different syndromes, in part depending on the nature and location of the insult to the cerebellum, and in part dependent on other genetic and environmental vulnerabilities.

Impact of Psychiatric Disturbances on Patients and Family

Little data are available concerning the extent to which psychiatric phenomena contribute to the overall burden faced by individuals with cerebellar diseases and their families. Anecdotally, and consistent with the findings in other neuropsychiatric disorders, both cognitive and noncognitive psychiatric syndromes have a significant impact on functional capacity and quality of life. Given the long history of emphasis on motor dysfunction, these factors are often not considered by clinicians, patients, or family members in the clinical management of cerebellar disorders. Although relatively infrequent, syndromes that include hallucinations and delusions may be particularly disruptive. Mild abnormalities in cognition (particularly executive dysfunction), personality, and mood may cause less overt disruption than psychotic disorders, but over time, especially if unrecognized, they can cause considerable problems in multiple spheres of life.

Treatment

Determining the cause of the cerebellar lesion or dysfunction is essential, because degeneration due to nutritional, dietary, and some metabolic disorders may be treatable and at least partially reversible (Perlman, 2004). Surgical intervention may be important for tumors and vascular malformations. There is no treatment for sporadic or genetic degenerative diseases of the cerebellum.

The neurologic evaluation of patients with cerebellar disease should include a psychiatric history and mental status examination as outlined in Chapter 1. This evaluation should include a bedside cognitive assessment, such as the Mini-Mental State Examination for overall cognitive performance (Folstein, Folstein, and McHugh, 1975), and a more focused test of executive function, such as EXIT 25 (Royall, Mahurin, and Gray, 1992). Opinions about the patient's cognition, mood and behavior should be sought from the family. There should be a low threshold for obtaining detailed cognitive testing, if possible performed under the auspices of a psychologist experienced in interpreting results from patients with neurodegenerative diseases. It is vital that the clinician not automatically accept the explanations offered by patients or families that emotional or cognitive disturbances merely reflect an understandable psychologic reaction to functional disability.

Cognitive Disorders

Treatments for cognitive deficits are supportive and educational, using approaches developed with the other dementias. In the case of cerebellar disease, education may be particularly important, because patients, families, and referring clinicians may not be aware of the association between cerebellar disease and cognitive deficits, and the relative sparing of memory and use of words may mask more subtle executive deficits, such as difficulty making decisions or planning future activities. As with any impairment affecting executive dysfunction, it is of great value to help family members avoid blaming the patient or each other for the patient's behavioral problems. The results of neuropsychologic testing may prove valuable in pinpointing cognitive strengths and weaknesses over time and in providing the patient and family with objective data that may explain difficulties otherwise attributed to "laziness" or a "bad attitude." Establishing routines, finding outside sources of support such as day programs, and adjusting cognitive demands on the patient to match his or her capacity can vastly improve quality of life for both patients and their families.

Noncognitive Disorders

Little data are available to guide the treatment of noncognitive psychiatric disorders in patients with diseases of the cerebellum. Supportive, interpersonal, and cognitive-behavioral psychotherapy are likely to be of help, both as specific treatments for psychiatric conditions such as depression or anxiety and to help the demoralized patient adapt to the psychiatric disorders and the underlying cerebellar disease.

Pharmacotherapy of noncognitive psychiatric disorders associated with cerebellar disease has not been systematically assessed. Given the apparent frequency of depression in cerebellar disease, and the relative safety of most antidepressants, it is reasonable for the neurologist to initiate and monitor pharmacologic treatment of depression, perhaps in conjunction with the primary care physician. Unfortunately, there is no empirical evidence to guide the choice of particular psychotropic medicines in patients with cerebellar disease. Doses appear to be in the usual range for each agent (see Chapter 15), although as in other brain diseases, it is prudent to start with a relatively low dose of medicine and increase the dose cautiously. Patients with cerebellar disease are already at increased risk of falling and are particularly vulnerable to medication-induced ataxia and orthostatic hypotension. Otherwise, standard practice for treatment with an antidepressant applies, including supportive psychotherapy and careful monitoring for side effects, nonadherence, suicidality, and worsening of symptoms. A somewhat arbitrary list of the first-line choices of antidepressants might include sertraline (start at 25 mg daily), bupropion (start at 37.5 mg daily), or venlafaxine (start at 37.5 mg daily). In younger patients with minimal neurologic impairment, starting at double these doses may be possible. Extended-release forms of bupropion (taken twice a day) and venlafaxine (taken once a day) may improve adherence, with the same total doses used in the normal release preparations. In some diseases involving the cerebellum or resulting in ataxia, additional caution is necessary because of cardiac or other systemic complications. For instance, in Friedreich's ataxia most patients have cardiac disease (Pandolfo, 2003), most commonly hypertrophic cardiomyopathy, although several case reports demonstrate that various psychotropic agents and electroconvulsive therapy (ECT) can be used safely. If the depressed patient worsens or does not improve over six to eight weeks, has trouble adhering to the medication regimen, has bipolar disorder or psychotic symptoms (hallucinations or delusions), or appears severely anxious, referral to a psychiatrist is warranted. For bipolar disorder, the consulting psychiatrist may prescribe lithium, valproic acid, or carbamazepine. Although these agents may increase ataxia, which means that close monitoring of gait by all treating physicians is warranted, they should not be considered contraindicated. For psychotic symptoms or irritability, neuroleptic agents may be useful, although again gait and orthostatic changes in blood pressure must be monitored carefully, initial doses should be low, and changes may be necessary in response to side effects. Despite these cautions, it is essential to avoid undertreatment, because psychiatric disorders may be life-threatening and lead to major morbidity, whereas medicines can be quickly stopped if untoward side effects develop.

Acknowledgments   This chapter is adapted from Margolis, R.L. (2006). The Psychiatry of the Cerebellum. In Jeste D. and Friedman R. (Eds.), *Psychiatry for Neurologists* (Totowa, NJ: Humana Press, with permission from the publisher.

References

Brandt, J., Leroi, I., O'Hearn, E., Rosenblatt, A., Margolis, R.L. (2004). Cognitive impairments in cerebellar degeneration: a comparison with Huntington's disease. *Journal of Neuropsychiatry and Clinical Neurosciences* 16: 176–84.

Burk, K., Globas, C., Bosch, S., Klockgether, T., Zuhlke, C., Daum, I., Dichgans, J. (2003). Cognitive deficits in spinocerebellar ataxia type 1, 2, and 3. *Journal of Neurology* 250: 207–11.

Durr, A. (2002). Friedreich's ataxia: treatment within reach. *Lancet Neurology* 1: 370–4.

Folstein, M., Folstein, S., McHugh, P.R. (1975). 'Mini mental state': a practical method for grading the cognitive state of patients for the clinician. *Journal of Psychiatric Research* 12: 189–98.

Hoffmann, M., Schmitt, F. (2004). Cognitive impairment in isolated subtentorial stroke. *Acta Neurologica Scandinavica* 109: 14–24.

Kuttesch, J.F., Ater, J.L. (2004). Brain tumors in childhood. In R.E. Behrman, R.M. Kliegman, and H.B. Benson (Eds.), *Nelson Textbook of Pediatrics.* Philadelphia, PA: WB Saunders, 1703–9.

Leroi, I., O'Hearn, E., Marsh, L., Lyketsos, C.G., Rosenblatt, A., Ross, C.A., Brandt, J., Margolis, R.L. (2002). Psychopathology in degenerative cerebellar diseases: a comparison to Huntington's disease and normal controls. *American Journal of Psychiatry* 159: 1306–14.

Liszewski, C.M., O'Hearn, E., Leroi, I., Gourley, L., Ross, C.A., Margolis, R.L. (2004). Cognitive impairment and psychiatric symptoms in 133 patients with diseases associated with cerebellar degeneration. *Journal of Neuropsychiatry and Clinical Neurosciences* 16: 109–12.

Margolis, R.L. (2003). The dominant spinocerebellar ataxias: a molecular approach to classification, diagnosis, pathogenesis, and the future. *Expert Review of Molecular Diagnostics* 3: 715–32.

Middleton, F.A., Strick, P.L. (2000). Basal ganglia and cerebellar loops: motor and cognitive circuits. *Brain Research Brain Research Reviews* 31: 236–50.

Pandolfo, M. (2003). Friedreich ataxia. *Seminars in Pediatric Neurology* 10: 163–72.

Perlman, S.L. (2004). Symptomatic and disease-modifying therapy for the progressive ataxias. *The Neuroloigst* 10: 275–89.

Pollack, I. (2001). Neurobehavioral abnormalities after posterior fossa surgery in children. *International Review of Psychiatry* 13: 302–12.

Raco, A., Caroli, E., Isidori, A., Salvati, M. (2003). Management of acute cerebellar infarction: one institution's experience. *Neurosurgery* 53: 1061–5.

Royall, D.R., Mahurin, R.K., Gray, K.F. (1992). Bedside assessment of executive cognitive impairment: the executive interview. *Journal of the American Geriatrics Society* 40: 1221–6.

Schmahmann, J.D. (2001). The cerebrocerebellar system: anatomic substrates of the cerebellar contribution to cognition and emotion. *International Review of Psychiatry* 13: 247–60.

Schmahmann, J.D. (2004). Disorders of the cerebellum: ataxia, dysmetria of thought, and the cerebellar cognitive affective syndrome. *Journal of Neuropsychiatry and Clinical Neurosciences* 16: 367–78.

Starkstein, S.E., Robinson, R.G., Berthier, M.L., Price, T.R. (1988). Depressive disorders following posterior circulation as compared with middle cerebral artery infarcts. *Brain* 111: 375–87.

White, M., Lalonde, R., Botez-Marquard, T. (2000). Neuropsychologic and neuropsychiatric characteristics of patients with Friedreich's ataxia. *Acta Neurologica Scandinavica* 102: 222–6.

Zawacki, T.,M., Grace, J., Friedman, J.H., Sudarsky, L. (2002). Executive and emotional dysfunction in Machado-Joseph disease. *Movement Disorders* 17: 1004–10.

13

Tourette's Syndrome

JOHN T. WALKUP
BENJAMIN N. SCHNEIDER

Tourette's syndrome (TS) is a neuropsychiatric disorder of childhood onset characterized by the presence of motor and vocal tics for a duration of at least 1 year. Tics are typically brief and stereotypical movements (eg, eye blinking, head jerks) or vocalizations (eg, throat clearing, grunting), but they can also be more complex movements involving multiple muscle groups and combinations of movements and sounds. There is a great range of tic severity. Tics can be so subtle or occur so infrequently as to be unnoticeable, even to the person with the tics. However, tics can also be so intense and frequent that they are readily noticeable by others, and they can be disruptive of daily activities. Indeed, in some cases (eg, severe head jerks), tics can cause pain or physical injury (eg, cervical disc and spine damage).

Tics usually begin in childhood; the average age at diagnosis is 7 years. They reach peak severity in the early teen years and then lessen in intensity and frequency during young adulthood (Leckman et al., 2001). Tics wax and wane in severity, worsening with excitement and stress and improving during calm, focused activities. Coprolalia and its motor counterpart copropraxia (uttering obscene words or making obscene gestures, respectively) are uncommon symptoms, occurring in less than 10% of patients with TS and are not required for a diagnosis of TS (Robertson and Stern, 1998). Many patients describe a sensation or urge prior to tic occurrence, commonly referred to as a *premonitory sensation* or *urge* (Miguel et al., 2000). Even though tics are considered involuntary, they can be voluntarily suppressed for short periods of time.

Prevalence estimates of TS have varied and depend a great deal on the threshold for diagnosis and setting in which cases are identified. A review of the many epidemiologic studies suggests that 0.1% to 1% of people are affected with TS (Scahill et al., 2005). Despite this variability in specific rates, epidemiologic studies have consistently identified that males are more commonly affected than females, children are more frequently affected than adults, and that milder forms of TS are more common than severe forms.

Evidence from twin and family studies suggest that TS is an inherited condition. However, the inheritance pattern is likely more complex than initially thought. Although it is possible that there are genes with major effects, multiple genes and environmental factors likely also play a role (Pauls, 2003). Efforts to identify the genes for TS have recently resulted in the identification of an abnormality in the *SLITRK1* gene (chromosome 13q31.1) (Abelson et al., 2005). Abnormalities in this gene are associated with less complex dendritic growth.

In addition to TS, a broader diagnostic group of tic disorders includes *chronic motor or vocal tic disorder* (CTD), characterized by either motor or vocal tics for a period of at least 1 year, and *transient tic disorder*, characterized by motor and or vocal tics for a period of greater than 4 weeks but less than 1 year. Although CTD has not been studied as extensively as TS, it is considered to be a variant expression of the same underlying pathophysiology. Because CTD shares many features with TS, including the risk of co-occurring psychiatric disorders, the identification of any tic disorder in a child, regardless of severity, should lead to an evaluation for psychiatric comorbidity.

Psychiatric Disorders Associated with Tourette's Syndrome

Nearly all psychiatric disorders, including disorders of attention, activity level, impulse control, and mood, have been described in people with TS. However, two conditions, attention deficit hyperactivity disorder (ADHD) and obsessive-compulsive disorder

(OCD) commonly co-occur with TS and share a genetic relationship with it. All patients with TS should be routinely screened for these disorders (Pauls et al., 1986b; Pauls et al., 1993). There is controversy regarding the genetic relationship between TS and other psychiatric disorders (Pauls, Leckman, and Cohen, 1994; Comings, 1995), but because depression and anxiety disorders are common in the general population, it is likely that neurologists will identify patients with TS who have other psychiatric disorders. Lastly, people with TS may experience problems coping with TS (ie, adjustment disorders), with resultant difficulties at home, school, and work.

Attention Deficit Hyperactivity Disorder

Studies of clinical populations suggest that 40% to 50% of children with TS have comorbid ADHD (Pauls et al., 1986a; Comings and Comings, 1987; Freeman et al. 2000). In assessing children with TS for ADHD, it is important to consider the differential diagnosis of inattention, impulsivity, and hyperactivity in patients with TS. The causes of impaired attention and concentration in patients with TS can include the tics themselves, learning difficulties, premonitory sensations, obsessions, anxiety, and depression. Hyperactivity in patients with TS may be a reflection of the motor restlessness and agitation commonly seen in children with learning disorders, anxiety disorders, and mood disorders who are unable to sit still or are impulsive in environments that are challenging for them. Neurologists should be particularly cautious in making the diagnosis of ADHD, inattentive subtype, until a full evaluation for other psychiatric disorders has been completed.

Although TS is commonly associated with learning disabilities, recent research suggests that learning problems in patients with TS are likely associated with ADHD rather than with TS alone (Denckla, 2006). A psychologic assessment may be helpful in identifying learning difficulties and planning treatment.

Obsessive-Compulsive Disorder

OCD is characterized by recurrent, stereotypical, intrusive and unwanted thoughts and behaviors. Factor analytic studies of obsessive-compulsive symptoms in patients with OCD suggest four subtypes of the disorder: a contamination group, an obsessions group, a symmetry/order group, and a hoarding group (Mataix-Cols, Rosario-Campos, and Leckman, 2005; Cullen et al., 2007). It is important that neurologists to be aware of these groups, because not all subtypes are as responsive to treatment with serotonin reuptake inhibitors (SRIs) and psychotherapy (Mataix-Cols et al., 1999; Mataix-Cols et al., 2002). Determining which OCD subtype a person with TS has ensures more appropriate expectations for treatment and minimizes the overuse of medication for symptoms that are not medication responsive.

The *contamination* subtype is characterized by obsessions about dirt and germs as well as by compulsive cleaning and grooming rituals. The contamination subtype is generally more distressing than the other subtypes; does not appear to be as highly comorbid with other psychiatric disorders, including TS; and appears moderately responsive to SRIs and cognitive behavioral therapy. The *obsessions* subtype is characterized by obsessive thoughts that include religious, sexual, and aggressive themes. The *symmetry/order* subtype is characterized by ordering, arranging, and aligning objects. Both the obsessions and symmetry/order subtypes are highly comorbid with other anxiety and mood disorders. People with TS and OCD consistently report obsessions of sexual and aggressive themes and symmetry/order compulsions. The *hoarding* subtype is characterized by the collection of and inability to discard objects of little apparent significance. Hoarding has repeatedly been identified as a distinct subtype, is associated with obsessive-compulsive personality (ie, perfectionism and rigidity), and appears less responsive to SRIs.

It can be difficult even for the seasoned clinician to differentiate correctly among the variety of repetitive thoughts (ie, obsessions, anxious worries, premonitory urges) and behaviors (ie, compulsions, tics, complex tics, stereotypies, other dyskinetic movements) that can be seen in patients with TS. For example, if a patient with TS shrugs his shoulder three times in a row, is that a complex tic or a compulsion? Studies comparing obsessive-compulsive symptoms in patients with TS and primary OCD offer some guidance as to whether repetitive mental experiences and rituals are tics or obsessive-compulsive symptoms. Obsessive-compulsive symptoms observed in patients with TS tend to be more sensorimotor in nature as opposed to such symptoms seen in patients with OCD alone, which are more cognitive and affective in nature (Miguel et al., 2000). Although commonly considered an obsessive-compulsive symptom, three successive shoulder shrugs associated to relieve a sensation are more appropriately considered a complex tic, because this symptom shares most features with tics (premonitory sensation and motor movement) and only one feature with compulsions (repetition). This is in contrast to cognitions (eg, worries that contamination may lead to death) associated with resulting in rituals that appear more purposeful (eg, hand washing). The implication of such distinctions for treatment is discussed below.

Other Clinically Important Psychiatric Disorders that can Co-Occur with Tourette's Syndrome

In addition to OCD and ADHD, patients with TS can present with developmental disorders (eg, Asperger's syndrome), anxiety disorders, depressive disorders and disruptive behavioral disorders (eg, oppositional defiant disorder, conduct disorder). ADHD and OCD can start early in life. Developmental disorders such as Asperger's syndrome also start early but when mild may not necessarily be impairing until the teenage years. Other anxiety disorders such as separation anxiety and generalized anxiety also have a childhood onset and may present suddenly with intense distress. Panic disorder is not likely to affect children with TS, because its earliest age of onset is the late teens and early 20s. Major depression and bipolar disorder are less common in childhood than in adolescence. Disruptive behavior disorders can appear at almost any time during development, but solidification of disruptive behavior into an antisocial pattern occurs in the late teens. There is little literature about substance abuse in patients with TS. Despite a lack of research, it is not uncommon for patients to describe short term benefit of either alcohol, marijuana, or tobacco on tic severity. Such an experience may put people with TS at risk for a substance use disorder (abuse or dependence).

Because TS, ADHD, and OCD commonly co-occur, the evaluation of patients with TS often stops after all three disorders are identified. It is particularly important that the evaluation of patients with refractory, complex, or atypical symptoms be extended so that the physician may inquire about other symptomatology described above. Patients with TS, ADHD, OCD plus either separation anxiety, depression, Asperger's syndrome, or bipolar disorder may require consultation with a psychiatrist who has experience evaluating and treating in these disorders.

Problems Related to Living with Tourette's Syndrome

It is not easy living with TS. For many patients, living with the disorder is not associated with any functional impairment, but even in the absence of impairment, patients may experience the lack of motor control as disturbing and may be uncomfortable with the reactions of others to their tics. The self-consciousness associated with TS may restrict social involvement or affect the choice of jobs and leisure activities. After patients with TS are diagnosed, it is possible for them to educate family, friends, and coworkers, but this, too, has a social cost. Not everyone will be supportive, and some will be skeptical or cynical (eg, "You should be able to control it"). Patients with TS may also be teased by peers and discriminated against by teachers or employers. Such discrimination can be a significant burden, even for patients who are not functionally impaired. Although most patients with TS do well over the long term, the social and occupational problems that occur because of TS may result in distorted self-concept, demoralization, interpersonal problems, maladaptive coping strategies, and financial difficulties.

Tourette's Syndrome Across the Life Span

Children with Tourette's Syndrome

Children with TS are undergoing identify formation at the time when tic symptoms are typically at their worst. Parents and teachers can provide support for appropriate identity development by encouraging children with TS to engage in those activities associated with good long-term outcome—academic achievement, positive family and peer relationships, behavioral and emotional self-control skills, and restful and restorative leisure activities. By having support for the development of appropriate lifelong skills, children with TS likely do better regardless of their illness severity. Although it is appropriate for children to know that they have TS and to advocate for themselves, there is some risk involved when TS becomes so central to a child's identity that it excludes other, more positive, components of self-concept (Hollenbeck, 2001). Children with TS can be more difficult to parent. It is not uncommon for parents to become confused about whether some of their children's behaviors are voluntary or not (eg, swearing versus coprolalia) and to become paralyzed in their parenting approach. After their child is diagnosed, some parents find it more difficult to set limits, or they become overprotective. Power struggles between parents and children may lead to the development of more serious and maladaptive behavior patterns such as severe oppositional behavior, tantrums, aggression (Patterson, DeBaryshe, and Ramsey, 1989). Ironically, some parenting advice provided by clinicians may inadvertently support the development of problem behaviors. Thus statements such as "ignore the behavior, it is probably TS-related" and "he probably can't control it, he has TS" may be attempts to educate the parents about how best to treat a child with TS, but they can backfire if parents interpret the advice too liberally and do not effectively address behavioral difficulties.

Teenagers with Tourette's Syndrome

TS often improves during later adolescence. Teenagers who have not laid the groundwork for a solid identity and good self-control skills may have significant problems with coping and adaptation during adolescence. Ironically, such problems may actually increase at a time when tic symptoms are decreasing. Teenagers who have not developed a complex sense of self with good coping and self-control skills may find themselves struggling to function without tic symptoms as an explanation for their difficulties.

Parenting strategies for teenagers differ from those for children. Some parents have difficulty making the transition from parenting a child with TS to parenting a teenager, and behavioral problems may result. Teenagers with TS, like all adolescents, respond better to parents who encourage increasing responsibility and facilitate increasing autonomy.

The pattern of onset for comorbid conditions also change during adolescence. New-onset anxiety disorders such as separation anxiety disorder are less common in adolescence than in childhood, and mood disorders, both depression and bipolar disorder, are more common. Substance abuse and consolidated patterns of defiant and antisocial behavior also increase during the teen years.

Young Adults with Tourette's Syndrome

Although tics are likely to decrease in severity during the young adult years, young adults are at risk for adult-onset psychiatric disorders or from continuing impairment from psychiatric difficulties in childhood. It is also not uncommon for young adults with TS to have difficulties living away from the family home, forming intimate relationships, and obtaining and maintaining a positive work experience.

Adults with Tourette's Syndrome

Adults older than 40 years of age with TS have gone through the period of risk for most psychiatric disorders, so there is less likelihood of new-onset disorders except, perhaps, major depression. However, psychiatric disorders that emerged earlier, problems with living, and the potential for discrimination continue for older adults. Also, older adults with TS did not grow up in a climate of understanding or acceptance of TS. When these individuals were children, little was known about TS or its treatment. They may have been misdiagnosed, mistreated, or simply misunderstood. Although most who have come to diagnosis later in life find the diagnosis helpful, some have the capacity for acceptance and some struggle to come to terms with their diagnosis. Some adults with TS may resist engaging in treatment "again," especially if previous treatments were ineffective or misguided.

Treatment

Treatment of patients with TS begins with education about TS, its symptoms and course, and the various approaches to treatment for both tics and psychiatric comorbidity. For many patients such educational efforts can be very helpful. It is not uncommon for patients to report decreased tic symptoms after a good diagnostic evaluation and learning more about the disorder. Given the limited time for patient education in most busy practice settings, printed and online materials from the Tourette Syndrome Association can address the myriad issues regarding TS and comorbid conditions for patients of all ages with TS. These materials are readily available at nominal cost at www.tsa-usa.org.

The following section will briefly review tic-suppressing treatments, both pharmacologic and behavioral, as well as treatment approaches to the commonly co-occurring psychiatric disorders.

Tic-suppressing Treatment

Pharmacologic treatments. The goal of pharmacologic tic suppression is a reduction in tic severity not an elimination of all tic symptoms (Scahill et al., 2006a). The gold-standard treatment for tic suppression is low-dose antipsychotic medication. A number of antipsychotics have demonstrated efficacy (e.g. haloperidol, pimozide, risperidone), but there have been few comparative clinical trials to guide the choice between them (Shapiro, Shapiro, and Eisenkraft, 1983a; Shapiro, Shapiro, and Eisenkraft, 1983b; Sallee et al., 1997; Sallee et al., 2000; Scahill et al., 2003). Our clinical experience suggests that the fluphenazine is as effective and perhaps better tolerated than haloperidol, with fewer cardiac and drug-drug interaction concerns than pimozide. A typical starting dose of fluphenazine is 0.5–1 mg/day. Weekly increases in dose up to 3–5 mg/day may be required for good tic control.

Of the atypical antipsychotics (eg. aripiprazole, clozapine, olanzapine, quetiapine, risperidone, ziprasidone), only risperidone (daily dose 1–3 mg) has demonstrated efficacy in TS (Scahill et al., 2003). Although atypical antipsychotics appear to have a lower risk of inducing extrapyramidal side effects, more recent concerns about weight gain and the development of type 2 diabetes have decreased enthusiasm for this group of agents. Among the atypical neuroleptics, ziprasidone (daily dose up to 80 mg) appears less likely to induce weight gain, but carries a warning regarding QTc prolongation, which may limit its acceptability to clinicians and families. Aripiprazole (daily dose 2.5–7.5 mg) has been promising in open trials and is undergoing randomized controlled trails for tic suppression. Tetrabenazine, which has been available in Canada and Europe for many years, will likely be available in the United States for the treatment of Huntington's disease. Open trials of tetrabenazine (daily dose 50–125 mg) suggest that it may be effective for tic suppression (Silay and Jankovic, 2005).

Side effects of the antipsychotics (eg, sedation, weight gain, cognitive changes, extrapyramidal symptoms) are common and often lead to medication discontinuation. Less common, but of obvious concern to patients and families, are tardive dyskinesia and antipsychotic malignant syndrome. Often unrecognized is the capacity for antipsychotics to induce depression or anxiety in patients with TS (Mikkelsen, Detlor, and Cohen, 1981; Bruun, 1988). Care should be taken not to attribute such worsening to TS but rather to evaluate whether any such worsening could be related to medication.

Given the limited tolerability of antipsychotics in patients with TS, many clinicians begin treatment with alpha-agonists such as clonidine or guanfacine. The alpha-agonists have benefits for both tics and ADHD symptoms (Scahill et al., 2001), but in our experience are less consistently effective than antipsychotics for tic suppression and stimulants for ADHD. Side effects commonly seen with alpha-agonists include sedation and irritability. Because of its short half-life, clonidine is dosed two to three times per day. Starting doses for clonidine are 0.05–0.075 mg/day, with weekly increases to 0.2–0.3 mg/day as tolerated. Guanfacine has a longer half-life but still requires a minimum of twice-daily dosing. Starting doses of guanfacine are 0.5–1 mg/day, with weekly increases to 2–3 mg/day.

For patients with treatment refractory tics there are two other treatment options: botulinum injections of affected muscles and deep brain stimulation (DBS). Open trials of botulinum toxin have demonstrated benefit for both motor and vocal tics (Marras et al., 2001; Porta et al., 2004). Case reports of DBS suggest that, for adults with severe tic disorders, DBS may offer short-term benefit (Temel and Visser-Vandewalle, 2004). Recommendations for patient selection have been developed by the Tourette Syndrome Association Scientific and Medical Advisory Boards (Mink et al., 2006).

Nonpharmacologic and behavioral treatments for tic suppression. Patients with TS describe a number of strategies they have learned through trial and error to manage their tic symptoms. These methods include relaxation techniques, camouflaging (ie, making tics appear as voluntary actions), voluntary suppression or blunting of tic severity, self-distracting techniques, and physical exercise. The goal of behavioral treatment development for tic suppression has been to take the best of these strategies and merge them with behavioral theory to develop a training program for patients to manage their tics more effectively. The behavioral model of tic suppression in no way implies that tics are voluntary or not of neurologic origin. Rather, it acknowledges that environmental factors and voluntary behaviors can influence tic severity, both in the short-term and the long-term (Himle et al., 2006).

The central component for the most effective behavioral interventions is competing response training. Competing response training attempts to break the reinforcement cycle that is hypothesized to maintain or enhance tic severity. That is, every time a premonitory sensation dissipates on completion of a tic, the tic is reinforced and is more likely to occur again when the premonitory sensation is experienced (ie, negative reinforcement). A competing response—essentially, an alternative behavior initiated by the patient voluntarily—interrupts this cycle by completing a voluntary activity, allowing the urge to dissipate prior to the tic's being completed. For example, a competing response for vocal tics is diaphragmatic breathing, a voluntary contraction of the diaphragm to exhale and relaxation to inhale. Other examples include voluntarily contracting an opposing muscle group of the tic (eg, holding the mouth closed for a "yawning" tic) or voluntarily initiating an action that hinders the expression of the vocal tic (eg, sitting down for a hopping movement).

With training and practice, competing responses training can be implemented inconspicuously, even "unconsciously." Interestingly, tics that are often the most difficult to address pharmacologically (ie, slow, complex motor movements and vocalizations) may be the most sensitive to competing response training (Himle et al., 2006).

Treatment of Psychiatric Disorders Commonly Co-Occurring with Tourette's Syndrome

An accurate diagnosis that focuses not only the patient's TS symptoms but also on any co-occurring conditions is central to appropriate treatment. The diagnostic assessment should lead to the development of a treatment hierarchy of the most impairing conditions. The development of a treatment hierarchy guards against the tendency of patients, their families, and even physicians to become focused on tic symptoms to the exclusion of other disorders, and to treat tic symptoms first, even if these are not the patient's most debilitating condition.

Many patients and families ask what specialist is best suited to treat patients with TS. The answer to this question is increasingly complicated. Historically, both neurologists and psychiatrists have had the expertise to treat both tics and the common comorbid conditions. However, the type of clinician who cares for patients with TS is best determined case by case according to each patient's treatment needs and each clinician's expertise with TS, rather than by specialty, for three reasons: (1) increasing awareness of the complexity of psychiatric comorbidity, (2) increasing use of behavioral interventions for tics as well as comorbid conditions, and (3) increasing use of invasive somatic treatments such as botulinum toxin and DBS. Because no single individual clinician is trained to address all the issues that TS patients present, it is likely that a team of clinicians will need to work collaboratively to address the needs of TS patients. It is prudent that the clinician who first contacts a patient with TS to discuss the potential need for other specialists to become involved over time.

Attention deficit hyperactivity disorder. There is an extensive history of case reports describing the development or worsening of tics in children treated with stimulant medications (Gadow and Sverd, 2006). Reassuringly, recent placebo-controlled trials of stimulants suggest good efficacy for ADHD in children with tic disorders, with minimal impact on tic severity (Gadow et al., 1995; Castellanos et al., 1997; Tourette's Syndrome Study Group, 2002). In the largest trial to date (Tourette's Syndrome Study Group, 2002), tic worsening was observed in the trial (the average dose of methylphenidate was 30 mg/day in divided doses); however, the extent of tic worsening did not differ in those on stimulants, clonidine, or placebo, suggesting that tic worsening observed in children with TS and ADHD treated with stimulants may be due not to stimulant treatment but more likely results from the waxing and waning of tic symptoms. These studies suggest that stimulants can be used safely for ADHD in children with TS.

With respect to other risks of stimulant medication, recent reports of deaths in children with known cardiac abnormalities taking stimulant medication have resulted in more extensive warnings in product information for these medications (Hirsch, 2006). Despite the demonstrated safety and efficacy of stimulants in children with tics and ADHD, safety concerns may still make families and clinicians reticent to use stimulant medications in this population. Reasonable alternative medications for ADHD in TS patients are available, including clonidine (Tourette Syndrome Study Group, 2002) and guanfacine (Scahill et al., 2001). Doses used to target ADHD with clonidine and guanfacine are similar to those used for tic suppression.

Psychosocial treatments have also proven to be beneficial for children with ADHD, especially for children with co-occurring anxiety and behavior problems (Swanson et al., 2001). A structured environment, good supervision, and a positive rewarding atmosphere can all help a child with TS who has ADHD. Disruptive behavior in children with TS and ADHD is also responsive to parental behavioral management strategies (Scahill et al., 2006b).

Neurologists may choose to seek psychiatric consultation for children with TS and ADHD who have: (1) additional symptoms of co-occurring psychiatric disorders (eg, Asperger's syndrome, anxiety and mood disorders) to determine what is the best first treatment—one that targets tics, ADHD or the co-occurring psychiatric disorder; (2) the inattentive subtype of ADHD, because inattention has a complex differential diagnosis and the choice of first treatment may not be obvious; and (3) an atypical response to pharmacologic treatment of ADHD. Neurologists should consider referral to a psychologist for any child with TS, ADHD, and behavioral problems for parent behavioral management training. Psychologists specializing in learning disabilities can assess and make recommendation for children with TS, ADHD, and learning disorders.

Obsessive-compulsive disorder. SRIs have consistently demonstrated efficacy for children and adults with OCD (Pigott and Seay, 1999). It is important to remember that complex tics may be confused with compulsions, and premonitory urges may be confused with obsessions. At this time, there is no reason to believe that SRIs medications will be helpful for tics or premonitory urges. The SRIs clomipramine, fluvoxamine, sertraline, and fluoxetine all have indications for OCD and appear to be similarly effective in children and adults. The use of SRIs for typical OCD symptoms is fairly straightforward, although there are several caveats. Even though children may be more sensitive to the activating side effects of the SSRIs than adults and thus only tolerate low doses (Hammad et al., 2006), it is not uncommon for children to benefit from and tolerate adult doses of the SSRIs.

Doses used in clinical trials were often the highest safe dose rather than the lowest effective dose. Usual effective doses for the U.S. Food and Drug Administration (FDA)–approved SRIs are clomipramine up to 3 mg/kg/day, or 200 mg maximum,; fluvoxamine 100–200 mg/day; fluoxetine 20–60 mg/day; and sertraline 50–200 mg/day. Patients are usually started with low doses, and doses are increased based on the benefits and side effects. The recent "black box" warning regarding an increased risk of suicidal ideation and behavior in child and adolescents that has been added to the product information for all antidepressant medications may make it less feasible for neurologists to use these medications; recommendations for starting and monitoring antidepressant treatment in children and adolescents may require more time than may be available in neurologic practice. For more information on the safe use of antidepressant in children and adolescents, please see the Parent Medication Guide (http://www.parentsmedguide.org) prepared by the American Academy of Child and Adolescent Psychiatry and endorsed by many family, mental health, and professional advocacy groups.

Cognitive-behavioral therapy (CBT), which includes exposure and response prevention (ERP), is arguably the treatment of choice for patients with TS and OCD (Pediatric OCD Treatment Study Team, 2004). ERP strategies consist of exposing the patient to the fear-inducing stimulus (eg, dirt) and preventing the corresponding compulsion (e.g., hand washing), which results in decreased obsessions and compulsions over time. It is unclear if ERP is equally effective for all the various subtypes of OCD, because most trials have not assessed outcome of specific subtypes. Psychologists trained in cognitive-behavioral techniques are best equipped to use these strategies. Increasingly, psychiatrists are being trained to implement these strategies also. Neurologists should counsel their patients in the basic tenets of CBT as applied to TS: obsessions and compulsions are to be addressed head-on, because accommodation to them typically makes them worse. Teaching this can be very helpful to patients and the psychiatrists or psychologists working with them.

Neurologists should consider consultation with a psychiatrist when obsessive-compulsive symptoms are atypical or are unresponsive to usual SRI doses. Patients who are partially responsive to SRI treatment may require multiple medications to achieve benefit. Consultation with a psychiatrist experienced with complex pharmacologic interventions maybe very helpful for these patients. Patients who have not benefited from standard CBT should see a psychologist who specializes in OCD treatment, because there are nuances to CBT that may require the experience and training of true specialist.

Other disorders. Because so many psychiatric disorders have been described in patients with TS, it is beyond the scope of this book to review treatments for each. Practically speaking, the treatment of developmental disorders, anxiety disorders, major depression, bipolar disorder, substance abuse and dependence, and behavior disorders should follow the treatment guidelines for those disorders in children and adults and preferably be implemented by clinicians with experience in those disorders.

References

Abelson, J.F., Kwan, K.Y., O'Roak, B.J., Baek, D.Y., Stillman, A.A., Morgan, T.M., Mathews, C.A., Pauls, D.L., Rasin, M.R., Gunel, M., Davis, N.R., Ercan-Sencicek, A.G., Guez, D.H., Spertus, J.A., Leckman, J.F., Dure, L.S. IV, Kurlan, R., Singer, H.S., Gilbert, D.L., Farhi, A., Louvi. A., Lifton, R.P., Sestan, N., State, M.W. (2005). Sequence variants in SLITRK1 are associated with Tourette's syndrome. *Science* 5746: 317–20.

Bruun, R.D. (1988). Subtle and underrecognized side effects of neuroleptic treatment in children with Tourette's disorder. *American Journal of Psychiatry* 5: 621–4.

Castellanos, F.X., Giedd, J.N., Elia, J., Marsh, W.L., Ritchie, G.F., Hamburger, S.D., Rapoport, J.L. (1997). Controlled stimulant treatment of ADHD and comorbid Tourette's syndrome: effects of stimulant and dose. *Journal of the American Academy of Child and Adolescent Psychiatry* 5: 589–96.

Comings, D.E. (1995). Tourette's syndrome: a behavioral spectrum disorder. *Advances in Neurology* 65: 293–303.

Comings, D.E., Comings, B.G. (1987). A controlled study of Tourette syndrome. I. Attention-deficit disorder, learning disorders, and school problems. *American Journal of Human Genetics* 5: 701–41.

Cullen, B., Brown, C.H., Riddle, M.A., Grados, M., Joseph Bienvenu, O., Hoehn-Saric, R., Yao Shugart, Y., Liang, K.Y., Samuels, J., Nestadt, G. (2007). Factor analysis of the Yale-Brown Obsessive Compulsive Scale in a family study of obsessive-compulsive disorder. *Depression and Anxiety* 24: 130–8.

Denckla, M.B. (2006). Attention deficit hyperactivity disorder: the childhood co-morbidity that most influences the disability burden in Tourette syndrome. *Advances in Neurology* 99: 17–21.

Freeman, R.D., Fast, D.K., Burd, L., Kerbeshian, J., Robertson, M.M., Sandor, P. (2000). An international perspective on Tourette syndrome: selected findings from 3,500 individuals in 22 countries. *Developmental Medicine and Child Neurology* 7: 436–47.

Gadow, K.D., Sverd, J. (2006). Attention deficit hyperactivity disorder, chronic tic disorder, and methylphenidate. *Advances in Neurology* 99: 197–207.

Gadow, K.D., Sverd, J., Sprafkin, J., Nolan, E,E., Ezor, S.N. (1995). Efficacy of methylphenidate for attention-deficit hyperactivity disorder in children with tic disorder. *Archives of General Psychiatry* 6: 444–55.

Hammad, T.A., Laughren,T., Racoosin, J. (2006) Suicidality in pediatric patients treated with antidepressant drugs. *Archives of General Psychiatry* 3: 332–9.

Himle, M.B., Woods, D.W., Piacentini, J., Walkup, J.T. (2006). Brief review of habit reversal training for Tourette syndrome. *Journal of Child Neurology* 8: 719–25.

Hirsch, G. (2006). ADHD medication and the FDA: an update and some background. Retrieved [2007] from http://www.aboutourkids.org/aboutour/articles/stimulants_fda.html.

Hollenbeck, P.J. (2001). Insight and hindsight into Tourette syndrome. *Advances in Neurology 85:* 363–7.

Leckman, J.F., Peterson, B.S., King, R.A., Scahill, L., Cohen, D.J. (2001). Phenomenology of tics and natural history of tic disorders. *Advances in Neurology* 85: 1–14.

Marras, C., Andrews, D., Sime, E., Lang, A.E. (2001). Botulinum toxin for simple motor tics: a randomized, double-blind, controlled clinical trial. *Neurology* 5: 605–10.

Mataix-Cols, D., Rauch, S.L., Manzo, P.A., Jenike, M.A., Baer, L. (1999). Use of factor-analyzed symptom dimensions to predict outcome with serotonin reuptake inhibitors and placebo in the treatment of obsessive-compulsive disorder *American Journal of Psychiatry* 9: 1409–16.

Mataix-Cols, D., Marks, I.M., Greist, J.H., Kobak, K.A., Baer, L. (2002). Obsessive-compulsive symptom dimensions as predictors of compliance with and response to behaviour therapy: results from a controlled trial. *Psychotherapy and Psychosomatics* 5: 255–62.

Mataix-Cols, D., Rosario-Campos, M.C., Leckman, J.F. (2005). A multidimensional model of obsessive-compulsive disorder. *American Journal of Psychiatry* 2: 228–38.

Miguel, E.C., do Rosario-Campos, M.C., Prado, H.S., do Valle, R., Rauch, S.L., Coffey, B.J., Baer, L., Savage, C.R., O'Sullivan, R.L., Jenike, M.A., Leckman, J.F. (2000). Sensory phenomena in obsessive-compulsive disorder and Tourette's disorder. *Journal of Clinical Psychiatry* 2: 150–6.

Mikkelsen, E.J., Detlor, J., Cohen, D.J. (1981). School avoidance and social phobia triggered by haloperidol in patients with Tourette's disorder. *American Journal of Psychiatry* 12: 1572–6.

Mink, J.W., Walkup, J., Frey, K.A., Como, P., Cath, D., Delong, M.R., Erenberg, G., Jankovic, J., Juncos, J., Leckman, J.F., Swerdlow, N., Visser-Vandewalle, V., Vitek, J.L., Tourette Syndrome Association, Inc. (2006). Patient selection and assessment recommendations for deep brain stimulation in Tourette syndrome. *Movement Disorders* 21: 1831–8.

Patterson, G.R., DeBaryshe, B.D., Ramsey, E. (1989). A developmental perspective on antisocial behavior. *The American Psychologist* 2: 329–35.

Pauls, D.L. (2003). An update on the genetics of Gilles de la Tourette syndrome. *Journal of Psychosomatic Research* 1: 7–12.

Pauls, D.L., Hurst, C.R., Kruger, S.D., Leckman, J.F., Kidd, K.K., Cohen, D.J. (1986a). Gilles de la Tourette's syndrome and attention deficit disorder with hyperactivity. Evidence against a genetic relationship. *Archives of General Psychiatry* 12: 1177–9.

Pauls, D.L., Towbin, K.E., Leckman, J.F., Zahner, G.E., Cohen, D.J. (1986b). Gilles de la Tourette's syndrome and obsessive-compulsive disorder. Evidence supporting a genetic relationship. *Archives of General Psychiatry* 12: 1180–2.

Pauls, D.L., Leckman, J.F., Cohen, D.J. (1993). Familial relationship between Gilles de la Tourette's syndrome, attention deficit disorder, learning disabilities, speech disorders, and stuttering. *Journal of the American Academy of Child and Adolescent Psychiatry* 5: 1044–50.

Pauls, D.L., Leckman, J.F., Cohen, D.J. (1994). Evidence against a genetic relationship between Tourette's syndrome and anxiety, depression, panic and phobic disorders. *British Journal of Psychiatry* 2: 215–21.

Pediatric OCD Treatment Study Team (2004). Cognitive-behavior therapy, sertraline, and their combination for children and adolescents with obsessive-compulsive disorder: the Pediatric OCD Treatment Study (POTS) randomized controlled trial. *Journal of the American Medical Association* 16: 1969–76.

Pigott, T.A., Seay, S.M. (1999). A review of the efficacy of selective serotonin reuptake inhibitors in obsessive-compulsive disorder. *Journal of Clinical Psychiatry* 2: 101–6.

Porta, M., Maggioni, G., Ottaviani, F., Schindler, A. (2004). Treatment of phonic tics in patients with Tourette's syndrome using botulinum toxin type A. *Neurological Sciences* 6: 420–3.

Robertson, M.M., Stern, J.S. (1998). Tic disorders: new developments in Tourette syndrome and related disorders. *Current Opinion in Neurology* 4: 373–80.

Sallee, F.R., Nesbitt, L., Jackson, C., Sine, L., Sethuraman, G. (1997). Relative efficacy of haloperidol and pimozide in children and adolescents with Tourette's disorder. *American Journal of Psychiatry* 8: 1057–62.

Sallee, F.R., Kurlan, R., Goetz, C.G., Singer, H., Scahill, L., Law, G., Dittman, V.M., Chappell, P.B. (2000). Ziprasidone treatment of children and adolescents with Tourette's syndrome: a pilot study. *Journal of the American Academy of Child and Adolescent Psychiatry* 3: 292–9.

Scahill, L., Chappell, P.B., Kim, Y.S., Schultz, R.T., Katsovich, L., Shepherd, E., Arnsten, A.F., Cohen, D.J., Leckman, J.F. (2001). A placebo-controlled study of guanfacine in the treatment of children with tic disorders and attention deficit hyperactivity disorder. *American Journal of Psychiatry* 7: 1067–74.

Scahill, L., Leckman, J.F., Schultz, R.T., Katsovich, L., Peterson, B.S. (2003). A placebo-controlled trial of risperidone in Tourette syndrome. *Neurology* 7: 1130–5.

Scahill, L., Erenberg, G., Berlin, C.M. Jr., Budman, C., Coffey, B.J., Jankovic, J., Kiessling, L., King, R.A., Kurlan, R., Lang, A., Mink, J., Murphy, T., Zinner, S., Walkup, J. (2006a). Contemporary assessment and pharmacotherapy of Tourette syndrome. *NeuroRx* 2: 192–206.

Scahill, L., Sukhodolsky, D.G., Bearss, K., Findley, D., Hamrin, V., Carroll, D.H., Rains, A.L. (2006b). Randomized trial of parent management training in children with tic disorders and disruptive behavior. *Journal of Child Neurology* 21: 650–6.

Scahill, L., Sukhodolsky, D.G., Williams, S.K., Leckman, J.F. (2005). Public health significance of tic disorders in children and adolescents. *Advances in Neurology* 96: 240–8.

Shapiro, A.K., Shapiro, E., Eisenkraft, G.J. (1983a). Treatment of Gilles de la Tourette's syndrome with clonidine and neuroleptics. *Archives of General Psychiatry* 11: 1235–40.

Shapiro, A.K., Shapiro, E., Eisenkraft, G.J. (1983b). Treatment of Gilles de la Tourette syndrome with pimozide. *American Journal of Psychiatry* 9: 1183–6.

Silay, Y.S., Jankovic, J. (2005). Emerging drugs in Tourette syndrome. *Expert Opinion On Emerging Drugs* 2: 365–80

Swanson, J.M., Kraemer, H.C., Hinshaw, S.P., Arnold, L.E., Conners, C.K., Abikoff, H.B., Clevenger, W., Davies, M., Elliott, G.R., Greenhill, L.L., Hechtman, L., Hoza, B., Jensen, P.S., March, J.S., Newcorn, J.H., Owens, E.B., Pelham, W.E., Schiller, E., Severe, J.B., Simpson, S., Vitiello, B., Wells, K., Wigal, T., Wu, M. (2001). Clinical relevance of the primary findings of the MTA: success rates based on severity of ADHD and ODD symptoms at the end of treatment. *Journal of the American Academy of Child and Adolescent Psychiatry* 2: 168–79.

Temel, Y., Visser-Vandewalle, V. (2004). Surgery in Tourette syndrome. *Movement Disorders* 1: 3–14.

Tourette's Syndrome Study Group. (2002). Treatment of ADHD in children with tics: a randomized controlled trial. *Neurology;* 4: 527–36.

14

Brain Tumors, Systemic Lupus Erythematosus, HIV/AIDS, and Wilson's Disease

CONSTANTINE G. LYKETSOS

This chapter deals with four diseases affecting the central nervous system (CNS) for which neurologists are primarily involved as consultants. It follows the same approach as the chapters that focus on single diseases but does so more briefly.

Brain Tumors

Brain tumors are estimated to have an incidence of 12/100,000 per year (Scharre, 2000). The incidence is highest in old age, peaking between 60 and 80 years of age. Almost 50% of intracranial tumors are gliomas, 10% to 15% are meningiomas, 5% to 7% are pituitary adenomas, and 5% to 6% are metastatic tumors. Brain tumors produce signs and symptoms in a variety of ways, including direct invasion, compression, hemorrhage, and edema. Motor, sensory, visual, and gait disturbances are frequent manifestations of brain tumors. In addition, headache and focal or generalized seizures are quite common.

Psychiatric Manifestations and Differential Diagnosis

The psychiatric manifestations of brain tumors reflect their location; the type of brain damage they produce; patients' reactions to their symptoms or diagnosis; and the effects of treatments such as steroids, chemotherapy, and radiation. Tumors in specific brain regions have been linked to specific psychiatric manifestations (Table 14–1). Frontal lobe tumors are most closely associated with behavioral changes, sometimes referred to as the *frontal lobe syndrome* or *executive dysfunction syndrome*. Temporal lobe tumors are most closely associated with personality change, irritability, and hallucinations (especially auditory), as well as with a variety of language disorders. Patients with lan-

Table 14.1. Brain Tumor Location and Associated Psychiatric Symptoms

Location of Tumor	Associated Psychiatric Symptoms
Frontal lobes	Apathy, disinhibition, impulsivity, or socially inappropriate behavior
Temporal lobes	Personality change, irritability, hallucinations (especially auditory), language disorders
Parietal lobes	Apraxia, neglect syndromes, unformed visual hallucinations (eg, streaks or flashes of light)

guage disorders associated with temporal lobe tumors can experience catastrophic reactions when their deficits interfere with communication. Parietal lobe tumors typically are associated with cognitive deficits such as apraxia, neglect syndromes of the contralateral body or space, and unformed visual hallucinations such as streaks or flashes of light.

When evaluating brain tumor patients with psychiatric symptoms and signs, careful evaluation and differential diagnosis are critical. In hospitalized and seriously ill patients, it is especially important to rule out delirium, particularly when the psychiatric phenomena are intermittent and vary in intensity. Serial observations and repeated mental status examinations are the basis for the diagnosis of delirium, but an electroencephalogram (EEG) is also helpful, because in most cases of delirium it reveals generalized slowing involving brain areas far from the location of the brain tumor.

Once delirium has been ruled out, the specific nature of the psychiatric disturbance must be carefully assessed. Many patients with brain tumors develop dementia. Their dementia syndromes are usually different from those associated with Alzheimer's disease and therefore are sometimes referred to as atypical dementia syndromes. For example, instead of having the classical "4As" of Alzheimer's disease—amnesia, agnosia, aphasia, and apraxia—patients with dementia from brain tumors may have forgetfulness (dysmnesia) with inattention and apraxia, or apraxia and aphasia but relatively preserved memory.

As many as a third of patients with brain tumors develop a major depression in the first few months after diagnosis (Wellisch et al., 2002). This depressive syndrome must be distinguished from dementia because it has a different prognosis and frequently responds to treatment. Major depression in patients with brain tumors usually takes its typical form with sadness, loss of interest, anhedonia, and disturbances in sleep and appetite. Major depression due to the tumor itself must be distinguished from depression due to corticosteroids used to treat the tumor. To resolve this, it helps if corticosteroid doses can be decreased. If the depression abates when the corticosteroids are reduced or discontinued, there is no need to prescribe an antidepressant. If corticosteroids must be continued, an antidepressant trial may be indicated, although it increases the risk of delirium. Corticosteroids can produce euphoria, anxiety, and depersonalization, in addition to delirium and depression.

Seizures are common in patients with brain tumors, affecting 30% to 40% in the first few months after diagnosis (Scharre, 2000), and these conditions frequently complicate the psychiatric differential diagnosis. The physician must be careful not to mistake psychologic manifestations of partial seizures for other psychiatric symptoms.

Given that the prognosis for many brain tumors is poor, the physician must also be careful to differentiate major depression from demoralization. Demoralized patients have sad moods and may have disturbed sleep and appetite, but they generally do not display impairments in self-attitude, with guilty or self-deprecating ideas, or suicidal ideation. If they are hopeless about recovering from a terminal illness, that is realistic; if they are hopeless about not being able to do anything for themselves or their family in the time remaining to them, that may not be realistic and may indicate a major depression. When the distinction between demoralization and major depression is difficult to make, a psychiatric consultation should be requested.

Treatment

If the psychiatric disturbances in a patient with a brain tumor are due to delirium, a careful search for all its causes should be undertaken, and appropriate treatment should be implemented. In patients with brain tumors, it important to address *all* treatable causes of delirium, including fever, infection, metabolic abnormalities and medications (eg, opioids, corticosteroids, anticholinergics, certain antiemetics). Careful attention should be given to maintaining the sleep–wake cycle of patients with delirium. Interactions with family members and other visitors should be encouraged as appropriate as a means of maintaining orientation and activity. When the delirium is complicated by delusions, hallucinations, or severe agitation, neuroleptic treatment is appropriate. High-potency conventional neuroleptics, such as haloperidol (starting dose of 1–5 mg per day), or atypical neuroleptics, such as risperidone (starting dose of 0.5–2 mg per day), should be considered as first-line agents and used as described later in this book. Benzodiazepines should generally not to be used in delirium, unless neuroleptics are contraindicated (eg, if the patient has a history of neuroleptic malignant syndrome).

For patients with brain tumors and dementia, there are no proven pharmacologic therapies. Treatment consists of supportive care targeted at helping patients adjust to their cognitive deficits and teaching caregivers how to help patients manage in every day life.

Patients with severe demoralization often benefit from psychotherapy to help them adjust to their diagnosis, especially if their condition is terminal. In the presence of major depression, antidepressant medication is indicated and can be quite effective, despite a grim prognosis. Given that patients with brain tumors are often frail and on multiple medications, the selective serotonin reuptake inhibitor (SSRI) antidepressants, such as sertraline (starting dose of 25–50 mg per day) and citalopram (starting dose of 10–20 mg per day), are preferred as first-line agents because of their generally benign side-effect profile.

Physicians should seek psychiatric consultation when a patient with a brain tumor has psychiatric signs and symptoms and the diagnosis is not clear or the psychiatric disturbance does not respond quickly to treatment. In general, it is a good idea to consult with psychiatrists when treating delirium in such a patient. Similarly, psychiatric referral for the treatment of dementia is a good idea, for this can make a difference in helping patients and caregivers adjust to the patient's cognitive deficits. A nonpsychiatric physician often initiates antidepressant medications for major depression, but if the case is complicated or if the response to initial therapy is not successful, psychiatric consultation should be requested.

Systemic Lupus Erythematosus

Systemic lupus erythematosus (SLE) is a multisystem immunologic disorder that affects the brain in a variety of ways. It has an incidence of 5/100,000 per year and a prevalence of 45/100,000 per year (Scharre, 2000). Women are affected twice as often as men. SLE is associated with a variety of systemic manifestations, including fever, rash, adenopathy, joint pain, heart disease, renal disease, alopecia, and hypertension. The main pathologic feature of the condition is a small vessel vasculopathy with fibrinoid degeneration of the walls of blood vessels, resulting in microinfarcts and microhemorrhages. SLE has been associated with of variety of neurologic manifestations, both central and peripheral. The most common CNS manifestations include headache, strokes, seizures, myelitis, and parkinsonism. The mechanisms underlying CNS involvement are poorly understood but are believed to be multiple and to include the effects of autoantibodies, microangiopathy, and centrally produced inflammatory cytokines.

Psychiatric Manifestations and Differential Diagnosis

The most common psychiatric disorders seen in patients with SLE, affecting about 75% of patients (Hermosillo-Romo and Brey, 2002), include delirium, dementia and milder cognitive disorders, mood disorders, and schizophrenia-like psychoses (with thought disorder, delusions, and hallucinations). Delirium is generally uncommon and is most likely to occur with lupus cerebritis, from organ failure, or from corticosteroid medication. Cognitive dysfunction has been estimated to affect 70% to 75% of patients, with approximately 25% to 30% having a dementia syndrome (Hermosillo-Romo and Brey, 2002). The most prominent cognitive disturbances are slow mental processing, inefficient thinking, difficulty with attention and concentration, forgetfulness, impaired cognitive flexibility, and difficulty with abstraction. Cognitive impairment can be nonprogressive for long time periods, but it tends to wax and wane in relationship to fluctuations in the primary disease. Over time, however, most SLE patients who develop cognitive impairment eventually have a slowly progressive decline leading to dementia. The cognitive impairment is typically not associated with impairments in level of consciousness, which generally makes its distinction from delirium straightforward.

SLE-associated cognitive impairments must be distinguished from mood disorders, which affect 60% to 70% of patients with lupus at some point in the course of their condition (Hermosillo-Romo and Brey, 2002). The most common mood disorder in SLE is major depression marked by sadness, anxiety, irritability, fatigue, insomnia, and anorexia. It is also associated with apathy and loss of interest in usual activities, which can make distinction from dementia more difficult. Although anxiety symptoms are common in SLE, isolated anxiety disorders in the absence of major depression are quite rare. Occasionally, patients with SLE develop euphoria or a mixed bipolar state with features of depression and mania at the same time. Finally, some patients with SLE develop prominent apathy without anxious or sad features, which can be very distressing to them and their caregivers.

Although some patients with lupus and major depression have typical depressive delusions, 5% to 10% of patients with SLE have isolated delusions and/or hallucinations without prominent mood symptoms. These isolated psychotic disturbances can resemble schizophrenia and occur both in association with lupus cerebritis, with corticosteroid use, and without an obvious medication precipitant or cause. When psychotic phenomena occur, it can be difficult to determine their cause, especially whether they have been caused by an exacerbation of SLE or by corticosteroid treatment. In all cases of psychiatric disturbances, laboratory markers for disease activity can be helpful in resolving the differential diagnosis.

Treatment

The treatment of the psychiatric aspects of SLE depends on their nature of these conditions. It is important to rule out delirium, especially in hospitalized and sicker patients. If delirium is present, it should be treated as discussed above for patients with brain tumors. Cognitive dysfunction and dementia are not responsive to cholinesterase inhibitors, and these agents are best avoided. The management of cognitive dysfunction consist of addressing the underlying disease to stop or delay its overall progression. Patients with cognitive dysfunction, especially those with dementia, should be given psychiatric referral to help them and their caregivers develop proper compensatory mechanisms to their impairments.

For some patients with apathy but without depression or anxiety, low doses of psychostimulants have been useful to increase motivation, energy, or interest. For example, methylphenidate up to 60 mg per day may be tried if tolerated. If major depression is evident, potentially causative medications such as corticosteroids should be minimized or discontinued if possible. Psychotherapy, especially supportive psychotherapy, should be attempted if available and appropriate, However, most patients with SLE and depressive disorders require antidepressant medication. SSRI antidepressants are first-line agents (eg, sertraline, starting dose of 25–50 mg per day, or citalopram, starting dose 10–20 mg per day). Psychiatric referral should be pursued if the initial treatment is not successful or if the illness is complex. If mania is present and corticosteroids are being prescribed, it is a good idea to discontinue the corticosteroids if possible, even least temporarily. Treatment of a manic syndrome typically requires a mood stabilizer (lithium or one of the mood-stabilizing anticonvulsants such as divalproex), a conventional or atypical neuroleptic, or a mood stabilizer and a neuroleptic. When patients with major depression or mania have delusions or hallucinations, neuroleptic medication is almost always indicated. (See Chapters 17 and 18 for typical doses of neuroleptics and mood stabilizers, respectively.) Such patients, as well as those with schizophrenia-like psychoses, should be treated by a psychiatrist.

HIV/AIDS

Human immunodeficiency virus (HIV) infection is estimated to affect one million people in the United States and close to 45 million worldwide (Treisman et al., 2005). The HIV virus is acquired through sexual contact, through the use of injection drugs, through a pregnant mother transmitting the virus to her off-spring, and through blood transfusion. The last means of transmission is quite rare because systematic screening of the blood supply began in the mid-1980s. After transmission of the virus, most infected individuals experience a transient flu-like syndrome. Because the virus has a long asymptomatic phase after initial infection, a substantial number of infections remain undetected, even though with careful surveillance at present most cases are detected in early stages, allowing for early intervention. Once infection has set in, the vast majority of patients experience a steady decline in CD4 lymphocytes, one of the key immune systems cells. Eventually this immunocompromised state (acquired immunodeficiency syndrome [AIDS]) leads to opportunistic infections or to the development of certain cancers. Patients eventually become debilitated from repeated infections, and the disease becomes terminal. Modern therapy with combinations of antiretroviral agents and aggressive prophylaxis or treatment for the opportunistic infections has substantially extended the life of patients with HIV/AIDS. Nevertheless, this remains a terminal illness for many individuals and a chronic disease for most.

Brain infection is known to be an early manifestation of HIV infection. The HIV virus is carried into the CNS through infected lymphocytes. In the CNS the virus causes neurotoxicity, probably mediated locally through activation of the immune system and the release of cytotoxic cytokines. Brain infection has been associated with other neurologic complications, including brain tumors and progressive multifocal leukoencephalopathy. Peripheral neurologic manifestations of HIV disease include painful neuropathy and generalized muscle atrophy.

Psychiatric Manifestations and Differential Diagnosis

The psychiatric manifestations of HIV infection are quite varied. Patients with certain psychiatric disorders, in particular injection drug use, schizophrenia, and bipolar disorder, are more likely to engage in behaviors associated with contracting the virus. Therefore, many patients have pre-existing psychiatric conditions that they bring with them to the infection. Additionally, in the United States most patients with the infection are poor and disadvantaged, both socially and educationally. In this context, chronic demoralization and chaotic lifestyles, as well as personality disorders, are quite prevalent. Finally, patients with HIV infection also develop psychiatric symptoms related to the brain infection. These include a mild "motor-cognitive" disorder and a characteristic subcortical HIV-associated dementia—both associated with varying degrees of forgetfulness, inattention, executive dysfunction, uncoordination, apathy, slowness, and nonspecific neurologic signs. These cognitive disorders are less common since the advent of highly active antiretroviral therapy (HAART), suggesting that effective antiviral treatment reduces the CNS effects of the virus.

More than 50% of HIV/AIDS patients develop depressive mood disorders, in particular major depression (Treisman et al., 2005). HIV-infected patients with major depression typically presents with sadness, anhedonia, fatigue, apathy, anorexia, and sleep disorders. It is at times difficult to decide whether the latter symptoms are part of the HIV/AIDS disease or part of a depression. In general, among patients whose HIV disease is not advanced or active, when depressed mood or anhedonia are present, fatigue and other constitutional symptoms are best considered to be part of a depression. Additionally, a condition referred to as "AIDS mania"—an atypical manic syndrome characterized by irritability rather than euphoria—has been associated with the later stages of HIV brain infection.

In the early stages of the HIV infection substance abuse, mood disorders (usually pre-existing) and personality disorders are the major psychiatric conditions encountered. Late in AIDS, delirium, dementia and mood disorders due to AIDS itself are quite common. It should be noted that in many cases, HIV/AIDS patients present with multiple psychiatric disorders (eg, substance use, personality disorders, mood disorders) all at the same time. This is in addition to the many complexities of the HIV disease itself, as well as to the frequent presence of social disadvantage, all of which make for very challenging care situations.

It is a good idea to involve psychiatrists early when HIV-infected patients, especially those with AIDS, present with psychiatric disorders for two reasons: (1) the complexities involved in the differential diagnosis and treatment, and (2) the frequent interaction between psychotropic medications and the HAART regimen. The physician confronted with a new HIV-infected patient who has mood symptoms should attempt to differentiate whether they are related to problems adjusting to the diagnosis; to the result of substance use or withdrawal—especially alcohol, cocaine, or heroin; to a preexisting psychiatric condition such as major depression; or to a secondary mood disorder brought about by brain infection or HIV/AIDS treatments (eg, zidovudine).

Treatment

Physicians should keep in mind that in many cities the Federal government provides funds through the Ryan White Comprehensive AIDS Resource Emergency (Care) Act for the treatment of HIV-infected patients. Because psychiatric disorders are included in that treatment, the physician should find out if there is a Ryan White–supported clinic in the area and refer patients with HIV infection requiring psychiatric care to such a clinic; in that setting, they can receive the full range of primary and specialized services they need.

Most HIV-infected patients with pre-existing psychiatric disorders, in particular schizophrenia and bipolar disorders, are already in psychiatric care. Physicians treating the HIV infection should work closely with the psychiatrists to ensure that the patients continue to receive the psychiatric care they need. For patients who have substance use disorders, the primary goal of treatment is to achieve abstinence, and a secondary goal is to reduce or eliminate harm associated with continued use. These objectives can be accomplished through inpatient or outpatient detoxification followed by short-term or long-term rehabilitation. The involvement of psychiatrists, social workers, or substance abuse counselors is necessary to help substance-using HIV-infected patients.

For patients with cognitive disorder—in particular dementia—the best approach is to ensure that their underlying viral disease is being properly treated by an infectious disease specialist. No specific dementia treatments are available. These patients also benefit from the institution of care interventions that help them and their caregivers adjust to their disabilities in cognition and functioning, and that provide support to the caregivers. These interventions have been discussed in Chapter 23 (with secondary references in Chapters 9 and 10) and typically involve psychiatric services. Hospitalized late-stage patients with delirium or dementia usually require psychiatric consultation and sometimes psychiatric hospitalization or nursing home placement.

For patients with major depression, antidepressant therapies can be very effective, despite the complexities of the patients and their situations. SSRIs such as citalopram (starting dose of 10–20 mg per day) or sertraline (starting dose of 25–50 mg per day) are the first-line agents because their side-effect profile is less of a problem than non-SSRI antidepressants, especially for patients with AIDS. For depressed patients who also manifest significant weight loss or chronic pain treatment, mirtazapine (starting dose of 7.5–15 mg per day), which stimulates appetite and helps with weight gain, or a tricyclic antidepressant,— which can be very effective for certain pain syndromes, should be considered (in that order). Patients with HIV infection and depressive disorders also may manifest prominent fatigue, apathy, or weight loss. Some reports (Treisman et al., 2005). suggest that these problems respond to psychostimulants, dehydroepiandrosterone (DHEA), or testosterone (for men) added to the antidepressants. Patients with persistent apathy, fatigue, or weight loss are best served by being seen in an HIV clinic that can help deal with all their problems at the same time.

For patients with AIDS mania, it is best to avoid lithium therapy because most such patients do not tolerate the drug very well. Instead, mood-stabilizing anticonvulsants, such as divalproex, or conventional and atypical neuroleptics are best used to treat the mood disorder. Here again treatment by a psychiatrist at an AIDS clinic is indicated. Hospitalized late-stage patients with AIDS mania require psychiatric consultation and sometimes psychiatric hospitalization.

Wilson's Disease

Wilson's disease (WD) is an autosomal recessive inherited inborn error of copper metabolism that results in copper deposition in the liver and brain due to a deficiency of the copper transport protein ceruloplasmin, an alpha-2 globulin. It occurs in approximately 1/15,000 individuals, and the gene frequency is approximately 1 in 90. WD most commonly presents in the second or third decades, although onset in the sixth or even seventh decades occurs rarely. The most common presentation is a subacute onset of extrapyramidal and cerebellar movement abnormalities such as dystonia, bulbar speech, and gait disorder, but "behavior change," school performance decline, and liver enzyme abnormalities can also be the first identified problems. In addition to the abnormalities in the neurologic examination described above, the Kayser-Fleischer ring, a deposition of copper around the edge of the cornea, can be detected by shining a light into the eye at an obtuse angle; however, it is best observed by slit lamp examination. Serum ceruloplasmin and total copper levels are low, and 24-hour urinary copper excretion is elevated. In the majority of cases of WD, brain magnetic resonance imaging (MRI) reveals basal ganglia lesions. Abnormal liver function tests are almost always present, and some cases are detected as a result of the evaluation of elevated liver enzymes of unknown etiology. Hepatic failure can result, and before treatments became available, hepatic encephalopathy (delirium) was a common occurrence.

Psychiatric Manifestations and Differential Diagnosis

Psychiatric symptoms are prominent in one-third of cases of WD. Cognitive impairments include executive dysfunction and inattention. Hallucinations and delusions, mood disorder, and dyssocial behavior are common. The combination of "unusual" dystonic movements; personality, comportment, and behavioral abnormalities associated with executive function impairments; and onset in adolescence and early adulthood can lead to a failure to recognize WD due to incorrect attribution of the symptoms to a primary psychiatric conditions.

Treatment

Copper chelating agents such as D-penicillamine are the primary mode of therapy of WD and can reverse many of the neurologic and hepatic symptoms. The cognitive and behavioral abnormalities can reverse gradually. The behavioral abnormalities associated with executive dysfunction may need to be addressed with behavioral reinforcement approaches. Symptomatic treatment of the delusions and mood symptoms with appropriate medications is often necessary, but caution must be exercised; liver failure is almost always present, and kidney function can also be impaired.

References

Hermosillo-Romo, D., Brey, R.L. (2002). Diagnosis and management of patients with neuropsychiatric systemic lupus erythematosus (NPSLE). *Best Practice and Research in Clinical Rheumatology* 16: 229–44.

Scharre, D.W. (2000). Neoplastic, demyelinating, infectious, and inflammatory brain disorders. In C.E. Coffey and J.L. Cummings (Eds.), *Textbook of Geriatric Neuropsychiatry* Washington, DC: American Psychiatric Press. pp. 669–97.

Treisman, G.J., Angelino, A.F., Hutton, H.E., Hsu, J., Lyketsos, C.G. (2005). Neuropsychiatric aspects of HIV infection and AIDS. In B.J. Sadock and V.A. Sadock (Eds.), *Comprehensive Textbook of Psychiatry* (8th ed.). Philadelphia, PA: Lippincott Williams & Wilkins. pp. 426–51.

Wellisch, D.K., Kaleita, T.A., Freeman, D., Cloughesy, T., Goldman, J. (2002). Predicting major depression in brain tumor patients. *Psychooncology* 11: 230–8.

PART III

PSYCHIATRIC TREATMENTS

15

Antidepressants

JOHN R. LIPSEY

Antidepressant drug therapy is the cornerstone of treatment for major depression and is usually successful (Rosenbaum et al., 2005). Fifty percent of patients respond to the first antidepressant used, and 75% respond to one of the first three agents chosen if these agents represent different antidepressant classes. Insufficient dosage and duration of therapy are the most common causes of treatment failure. The required duration for a full therapeutic trial of any antidepressant is 6 to 8 weeks, but some patients require 10 to 12 weeks to achieve maximum benefit.

Every patient being treated pharmacologically for depression should be educated about the course of recovery. Even if an antidepressant is ultimately successful, improvement in the first week or two may be minimal and involve primarily improved sleep or diminished anxiety. When more substantial improvements begin later, they may vary greatly on a day-to-day basis, and patients should be forewarned that the early course of recovery may be punctuated by unexpected brief dips in mood. Patients may also find that their energy, appetite, activity level, and social engagement improve before they notice a positive change in their moods. Thus, they look much improved to their friends and families before they feel better. Eventually, however, the full range of depressive symptoms resolves, and this improvement is sustained.

During the course of antidepressant treatment, all patients must be asked about new or recurrent suicidal ideas, and their families should be told to report any evidence of self-harming actions or thoughts. Suicidal ideas, perhaps held in check by lack of energy to carry them out, may potentially develop into suicidal impulses or actions if a patient's energy improves while severely depressed mood or hopelessness persist.

Five classes of antidepressants will be described below: selective serotonin reuptake inhibitors (SSRIs), the serotonin-norepinephrine reuptake inhibitor (SNRI) venlafaxine, the alpha$_2$-adrenergic antagonist mirtazapine, the norepinephrine-dopamine reuptake inhibitor (NDRI) bupropion, and tricyclic antidepressants (TCAs). There is little evidence that any individual antidepressant (or antidepressant class) is generally superior to another, so the sequence of drug selection is determined primarily by tolerability and safety considerations.

Selective Serotonin Reuptake Inhibitors

The SSRIs are commonly used in the initial treatment of major depression. They have a potent and selective blocking effect on the reuptake of serotonin by central nervous system presynaptic nerve terminals. They have weak, if any, effects at noradrenergic, dopaminergic, histaminergic, and muscarinic cholinergic receptors, and they do not cause orthostatic hypotension or cardiac conduction abnormalities. Frequently used SSRIs include fluoxetine, sertraline, citalopram, and paroxetine.

Potential side effects include nausea, anorexia, more frequent or loose stools, anxiety, restlessness, sleep disturbance (insomnia or hypersomnia), apathy, diminished sexual drive, and orgasmic dysfunction. Sinus bradycardia is an uncommon side effect but is rarely symptomatic. Most of these adverse effects are mild or transient, and thus SSRIs are initially well tolerated by most patients. Eventually, however, up to 20% of patients discontinue treatment because of sexual dysfunction, and a smaller number discontinue use because of apathy, diminished energy, gastrointestinal side effects, or sleep disturbance.

No strong correlation between serum levels of SSRIs and treatment outcome has been demonstrated. Thus, routine monitoring of such levels is unnecessary.

Fluoxetine has a half-life of 3 days or more for the parent drug and a week or more for the active metabolite. Paroxetine, sertraline, and citalopram have half-lives of 21 hours, 26 hours, and 36 hours respectively.

Fluoxetine is generally begun at 10 mg PO every morning in the elderly, increasing to 20 mg PO every morning after a week if the drug is well tolerated. Younger patients can usually take 20 mg PO every morning from the outset of treatment. Most patients begin to respond to such doses within the first several weeks. An increase to 30 mg PO every morning for the elderly or 40 mg PO every morning in younger patients is indicated if there is no response by 6 weeks. Few patients require more than 40 mg per day. If improvement is attained but intolerable side effects develop, a return to a lower dosage often solves the problem without a relapse. The patient's clinical state and fluoxetine's long half-life may have led to dosage changes before plateau levels were reached, so dose reductions because of adverse effects may still keep the patient at an effective antidepressant level.

Sertraline is generally begun at 50 mg PO every morning and increased to 100 mg PO every morning after the first week. A subsequent increase to 150 mg PO every morning is made if there is no improvement by 4 weeks. The maximum dose is 200 mg per day.

Citalopram is begun at 10 mg PO every morning in the elderly and 20 mg PO every morning in younger patients. Doses may be increased to 40 mg daily over the next 3 to 4 weeks for patients who are not improving.

Paroxetine is begun at 10 mg PO QHS in elderly patients and 20 mg PO QHS in others. Dose increases are made to 20 or 30 mg PO QHS, respectively, if there is no response in the early weeks of treatment. The maximum dose is 40 mg PO QHS in elderly patients and 50 mg PO QHS in younger ones. Some patients find paroxetine sedating and tolerate it best when taken at bedtime. The relatively short half-life of paroxetine may lead to an uncomfortable withdrawal syndrome if the drug is stopped abruptly. Withdrawal symptoms may include dysphoria, anxiety, dizziness, and complaints of peripheral "electrical" sensations. When beginning patients on SSRIs, the potential for sexual dysfunction should be specifically discussed. Other side effects (eg nausea, sleep disturbance, anxiety) should also be discussed, but have far less potential to disrupt treatment. The potential for withdrawal symptoms should be discussed with patients taking paroxetine.

The SSRIs have a wide range of potential drug interactions because of their varying inhibitory effects on the cytochrome p450 system. Although many of these pharmacokinetic drug interactions are minor, some are dangerous, particularly when an SSRI significantly inhibits the metabolism of a drug with a narrow therapeutic margin.

Fluoxetine and paroxetine are strong inhibitors of cytochrome p450–2D6, whereas sertraline and citalopram are mild inhibitors of this isoenzyme. Cytochrome p450–2D6 metabolizes TCAs, and inhibition of this metabolism can lead to toxic TCA levels on low TCA doses. Cytochrome p450–2D6 is also important in the metabolism of certain beta-adrenergic blockers (propranolol, metoprolol, timolol, carvedilol) and antiarrhythmic agents (encainide, flecainide, propafenone, mexiletine). Prudence would dictate that all SSRIs be carefully prescribed to patients taking drugs metabolized by cytochrome p450–2D6, especially if such coprescribed drugs have a significant clinical toxicity with elevated serum levels. It should be noted that the prolonged half-life of fluoxetine may be associated with significant inhibition of cytochrome p450 isoenzymes for weeks following discontinuation of this drug.

The SSRIs may also inhibit cytochrome p450–3A4, but this inhibition appears to be only clinically significant for fluoxetine. Inhibition of this isoenzyme by fluoxetine and its metabolite may lead to elevated levels of coadministered alprazolam, triazolam, midazolam, diazepam, carbamazepine, quinidine, and calcium channel blockers.

The previously mentioned list of potential cytochrome p450–mediated SSRI drug interactions is by no means all-inclusive. Electronic data base drug interaction references, available now in all hospitals, are most useful for obtaining current information on drug-drug interactions.

Venlafaxine

The SNRI venlafaxine primarily blocks the reuptake of serotonin at low doses; at higher doses it blocks the reuptake of norepinephrine as well. Like the SSRIs, it has little anticholinergic or antihistaminergic effects, does not block peripheral vascular alpha receptors, and does not slow cardiac conduction.

Common side effects of venlafaxine include nausea, dizziness, sleep disturbance, and anxiety. The majority of these side effects are transient and mild. Patients may also develop the sorts of sexual dysfunction seen in patients treated with SSRIs. Five to seven percent of patients develop dose-related hypertension, which is usually mild to moderate. Thus, patients treated with venlafaxine should have their blood pressures monitored regularly.

Venlafaxine has relatively few significant drug interactions. Its short half-life (4 hours for the parent drug and 10 hours for the active metabolite) is associated with a withdrawal syndrome (similar to that described for paroxetine) if the drug is suddenly discontinued.

Sustained-release venlafaxine is taken once a day, at mealtime. Dosage begins at 37.5 mg PO daily for several days, then 75 mg PO daily, with a goal of 150 mg PO daily by 2 to 3 weeks. If there is no response to treatment by the fourth or fifth week, an increase up to 225 mg PO daily is indicated.

In addition to discussing common side effects and the potential for hypertension, all patients should be informed about uncomfortable withdrawal reactions if they suddenly discontinue the drug. Whenever possible, venlafaxine should be tapered over several weeks before it is stopped.

Mirtazapine

Mirtazapine blocks central alpha$_2$ receptors and thereby enhances noradrenergic and serotonergic neurotransmission. Although it does not block muscarinic cholinergic or peripheral alpha$_1$-adrenergic receptors, it does block histamine receptors. Sedation, appetite stimulation, weight gain, and dizziness are frequent side effects, but sedation is less common in the elderly. There are no significant cardiac adverse effects. Sexual dysfunction and nausea are less common than with SSRIs and SNRIs. Neutropenia has been rarely reported.

Mirtazapine is most effective at daily doses between 30 mg and 45 mg. The drug is usually taken at bedtime because of the sedative effects. An initial dose of 15 mg QHS is usually well tolerated, raising the dose to 30 mg QHS after a week. Lack of response by 3 or 4 weeks justifies increasing the dose to 45 mg QHS. In patients sensitive to side effects, dosage increases may be made in increments of 7.5 mg.

The weight gain associated with mirtazapine use may be helpful in anorexic elderly patients who may not develop problems with sedation.

Bupropion

Bupropion appears to inhibit the reuptake of both norepinephrine and dopamine and therefore is classified as an NDRI.

Sustained-release bupropion is begun at 150 mg PO every morning for 4days, and then increased to 150 mg BID, with at least
8 hours between doses. Lack of any response by 6 weeks indi-
cates a dosage increase to 200 mg PO BID (the maximum dose).
Occasional patients become overly stimulated or agitated
on bupropion, and insomnia or nausea may occur. In these instances, doses may have to be increased more slowly. For example, some patients may have to take 100 mg PO BID for a
week in order to tolerate an eventual dose increase to 150 mg
BID. For most patients, the drug is weight-neutral, and sexual
side effects are very uncommon.

Hypertension may rarely occur. The major significant adverse effect is seizures, which may develop in 0.4% of patients
taking the highest dosage of bupropion. To avoid excessively
high peak levels that increase seizure risk, no individual dose
of sustained-release bupropion should exceed 200 mg, and a
maximum dose of 200 mg PO BID should generally be observed.
Moreover, patients should be reminded to maintain at least 8-
hour intervals between doses.

Patients with anorexia nervosa or bulimia have a higher risk
of seizures on bupropion treatment. Patients with other medical
risks for lowered seizure threshold should generally be treated
with a different class of antidepressant. Bupropion is a moderate
inhibitor of cytochrome p450–2D6.

Tricyclic Antidepressants

The TCAs, which have been available for decades, block presynaptic reuptake of norepinephrine and serotonin in the brain.
They also cause, to a varying degree, orthostatic hypotension
(due to alpha$_1$-adrenergic blockade), anticholinergic effects
(secondary to antagonism of muscarinic receptors), sedation
(from antihistamine action), and slowed cardiac conduction (a

quinidine-like mechanism). They do not affect cardiac output in therapeutic doses but may be proarrhythmic in patients with ischemic heart disease (Nelson et al., 1999).

Despite their potential side effects, TCAs are not difficult to use if the best-tolerated agents are chosen and doses are increased gradually. Before the development of the newer antidepressants, TCAs were the treatment standard and successfully used—with appropriate precautions—even in the elderly and the medically frail. There is some evidence that TCAs may be more effective than newer antidepressants in the most severe major depressive episodes (Roose et al., 1994).

Nortriptyline is generally the best tolerated of the TCAs. It has low sedative potency, relatively mild anticholinergic effects, and causes less orthostatic hypotension than other TCAs. Another advantage is that it has a well-established "therapeutic window" of effective serum levels. These are reliably measured by many clinical laboratories and should be used to help guide treatment. A steady state serum nortriptyline level between 50 and 140 ng/ml, measured 12 hours after the last dose, optimizes therapeutic response (Asberg et al., 1971). Higher levels increase toxicity without enhancing antidepressant efficacy.

An electrocardiogram should be obtained before beginning nortriptyline to screen for conduction abnormalities that could be exacerbated by the drug's quinidine-like effect. The presence of such abnormalities or ischemic heart disease would favor the use of a different class of antidepressants (Nelson et al., 1999). Patients with a recent myocardial infarction, preexisting significant hypotension, bladder outlet obstruction, narrow angle glaucoma, or a tendency to become sedated should generally not be treated with nortriptyline. Falls from sedation and orthostatic hypotension are a potentially hazardous complication, especially in patients with concurrent neurologic disorders. However, careful monitoring of blood pressure and serum nortriptyline levels, and gradual dose escalation allow effective use of nortriptyline in many patients.

Elderly patients should begin nortriptyline at 10 mg PO QHS; if this is tolerated the first three nights, the dose is then increased to 25 mg PO QHS for 1 week. In patients middle-aged or younger, the initial does is 25 mg PO QHS for three nights, followed by 50 mg PO QHS for a week. Giving all of the medication at bedtime minimizes daytime sedation and often improves insomnia. The low doses in the first several days help detect patients who are extremely sensitive to sedative or hypotensive effects of the drug, which they may metabolize slowly.

After elderly patients have been taking 25 mg PO QHS for a week, and younger patients have been taking 50 mg PO QHS for the same period, a serum nortriptyline level should be drawn in the morning, 12 hours after the last dose. A goal level of 90–100 ng/ml is appropriate for most patients, if they can tolerate it, and doses are adjusted to attain it. Dosage changes are made in increments of 10–25 mg per week, depending on the last level, the age of the patient, and tolerance of side effects. Steady state levels are generally attained by seven days following a dosage change.

Although most patients require 50–100 mg of nortriptyline per day to attain therapeutic serum levels, the occasional patient needs as little as 10 mg per day or as much as 150 mg per day. The elderly usually have requirements lower in this range, but variability is great within all age groups. Serum levels should be obtained about a week after dosage changes to lessen the risk of unnecessary side effects. Repeat postural blood pressure measurements are also indicated with dosage changes.

The side effects of TCAs should be discussed with every patient before treatment is initiated. Patients should be told to contact their physician for severe sedation, palpitations, dizziness, severe constipation, or urinary hesitancy. They should also be advised to arise slowly from recumbent postures, at least initially, to reduce the risk of orthostatic hypotension.

Choosing an Antidepressant

All of the antidepressants discussed above are equally effective when used in general patient populations. Potential side effects, individual patient acceptance of those side effects, comorbid medical conditions, and concurrent medications should determine which agent to use initially. Individual patients may respond preferentially to one or two types of antidepressants, but this cannot be predicted by the clinician, so the sequence of drug trials is perforce a trial-and-error process (Rush et al., 2006).

Nortriptyline is generally not used early, given its greater potential for more severe side effects. An SSRI might be ideal for a patient with severe constipation but would be poorly accepted by a patient intolerant of any potential disruption of sexual function. Venlafaxine might be easier to give to patients on several other medications but would predictably lead to withdrawal symptoms in those prone to skip drug doses. Mirtazapine would be poorly tolerated by an obese patient with hypersomnia but might be ideal for a malnourished patient with difficulty falling asleep. Bupropion could provoke seizures in a patient intermittently abusing alcohol but might help activate a patient whose depression was accompanied by inactivity and diminished energy.

Patients who fail to respond to a full therapeutic trial of one class of antidepressants should be tapered from that medication and started on another drug class. Because the physician cannot predict which drug will work best, neither the physician nor the patient should become pessimistic if the first treatment efforts fail. Of course, the patient requires significant reassurance in this regard.

Transitions from one antidepressant to another must also take into account potential drug–drug interactions when residual levels of a discontinued or tapered medication may interact with the newly initiated agent. For instance, the transition from nortriptyline to an SSRI, or the reverse, may lead to elevated nortriptyline levels. If nortriptyline is tapered to zero over 5 or 6 days, and an SSRI is then slowly introduced, the potential for elevated nortriptyline levels is minimized. However, if nortriptyline is started and rapidly increased in dosage in close proximity to SSRI treatment, nortriptyline levels may become toxic. This is particularly likely to occur in transition from fluoxetine to nortriptyline, because fluoxetine may sustain significant serum levels for weeks after its discontinuation.

References

Asberg, M., Cronholm, B., Sjoqvist, F., Tuck, D. (1971). Relationship between plasma level and therapeutic effect of nortriptyline. *British Medical Journal* 3: 331–4.

Nelson, J.C., Kennedy, J.S., Pollock, B.G., Laghrissi-Thode, F., Narayan, M., Nobler, M.S., Robin, D.W., Gergel, I., McCafferty, J., Roose, S. (1999). Treatment of major depression with nortriptyline and paroxetine in patients with ischemic heart disease. *American Journal of Psychiatry* 156: 1024–8.

Roose, S.P., Glassman, A.H., Attia, E., Woodring, S. (1994). Comparative efficacy of selective serotonin reuptake inhibitors and tricyclics in the treatment of melancholia. *American Journal of Psychiatry* 151: 1735–9.

Rosenbaum, J.F., Arana, G.W., Hyman, S.E., Labbate, L.A., Fava, M. (2005). *Handbook of Psychiatric Drug Therapy* (5th ed.). Philadelphia, PA: Lippincott Williams & Wilkins. pp. 55–120.

Rush, A.J., Trivedi, M.H., Wisniewski, S.R., Stewart, J.W., Nierenberg, A.A., Thase, M.E., Ritz, L., Biggs, M.M., Warden, D., Luther, J.F., Shores-Wilson, K., Niederehe, G., Fava, M., STAR*D Study Team. (2006). Bupropion-SR, sertraline, or venlafaxine-XR after failure of SSRIs for depression. *New England Journal of Medicine* 354: 1231–42.

16

Stimulants and
Dopamine Augmenters

CHIADI U. ONYIKE

Stimulants are typically prescribed for their positive effects on mood, motivation, alertness, arousal, and energy. They are believed to exert their pharmacologic effects by increasing synaptic release of endogenous catecholamines (norepinephrine and dopamine) while simultaneously blocking catecholamine reuptake at the nerve terminals. The most commonly used "traditional" agents are methylphenidate and dextroamphetamine. Methylphenidate reaches peak blood levels in 1 to 3 hours and has an elimination half-life of 2 to 3 hours. Dextroamphetamine reaches peak levels in 2 to 4 hours and has an elimination half-life of 3 to 6 hours. Controlled-release formulations are available, allowing for dosing once daily. Dextroamphetamine is excreted primarily in the urine in unchanged form, whereas methylphenidate is excreted mainly as ritalinic acid.

The newer generation stimulant modafinil has been marketed in the United States since 1998. Initially used in the treatment of narcolepsy, it is now prescribed for a wider range of conditions because of its positive effects on wakefulness, vigilance, cognitive performance, and mood. Its pharmacologic effects are thought to result primarily from the stimulation of wakefulness-promoting orexinergic neurons in the anterior hypothalamus. Inhibition of norepinephrine reuptake in the ventrolateral preoptic nucleus and of dopamine reuptake (by binding to the transporter) may contribute to its action. Modafinil is administered orally, achieves peak plasma concentrations in 2 to 4 hours, and has an elimination half-life of 12 to 15 hours. It is 90% metabolized in the liver, and its metabolites are excreted in the urine.

The ergot alkaloids bromocriptine and pergolide are familiar to most neurologists in their use in the treatment of Parkinson's disease (PD) and migraine headache. These dopamine receptor agonists are also used in neuropsychiatry in the treatment of apathetic states in patients recovering from brain trauma, cerebral anoxia, and strokes.

Amantadine is another familiar agent used in the treatment of PD and drug-induced parkinsonism. In addition to other effects in the central nervous system (CNS), amantadine facilitates dopamine release and inhibits its reuptake. It thus has modest "stimulant-like" effects useful in the treatment of executive dysfunction syndromes, particularly in patients with dementia.

Bupropion is a dopamine and norepinephrine reuptake inhibitor. It usually is prescribed as a "nonsedating" antidepressant, but its potentiation of catecholamine neurotransmission results in modest stimulant-like clinical effects. Bupropion is more fully described in Chapter 15 on antidepressants.

Clinical Uses

Traditional stimulants have been used most frequently in the treatment of attention deficit hyperactivity disorder (ADHD), narcolepsy, and shift work sleep disorder. Modafinil has largely supplanted these agents in the latter two conditions, and it is also used in the treatment of daytime somnolence associated with obstructive sleep apnea. Generally behavioral interventions such as formal sleep regimens, dietary interventions, and exercise programs are effective for sleep disorders (other than narcolepsy), and many specialists have recommended that patients undergo a trial of these interventions before taking stimulants.

The conditions in which neurologists find traditional stimulants, modafinil, and dopamine augmenters most useful are listed in Table 16–1. Stimulants are not routinely used in the treatment for major depression. Some neuropsychiatrists still recommend bromocriptine and pergolide as alternatives to stimulants for the treatment of apathetic states, but prescription of these agents has become rare because of their limited effectiveness and their toxicity. On the other hand, there are

Table 16.1. Indications for Stimulants and Dopamine Augmenters

Condition	Context	Treatments
Attention deficit hyperactivity disorder	Poorly focused and/or sustained attention, impulsiveness and excessive motor activities in children and adults	Traditional stimulants, bupropion
Narcolepsy	Uncontrolled daytime sleep attacks	Traditional stimulants, modafinil
Obstructive sleep apnea	Daytime somnolence	Modafinil
Shift work sleep disorder, jet lag, and related conditions	"Inconvenient" sleepiness from sleep deprivation	Modafinil
Apathetic states	Mental dullness, apathy, and lack of initiative and vitality in patients who have suffered closed head injury, stroke, AIDS, and neurodegenerative diseases	Traditional stimulants, dopamine augmenters
Executive dysfunction syndromes	Apathy, slowness, disorganization, disinhibition, perseveration, and stimulus-bound behaviors observed in patients with brain injuries or neurodegeneration involving the frontal and subcortical structures	Traditional stimulants, amantadine, bupropion
Fatigue	Low energy and vitality in multiple sclerosis	Modafinil, traditional stimulants
Treatment-refractory major depression	Cases of major depression that have failed to respond to standard antidepressant therapy. Stimulants are prescribed for pharmacologic augmentation of an antidepressant regimen.	Traditional stimulants

indications that executive dysfunction syndromes, especially disinhibition, respond to treatment with amantadine (Kraus and Maki, 1997; Drayton et al., 2004).

The neuropsychiatry team at Johns Hopkins University has successfully treated some cases with bupropion. Bupropion has also proved useful in the treatment of apathetic states and ADHD.

Administration

At the beginning of therapy, traditional stimulants should be prescribed at low dosage, especially in the elderly, with the expectation of increases at 5- to 7-day intervals until an effective dose is reached. Dosage titration ensures that adverse effects are minimized and facilitates identification of the optimal dose for the patient. The range of effective doses for the traditional stimulants is wide, with some patients requiring a four-fold increase over the starting dose to achieve a clinical response.

Table 16–2 provides a dosing schedule for the more commonly prescribed stimulants. Most stimulants require twice-daily dosing, although some long-acting formulations are available. To avoid insomnia, patients should always take the medication in the morning, and if twice-daily dosing is necessary, they should take the second dose early in the afternoon.

Amantadine for apathy, disinhibition and distractibility (features of the executive dysfunction syndromes) is usually started at 50 mg twice daily and slowly increased as needed to a maximum of 400 mg daily in divided doses. Low initial doses are used to watch for intolerance (eg, hallucinations). Bupropion use in such patients is similar to its use to treat depression. The daily therapeutic doses range is 0.75 to 3 mg for pergolide and 2.5 to 40 mg for bromocriptine.

Table 16.2.   Stimulant Dosing Schedules

Medication	Starting Daily Dose (mg)	Usual Daily Dosage (mg)	Frequency of Dosing (mg)	Maximum Daily Dosage (mg)
Dextroamphetamine (Dexedrine)[a]	2.5–5	10–40	Twice daily	40–60
Amphetamine/ dextroamphetamine (Adderall)[a]	5–10	5–60	Twice daily	60
Methylphenidate (Concerta, Ritalin)[a]	5–10	20–40	Twice daily	60–80
Modafinil (Provigil)	100	200	Once daily	400

[a]Sustained release formulations allow for once-daily dosing.

Adverse Effects

On account of their CNS and peripheral effects, traditional stimulants can elevate the blood pressure—particularly in individuals who already have hypertension. In patients with pre-existing cardiovascular disease, high doses may precipitate cardiac arrhythmias and angina.

At clinically appropriate doses, the traditional stimulants are usually well tolerated, but they may produce dyspepsia, anorexia, insomnia, dry mouth, headache, tics, restlessness, and palpitations. Confusion, delirium, and agitation have been reported but are unusual—particularly with cautious dose titration. Tiredness, somnolence, and depression may follow stimulant discontinuation in patients taking high doses, and abrupt discontinuation of such doses may bring about a suicidal state in some patients. In yet other cases, tolerance to a dose develops, resulting in a "rebound" of the condition for which the stimulant has been prescribed. Adverse reactions of mild or moderate

Table 16.3. Management of Common Adverse Effects of Stimulants

---

1. For mild complaints, wait 1 week for tolerance to develop, or adjust dosages or dosing intervals.
2. Dyspepsia may be relieved by administering the drug before meals and anorexia by administration during or after meals. In some cases, a drug holiday or substitution with a different formulation may be necessary.
3. Insomnia can be managed by having the patient take the medicine earlier in the day, reducing the dose, or substituting a sustained-release formulation for a shorter-acting one.
4. If depression develops, first evaluate whether it has a relationship to the time course or dose of stimulant treatment. If the depression can be attributed to stimulant treatment, reduce the dose or switch to a sustained-release formulation. If the depression is not attributable to stimulant treatment, the options are to increase the dose, switch to a sustained-release formulation, or prescribe an antidepressant.
5. If delusions or hallucinations develop, reduce the dose or discontinue treatment and consider an alternative from a different pharmacologic class.

---

severity can often be ameliorated by adjusting the amount, timing or frequency of doses (Table 16–3).

Traditional stimulants promote euphoria and increased self-confidence. These behavioral effects have rapid onset of action and a high potential for tolerance from prolonged or repeated usage; thus, stimulants are subject to recreational use and abuse. When traditional stimulants are taken in very large doses, usually in the course of recreational abuse, extreme euphoria, anxiety and tension, severe dryness of the mouth, rapid and slurred speech, jitteriness, restlessness, and irritability may occur. On physical examination of these patients, dilated pupils, a fine tremor, tachycardia, and brisk reflexes are usually observed. Many stimulant-intoxicated patients develop hallucinations, acute confusion and paranoia, whereas others may suffer cardiac arrhythmias, myocardial infarction, or stroke. On the other hand, large doses or prolonged use are almost always followed by fatigue and depression. Traditional stimulants should not be given to patients who are taking monoamine oxidase inhibitors because their coadministration has been associated with deaths from fulminant hypertension and hyperthermia.

Modafinil is better tolerated than the traditional stimulants, although headache is not uncommon. It rarely causes dyspepsia or anorexia. Because it is not a CNS sympathomimetic and has limited peripheral sympathetic activity, it is much less likely to cause anxiety and tension, restlessness, tremor, hallucinosis, or paranoia; it is also much less likely to produce blood pressure increases, tachycardia, and arrhythmias. Modafinil has mood-brightening effects, but this effect is neither rapid nor dramatic. The development of tolerance has not been reported. Thus, modafinil has a considerably lower potential for abuse than do the traditional stimulants.

Up to 15% of patients prescribed bromocriptine or pergolide cannot tolerate these medicines at therapeutic doses. Nausea and vomiting are not uncommon, and profound hypotension may occur after the initial dose, especially if the patient is taking an antihypertensive or has orthostatic hypotension. In addition, adverse effects typical of ergot alkaloids such as pleuropulmonary (or retroperitoneal) fibrosis may also occur.

Amantadine is generally well tolerated with conservative starting doses and slow dose escalation. However nausea, vomiting, dry mouth, lightheadedness, dizziness, lethargy, and insomnia occur in 5% to 10% of cases. Tremulousness, gait disorder, confusion, irritability, agitation, hallucinations, and delirium are less common. Usually the adverse effects of amantadine appear within days of initiation of treatment (or dosage adjustment) and may resolve spontaneously within a few days—particularly if the dosage has been reduced or discontinued. Renal impairment significantly reduces excretion, an important consideration in the elderly or acutely ill. The adverse effects of bupropion are described in Chapter 15.

References

Drayton, S.J., Davies, K., Steinberg, M., Leroi, I., Rosenblatt, A., Lyketsos, C.G. (2004). Amantadine for executive dysfunction syndrome in patients with dementia. *Psychosomatics* 45: 205–9.

Kraus, M.F., Maki, P.M. (1997). Effect of amantadine hydrochloride on symptoms of frontal lobe dysfunction in brain injury: case studies and review. *Journal of Neuropsychiatry and Clinical Neurosciences* 9: 222–30.

17

Neuroleptics

DEIRDRE JOHNSTON

The "neuroleptic" antipsychotic group of pharmacologic agents was so named because the original agents, now called "conventional" antipsychotics, produced significant neurologic side effects in the form of extrapyramidal symptoms (EPS). However, neuroleptics were the first drugs to be effective in treating psychosis and remain the cornerstone of pharmacologic management of psychotic symptoms, whether such symptoms are primary or arise in the context of neurologic disorders.

Although the only U.S. Food and Drug Administration (FDA)–approved use of antipsychotic agents is for the treatment of schizophrenia, mania, and "psychosis," there is strong agreement among dementia experts that both the conventional antipsychotics and the newer "atypical" agents have a place in the management of several behavioral symptoms in persons with dementia (Small et al., 1997). Concerns have been raised regarding increased risk of stroke and increased mortality in the elderly, and a recent meta-analysis found the use of both conventional and atypical antipsychotics in dementia to be associated with a small increased risk for death compared with placebo (Schneider, Dagerman, and Insel, 2005). When choosing an antipsychotic medication, these and other risks should be considered within the context of an individual patient's medical need for the drug, medical comorbidity, and the efficacy and safety of alternatives.

In psychiatric disorders complicating neurologic diseases, antipsychotic drugs are used to treat specific syndromes (mania, delusional depression, schizophrenia) and target symptoms (hallucinations, delusions, tics in Tourette's syndrome, chorea in Huntington's disease). They are also used to ameliorate severe agitation or other behavioral problems that threaten the safety of the patient or others and have not responded to alternative interventions. These indications for antipsychotic drug use are further detailed in the chapters on specific neurologic diseases.

Antipsychotic medications should not be used for milder behavioral disturbances, such as the wandering, disinhibited social intrusiveness, or frustration-induced emotional lability seen in some patients with cognitive impairment. In these instances, nonpharmacologic methods such as environmental manipulation should be tried first. For example, gentle redirection of the patient, assistance with activities of daily living, a night light in the bedroom, structured schedules of activities, and caregiver education about such strategies may alleviate some problem behaviors. Furthermore, antipsychotic medications should not be used as general sedatives when a more specific treatment is indicated. Antidepressants, mood stabilizers, and anxiolytics are far more effective for depression, mania, and anxiety disorders, and these agents should be used as initial treatments for these disorders when they occur in the context of neurologic disease. Patients with pain and other physical discomforts (perhaps unknown to the physician and arising from conditions as simple as a urinary tract infection or fecal impaction) should have their medical problem treated first rather than being treated for their secondary distress.

Most importantly, delirium must always be considered in the differential diagnosis of any psychiatric disturbance and its etiology determined. Although antipsychotics may be symptomatically useful in delirium, the first order of business is to discover and treat the medical condition that has provoked the delirium.

In long-term care facilities, the use of all psychotropic medication, including antipsychotics, is governed by the "unnecessary drug" provision of Omnibus Budget Reconciliation Act of 1987 (OBRA). This requires that any psychotropic medications prescribed for nursing home residents be medically necessary, that the necessity be documented, that the response to the medications be monitored and documented, and that they be used for a limited amount of time with documentation of appropriate attempts to reduce them within specified intervals. The medications may be continued, with monitoring, if it is documented that attempts to reduce them resulted in deterioration of the patient. Consideration of the appropriate indications for antipsychotic drugs, described above, should make adherence to these regulations straightforward in the context of good clinical care.

Types of Antipsychotic Agents

Conventional antipsychotics, listed in order of increasing potency, include chlorpromazine, thioridazine, loxapine, perphenazine, trifluoperazine, thiothixene, fluphenazine, haloperidol, and pimozide. Higher potency drugs (eg, haloperidol and thiothixene) require lower doses to achieve antipsychotic efficacy, and they are more likely to cause EPS and less likely to cause sedation. Lower potency drugs (eg, chlorpromazine and thioridazine) cause more sedation, orthostatic hypotension, and anticholinergic effects, but induce less EPS. Long-term use of the conventional agents can lead to tardive dyskinesia (TD), which develops in at least 20% of patients on maintenance treatment with these drugs. Because of its potential for cardiac toxicity, thioridazine use is restricted to treatment-resistant schizophrenia (see note on Table 17–1).

The atypical antipsychotic drugs, widely in use since the 1990s, have supplanted conventional antipsychotics as the first-line treatment of psychotic disorders. These newer drugs include clozapine, risperidone, olanzapine, quetiapine, ziprasidone, and aripiprazole. With the exception of clozapine, they are better tolerated than conventional agents. In addition, they all have a lower burden of EPS (especially severe parkinsonism and acute dystonic reactions) and appear in limited longitudinal studies to induce less TD compared with the earlier antipsychotics.

Table 17.1. Efficacy and Side Effects of Conventional and Atypical Antipsychotic Agents

Property	Conventional High Potency (eg, Haloperidol Trifluoperazine Perphenazine Pimozide[a])	Conventional Medium Potency (eg, Loxapine)	Conventional Low Potency (eg, Chlorpromazine Thioridazine[b])	Ziprasidone	Risperidone	Quetiapine	Olanzapine	Aripiprazole	Clozapine
Efficacy	+++	+++	+++	+++	+++	++	+++	++	++++
ADVERSE EFFECTS									
Sedation	+	++	+++	+	+	++	++	+	+++
Anticholinergic	+	++	+++	0	0	0	+	0	+++
QT interval prolongation	0	0	++	+	0	0	0	0	0
Hypotension	+	++	+++	+	+++	++	++	+	+++
Hyperprolactinemia	++	++	++	+	++	0	+	0	0

(continued)

Table 17.1. (*continued*)

Property	Conventional High Potency (eg, Haloperidol Trifluoperazine Perphenazine Pimozide[a])	Conventional Medium Potency (eg, Loxapine)	Conventional Low Potency (eg, Chlorpromazine Thioridazine[b])	Ziprasidone	Risperidone	Quetiapine	Olanzapine	Aripiprazole	Clozapine
Type 2 diabetes mellitus	+	+	+	+	+	+	++	+	++
Sexual dysfunction	++	++	+++	+	++	+	++	+	++
Weight gain	+	+	++	0	+	++	+++	0	+++
EPS	++++	+++	++	+	++	0	+	+	0
NMS	+++	++	+	+	+	+	+	?	+
Dyslipidemia	+	+	++	+	+	++	+++	+	++

[a]Pimozide is an exception among the high-potency antipsychotics: it can cause QT prolongation.

[b]Thioridazine may cause hypotension, prolonged QT intervals, change T wave morphology, and induce prominent U waves, premature ventricular contractions, and ventricular arrhythmias, with related syncope, seizure, and even sudden death. It is comparable to quinidine in its antiarrhythmic and arrhythmogenic qualities. Thioridazine and other quinidine-like drugs may produce torsade de pointes.

Source: Adapted from Gardner, D.M., Baldessarini, R.J., Waraich, P. (2005). Modern antipsychotic drugs: a critical overview. *Canadian Medical Association Journal* 172: 1703–11.

Clozapine is used mainly for the treatment of refractory schizophrenia and requires close monitoring, particularly in elderly patients. Unless white blood cell (WBC) counts are regularly monitored, 1% to 2% of patients develop agranulocytosis, which may be fatal. The risk decreases once the patient has been on the drug for about 6 months. All patients on clozapine must be registered with the Clozaril Patient Monitoring Service. They require a WBC count and differential, including absolute neutrophil count, before treatment and weekly for the first 6 months and biweekly measurements thereafter. After a year, the frequency may be reduced to every 4 weeks if prior WBC counts and absolute neutrophil counts are acceptable. Hematologic monitoring must also continue for at least a month after drug discontinuation. All physicians prescribing clozapine must be familiar with its use and the detailed requirements for hematologic monitoring provided by its manufacturer.

The risk of agranulocytosis increases with age, and commencement of clozapine treatment in geriatric patients should be initiated cautiously. Clozapine is best avoided in patients with psychosis associated with neurologic conditions, because it is very sedating, causes substantial weight gain, provokes postural hypotension, and lowers the seizure threshold. However, clozapine appears to be highly effective for psychotic symptoms associated with longstanding L-dopa treatment of Parkinson's disease. In these cases, it is often beneficial in low doses and does not exacerbate EPS.

The other atypical antipsychotics (risperidone, olanzapine, quetiapine, ziprasidone, and aripiprazole) are fairly equivalent in efficacy. Risperidone is most likely to provoke EPS, olanzapine causes the most weight gain, quetiapine causes the least EPS but the most initial sedation, ziprasidone causes the most (but still modest) QT prolongation, and aripiprazole has the longest half-life.

Table 17.2. Clinical Equivalency and Dose Ranges of Antipsychotic Agents

Drug Name	Clinical Equivalency (mg)	Dose as Usual Range/day (mg) Geriatric	
		Geriatric	Adult
Olanzapine	5	2.5–15	10–20
Quetiapine	75	12.5–200	50–600
Risperidone	2	0.25–2.5	2–6
Ziprasidone	60	10–80	80–160
Aripiprazole	7.5	10–15	10–15
Chlorpromazine	100	25–200	50–800
Thioridazine	100	25–200	50–800
Perphenazine	8	2–12	16–48
Trifluoperazine	6	2–12	5–20
Haloperidol	2–6	0.5–6	2–64
Loxapine	15	2.5–20	5–100
Clozapine	50	50–100[a]	100–600[a]
Fluphenazine	2	6–12	6–20
Thiothixene	5	15–30	15–50
Pimozide	2	2–6	2–10

[a]Start at 12.5 mg daily.

Table 17–1 summarizes the efficacy and side effects of conventional and atypical antipsychotic agents.

Table 17–2 provides a guide to equivalent doses, and dose ranges, of commonly used conventional and atypical antipsychotic medications, as well as the geriatric dose ranges. In elderly or medically frail patients *the smallest possible dose* should be given as a starting dose.

Adverse Effects Monitoring

Because prolonged use of antipsychotics can lead to the development of TD, patients taking long-term antipsychotic regimens should be monitored regularly for the development of this movement disorder. Athetoid movements of the tongue, face, neck, limbs, and trunk occur; less frequently, there is involvement of diaphragmatic and swallowing function. Standardized assessments such as the Acquired Involuntary Movement Scale (AIMS) (Guy, 1976) may be helpful. There is no universally effective treatment for TD; the risk of developing it should be kept to a minimum by using (1) the lowest therapeutic dose of antipsychotic for the shortest possible time and (2) atypical agents in preference to conventional antipsychotics.

Neuroleptic malignant syndrome (NMS), a rare but potentially fatal side effect of all antipsychotic medications, is characterized by delirium, rigidity, fever, and autonomic instability. Fevers may surpass 41 C, and lead-pipe rigidity may lead to myonecrosis, myoglobinuria, and renal failure. Cardiac dysrhythmias and seizures may occur. Creatine kinase is usually markedly elevated, and elevations of the WBC count and hepatic transaminases may be found. Early recognition of NMS, discontinuation of neuroleptics, hydration, and meticulous supportive care, are the mainstays of initial treatment. Subsequent treatment generally requires an intensive care unit. Risk factors for NMS include dehydration, higher doses of neuroleptics, and rapid dose escalation (Hales and Yudofsky, 2003).

Metabolic Concerns and Recommendations

Recent evidence suggests that the atypical antipsychotic drugs (especially clozapine and olanzapine) are associated with an increased risk of metabolic syndrome in both adult and geriatric populations (Newcomer, 2005). Although as many as one-fourth of patients developing diabetes during treatment with atypical antipsychotics may not have other risk factors, in most, the risk of developing metabolic syndrome appears to be

Table 17.3.   ADA, APA, AACL, and NAASO Consensus Recommendations, 2004

Measurement	Baseline	4 weeks	8 weeks	12 weeks	Quarterly	Every 6 months	Yearly	Every 5 years
Weight	X	X	X	X	X			
Waist circumference	X						X	
Blood Pressure	X			X	X (if high risk)		X	
Fasting Plasma glucose	X			X	X (If high risk)		X	
Fasting lipid profile	X			X	X (if high risk)			X

Source: American Diabetes Association; American Psychiatric Association; American Association of Clinical Endocrinologists; North American Association for the Study of Obesity (2004). Consensus Development Conference on antipsychotic drugs and obesity and diabetes. *Diabetes Care 27*: 596–601.

associated with weight gain and other factors that contribute to weight gain. The American Diabetes Association (ADA), American Psychiatric Association (APA), the American Association of Clinical Endocrinologists (AACE), and the North American Association for the Study of Obesity (NAASO) recommend that before starting therapy, personal and family history should be evaluated for obesity, diabetes, dyslipidemia, hypertension, or cardiovascular disease. Then, the following monitoring protocol should be undertaken in patients being treated with atypical agents (Table 17–3).

Although these concerns for the metabolic syndrome have focused on the atypical agents, weight gain and diabetes have also been associated with conventional antipsychotics.

Use of Antipsychotics in Emergency Situations

Acute aggression associated with neurologic disorders at times requires intervention with intramuscular medications to avoid injury to the patient or others. In an elderly patient, 1 mg of haloperidol can be given as a "stat" dose, accompanied by 1 mg of lorazepam, orally or intramuscularly. In younger patients, depending on weight, 5 mg of haloperidol can be given, combined with 2 mg of lorazepam. Alternatively, if there are concerns about extrapyramidal side effects, and the QTc is normal, ziprasidone is available in injectable form and can be given intramuscularly, at a dose of 10 mg (geriatric) or 20 mg (adult). Once the patient is calmer, oral antipsychotics may be used if the need for treatment continues.

In agitation occurring in delirium (often associated with hallucinations or delusions), the higher potency antipsychotic agents, such as risperidone or haloperidol, are most effective, often in low doses (risperidone 0.25–1 mg BID; haloperidol 0.5–1 mg BID), titrating up from the lowest dose until the target symptoms are controlled. It is best not to exceed 4 mg of either medication in older patients. Once symptoms are controlled and the underlying cause of the delirium has resolved, attempts should be made to taper the neuroleptic.

References

American Diabetes Association; American Psychiatric Association; American Association of Clinical Endocrinologists; North American Association for the Study of Obesity (2004). Consensus Development Conference on antipsychotic drugs and obesity and diabetes. *Diabetes Care* 27: 596–601.

Guy, W. (1976). *ECDEU Assessment Manual for Psychopharmacology.* Washington, DC: US Department of Health, Education and Welfare. pp. 534–7.

Hales, R.E., Yudofsky, S.C. (2003). Antipsychotic drugs. In *Textbook of Clinical Psychiatry* (4th ed.). Washington, DC: American Psychiatric Publishing.

Newcomer, J.W. (2005). Second-generation (atypical) antipsychotics and metabolic effects: a comprehensive literature review. *CNS Drugs* 19 Suppl 1: 1–93.

Schneider, L.S., Dagerman, K.S., Insel, P. (2005). Risk of death with atypical antipsychotic drug treatment for dementia: meta-analysis of randomized placebo-controlled trials. *Journal of the American Medical Association* 294: 1963–5.

Small, G.W., Rabins, P.V., Barry, P.P., Buckholtz,, N.S., DeKosky, S.T., Ferris, S.H., Finkel, S.I., Gwyther, L.P., Khachaturian, Z.S., Lebowitz, B.D., McRae, T.D., Morris, J.C., Oakley, F., Schneider, L.S., Streim, J.E., Sunderland, T., Teri, L.A., Tune, L.E. (1997). Diagnosis and treatment of Alzheimer disease and related disorders. Consensus statement of the American Association for Geriatric Psychiatry, the Alzheimer's Association, and the American Geriatrics Society. *Journal of the American Medical Association* 278: 1363–71.

18

Mood Stabilizers

SUSAN W. LEHMANN

The term "mood stabilizers" refers to a heterogeneous group of medications that are effective in the treatment of bipolar disorder, an illness characterized by recurrent episodes of mania and major depression. The list of mood stabilizers includes lithium, several anticonvulsant medications, and atypical antipsychotic medications. For some of these medications, there have been randomized, placebo-controlled studies demonstrating efficacy in reducing the severity and frequency of illness episodes (Kahn et al., 2000). For other medications, the evidence supporting therapeutic use in mood disorders is more anecdotal or preliminary.

Late-onset bipolar disorder beginning after 50 years of age is more likely to be associated with comorbid medical or neurologic condition, or their treatments (McDonald, 2000; Depp and Jeste, 2004). A number of medications have been known to precipitate manic episodes. These include antiparkinsonian medications, corticosteroids, anticholinergic agents, and antidepressants. In addition, manic episodes may develop in patients with Huntington's disease, multiple sclerosis, brain tumors, seizure disorders, dementia, neurosyphilis, human immunodeficiency virus (HIV), and some poststroke syndromes.

The goal of long-term psychiatric management is to minimize affective upheaval and to diminish frequency of mood cycling. Psychotic symptoms are common in bipolar disorder, and severe behavioral disturbances such as physical aggression can occur as well during manic episodes. Depressive episodes are accompanied by a risk of suicide. Given the potential for these severe complications, and the need for continual medication reassessment and adjustment, the long-term pharmacologic and psychologic treatment of bipolar disorder is best managed by a psychiatrist.

Lithium

Lithium, the oldest of the mood-stabilizing medications, is also considered to be the "gold standard" of treatment against which all other potentially mood-stabilizing medications are compared. It is still the treatment of choice for many patients with bipolar disorder, and it has been approved by the U.S. Food and Drug Administration for treatment of manic episodes and for maintenance therapy. At least eight placebo-controlled, randomized trials have shown lithium to have efficacy in maintenance treatment of bipolar disorder (Goodwin, 2002). Lithium is effective in reducing risk of recurrent episodes of both mania and depression, although studies have suggested greater superiority in reducing risk of manic episodes.

For lithium to be effective, it must be both carefully monitored by a psychiatrist and taken reliably by the patient. Not only does it have a narrow therapeutic index, but adverse effects are often experienced at therapeutic serum levels. This is especially true for older patients, who may experience hand tremors or gastrointestinal distress at even subtherapeutic serum levels. These adverse effects may limit the patient's compliance with lithium therapy but may not necessarily be a cause for discontinuation of lithium, especially if it has been effective as a mood stabilizer. In such cases, the addition of a low dose beta-blocker such as propranolol may reduce tremors associated with lithium. Changing the preparation of lithium to a slow-release form may reduce nausea, and aiming for a serum level at the lower limits of therapeutic efficacy may help minimize loose stools.

For stable patients on maintenance treatment, serum lithium levels should be obtained (12 hours postdose) every 3 or 4 months. In addition, serum creatinine and thyroid-stimulating hormone levels should be followed every 6 months to monitor for renal dysfunction and lithium-induced hypothyroidism.

Laboratory testing is done much more frequently when lithium is initiated, when doses are adjusted, or if there has been a recent addition or deletion of a medication that affects lithium clearance by the kidney. Lithium use has been associated with sinoatrial node dysfunction, and this occasionally is a cause for discontinuation of treatment. Patients should have an electrocardiogram (EKG) before lithium is begun, and patients with sick sinus syndrome should not take lithium.

Because lithium is excreted exclusively by the kidney, it is exquisitely sensitive to changes in creatinine clearance. Patients with long histories of lithium treatment usually require lower lithium dosages with age as a consequence of physiologic decrements in glomerular filtration rates associated with normal aging. Lithium treatment sometimes leads to nephrogenic diabetes insipidus resulting in polyuria of greater than three liters per day. In such situations, lithium should be replaced with another mood-stabilizing agent. However, studies of patients with long-term lithium treatment indicate that for many people lithium continues to provide therapeutic benefit over decades of use and without significant adverse renal effects (Gitlin, 1999; Geddes et al., 2004).

Nonsteroidal anti-inflammatory drugs, thiazide diuretics, and angiotensin-converting enzyme inhibitors can cause elevated lithium levels. All patients taking lithium should be advised to not take it when dehydrated, and to discuss all new medications with their physicians. The therapeutic lithium level for acute episodes of mania is considered to be 0.8 to 1.2 mEq/l for young to middle age adults. For maintenance treatment, somewhat lower lithium levels of 0.6 to 0.8 mEq/l may be appropriate. In older patients (older than 60 years of age) therapeutic lithium levels are considered to be lower: about 0.6 to 0.8 mEq/l for acute episodes of illness and 0.4 to 0.6 mEq/l for maintenance treatment. Lithium toxicity is a frequent cause of change in mental status (ie, delirium), especially in older patients and in patients with medical comorbidity.

For many patients, lithium alone is either insufficient to maintain mood stability or cannot be tolerated due to its adverse effects. As a result, there has been considerable interest in finding alternative mood-stabilizing medications that may be used either in place of lithium or as an adjunct to lithium. Over the past 20 years, anticonvulsant medications have been increasingly used in the treatment of mood disorders, especially bipolar disorder, and have been found to have efficacy as mood stabilizers.

Carbamazepine

Carbamazepine was the first anti-epileptic drug studied as a treatment for bipolar disorder. Placebo-controlled studies have demonstrated its effectiveness in treating acute mania when used as a single mood-stabilizing agent (Weisler, Kalili, and Ketter, 2004). A number of open and controlled studies have suggested that it is less successful in treating the depressive phases of bipolar disorder. For some patients, however, combined therapy of carbamazepine and lithium provides good efficacy and mood stability. When used in the treatment of bipolar disorder, serum blood levels of 8.0 to 12.0 microg/ml are usually recommended. However, at dosages which produce therapeutic serum levels, carbamazepine may cause daytime sedation, nausea, mental confusion, and gait ataxia. Severe blood dyscrasias and hepatitis rarely occur. Sedation and gait ataxia may be particularly problematic for older patients.

As is the case for epileptic patients treated with carbamazepine, complete blood counts and liver function testing should be followed regularly, and more frequently early in treatment. An extended-release preparation of carbamazepine is now available as an U.S. Food and Drug Administration (FDA)–approved agent for bipolar disorder (Ginsberg, 2006).

Valproate

Studies of valproate have shown it to be superior to placebo for treatment of acute mania. Valproate is more effective in treating the manic phase of bipolar disorder than the depressed phase of the illness, and it has been approved by the FDA for the treatment of manic episodes associated with bipolar disorder (Weisler et al., 2006). In the elderly it has been found to be better tolerated than carbamazepine and has become the most common second-line mood-stabilizing agent, after lithium. It is also frequently prescribed in combination with lithium in patients for whom lithium alone is insufficient in maintaining mood stability. The recommended therapeutic plasma concentration for bipolar disorder is 50 μg/l–100 μg/l. Patients who are acutely manic may benefit from higher serum levels of up to 125 μg/l.

Adverse side effects are less commonly seen than with either lithium or carbamazepine but do include mild tremor and nausea. In addition, valproate may cause thrombocytopenia and sometimes causes hyperammonemic encephalopathy. Pharmaceutical labeling of valproate includes a "black box" warning for pancreatitis as well as for hepatotoxicity. Routine monitoring for stable patients on valproate should include drug serum level measurements every 3 to 4 months as well as liver function tests and complete blood counts.

Lamotrigine

Over the past 10 years there has been considerable interest in the use of lamotrigine as a mood-stabilizing agent for bipolar disorder. This interest developed out of observations in lamo-trigine trials for patients with epilepsy in which patients bene-fited from improved mood and sense of well-being that were separate from reductions in seizure frequency. Numerous stud-ies have indicated that it has antidepressant efficacy as well as delaying the time to occurrence of episodes of depression and mania (Gao and Calabrese, 2005). In 2003 the FDA approved lamotrigine for maintenance treatment in bipolar I disorder. Its efficacy as an acute treatment for mania has not been estab-lished. Although lamotrigine monotherapy may work well for some patients, others may benefit more from combined treat-ment with lithium.

The most significant adverse effect of lamotrigine is a rash, which may be benign or serious, and the package insert includes a "black box" warning about this risk. On rare occasions, the rash has taken the form of Stevens-Johnson syndrome. How-ever, in clinical trials of bipolar disorder, the incidence of these rashes was quite low at 0.08%. Nonetheless, because it is not possible to predict which rashes will become serious, the med-ication should be discontinued if any rash occurs. To minimize the risk of rash, it is recommended that the dosing schedule start at 25 mg/day for the first 2 weeks before slowly increasing the dose up to a final dose of 200 mg/day at 6 weeks.

It must be noted that valproate decreases the clearance of lamotrigine by about 50%. Thus, if lamotrigine is prescribed to a patient on valproate, the lamotrigine must be started at half the usual starting strength and increased more slowly to a final dose of 100 mg/day. On the other hand, lamotrigine is eliminated more rapidly in patients who are concurrently taking other anti-epileptic drugs such as carbamazepine, phenytoin, and primi-done. In these patients, the starting dosage strength of lamo-trigine should be 50 mg/day, and the dose should be gradually increased to a total of 300 to 400 mg/day by 6 or 7 weeks.

Other Anti-Epileptic Agents

A number of open-label studies have indicated that topiramate
(McIntyre et al., 2005) and gabapentin (Vieta et al., 2006) may
also have mood-stabilizing properties for patients with bipolar
disorder. Usually in these studies, topiramate and gabapentin
have been agents that have been added to other mood stabilizers. The results to date, however, are both preliminary and
inconsistent. At the present time, there is insufficient evidence
to support using either gabapentin or topiramate as mood-
stabilizing medication, and further controlled trials are needed
to establish whether these anticonvulsants will have a useful
role in the mood-stabilizer armamentarium.

Atypical Antipsychotic Medications

Psychiatrists have long used antipsychotic medications as adjunctive agents in the treatment of acute manic episodes. Antipsychotic medications are especially useful in the treatment of
severe agitation, hallucinations, and delusions associated with
mania. Over the past decade, atypical antipsychotic medications
have become preferred treatment choices over older neuroleptics because of their reduced tendency to induce extrapyramidal
side effects and tardive dyskinesia. Olanzapine, risperidone,
quetiapine, ziprasidone and aripriprazole have all been studied
as possible mood-stabilizing agents, and all appear effective in
the treatment of mania (Vieta and Goikolea, 2005; Ketter,
Nasrallah, and Fagiolini, 2006). Olanzapine is usually prescribed
as a once daily dose in the evenings, beginning at 2.5 to 5
mg/day and increasing up to 15 to 20 mg/day. The higher
dosages are usually needed for patients with agitation and/or
hallucinations or delusions in the context of mania. Common

adverse effects include sedation, weight gain, and orthostatic hypotension.

In placebo-controlled trials in which quetiapine has been used for treatment of mania, most patients were effectively treated with 400 to 800 mg/day in divided doses. However, slow titration of quetiapine is indicated (starting at 25 mg/day) to minimize potentially severe initial sedation and hypotension. Some older patients show improvement on low doses. Quetiapine is often a good choice for elderly patients with mania and Parkinson's disease because of its low incidence of extrapyramidal side effects.

Aripriprazole is usually begun at 10–15 mg/day in the treatment of mania with eventual escalation to 20–30 mg/day if needed. Plateau blood levels are reached slowly, because the drug has a half-life of 75 hours. Common adverse side effects of Aripriprazole include mild orthostatic hypotension and sedation, as well as occasional anxiety.

See Chapter 17 for further discussion of atypical antipsychotic medications and risks associated with them, including the risks of weight gain and diabetes.

Summary

Bipolar disorder is a complex disorder requiring close monitoring and on-going psychiatric treatment. Successful treatment often necessitates combined therapy with multiple mood-stabilizing agents. The importance of adjunctive psychotherapy cannot be underestimated; it assists patients and their families with coping with mood cycling and troublesome symptoms and ensures adherence with medications regimens. When bipolar disorder occurs in patients with comorbid neurologic disorders, it is important to establish an active partnership with a treating psychiatrist in the care of the patient. Patients who express suicidal thoughts or psychotic symptoms, or who are significantly impaired in their functioning should be referred for immediate psychiatric consultation and possible psychiatric hospitalization.

References

Depp, C.A., Jeste, D.V. (2004). Bipolar disorder in adults: a critical review. *Bipolar Disorders* 6: 343–67.

Gao, K., Calabrese, J.R. (2005). Newer treatment studies for bipolar depression. *Bipolar Disorders* 7: 13–23.

Geddes, J.R., Burgess, S., Hawton, K., Jamison, K., Goodwin, G.M. (2004). Long-term lithium therapy for bipolar disorder: systematic review and meta-analysis of randomized controlled trials. *American Journal of Psychiatry* 161: 217–22.

Ginsberg, L.D. (2006). Carbamazepine extended-release capsules in bipolar disorder: efficacy and safety in adult patients. *Annals of Clinical Psychiatry* 18: 9–14.

Gitlin, M. (1999). Lithium and the kidney: an updated review. *Drug Safety* 20: 231–43.

Goodwin, F.K. (2002). Rationale for long-term treatment of bipolar disorder and evidence for long-term lithium treatment. *Journal of Clinical Psychiatry* 63: 5–12.

Kahn, D.A., Sachs, G.S., Printz, D.J., Carpenter, D., Docherty, J.P., Ross, R. (2000). Medication treatment of bipolar disorder 2000: a summary of the expert consensus guidelines. *Journal of Psychiatric Practice* 6: 197–211.

Ketter, T.A., Nasrallah, H.A., Fagiolini, A. (2006). Mood stabilizers and atypical antipsychotics: bimodal treatments for bipolar disorder. *Psychopharmacology Bulletin* 39: 120–46.

McDonald, W.M. (2000). Epidemiology, etiology, and treatment of geriatric mania. *Journal of Clinical Psychiatry* 61: 3–11.

McIntyre, R.S., Riccardelli, R., Binder, C., Kusumake, V. (2005). Open-label adjunctive topiramate in the treatment of unstable bipolar disorder. *Canadian Journal of Psychiatry* 50: 415–22.

Vieta, E., Goikolea, J.M. (2005). Atypical antipsychotic: newer options for mania and maintenance therapy. *Bipolar Disorders* 7: 21–33.

Vieta, E., Manuel Goikolea, J., Martinez-Aran, A., Comes, M., Verger, K., Masramon, X., Sanchez-Moreno, J., Colom, F. (2006). A double-blind randomized, placebo-controlled, prophylaxis study of adjunctive gabapentin for bipolar disorder. *Journal of Clinical Psychiatry* 67: 473–7.

Weisler, R.H., Kalili, A.H., Ketter, T.A. (2004). A multi-center, randomized, double-blind, placebo-controlled trial of extended-release carbamazepine capsules as monotherapy for bipolar disorder patients with manic or mixed episodes. *Journal of Clinical Psychiatry* 65: 478–84.

Weisler, R.H., Cutler, A.J., Ballenger, J.C., Post, R.M., Ketter, T.A. (2006). The use of antiepileptic drugs in bipolar disorders: a review based on evidence from controlled trials. *CNS Spectrums* 11: 788–99.

19

Anxiolytics

DEIRDRE JOHNSTON

Anxiety disorders may occur as primary conditions (generalized anxiety, panic disorder); or may be associated with other psychiatric syndromes such as major depression or dementia. Benzodiazepines are the most widely prescribed anxiolytics. However, antidepressants such as selective serotonin reuptake inhibitors (SSRIs), serotonin-norepinephrine reuptake inhibitors (SNRIs), and tricyclic antidepressants (TCAs) also have potent anxiolytic properties; these agents are often safer and more effective in the long-term treatment of generalized anxiety and panic attacks. Buspirone is occasionally effective for relatively milder forms of generalized anxiety.

Neurologists evaluating anxious patients should have a high suspicion for the diagnosis of depression, because major depression can present with predominant anxiety symptoms, particularly in the elderly in whom agitation associated with depression may mimic severe anxiety (Schoevers et al., 2003). The neurologist may also encounter anxiety symptoms in patients with Alzheimer's disease, vascular dementia, or following stroke. General medical causes of anxiety symptoms should be included in the differential diagnosis before anxiolytic treatment is begun. Such medical etiologies include hyperthyroidism, respiratory distress, cardiac arrhythmias, hypoglycemia, and pheochromocytoma. Moreover, physical discomfort may provoke anxiety symptoms in cognitively impaired patients who cannot express their physical symptoms to caregivers.

Antidepressants as Anxiolytics

Generalized anxiety, especially if accompanied by depression, is best treated with antidepressant agents. Benzodiazepines may produce benefits in the short term, if distress is great, but the long-term use risks the induction of physiologic dependence.

The SSRIs sertraline and paroxetine, as well as the SNRI venlafaxine, are effective for generalized anxiety. Each drug should be started at low doses (sertraline 25 mg daily, paroxetine 10 mg QHS, extended-release venlafaxine 37.5 mg daily) and slowly increased as tolerated. Final doses are similar to those required for the treatment of major depression, and slow dose escalation minimizes early exacerbation of anxiety symptoms. See Chapter 15 for further description of these agents, including side effects.

TCAs are second-line agents for the treatment of generalized anxiety. Nortriptyline is the best tolerated TCA. It should be started at low doses (10 mg QHS) and slowly increased as tolerated. Final doses generally need to achieve serum levels similar to those required for the treatment of major depression. Details of nortriptyline use can be found in Chapter 15.

Panic disorder is also effectively treated by sertraline, paroxetine, extended-release venlafaxine, and nortriptyline. Initial doses, dose escalation, and maintenance doses are similar to those used in the treatment of generalized anxiety. Again, nortriptyline should be used only if prior interventions have failed, because the other drugs are generally safer and better tolerated. Serum nortriptyline levels must be monitored as the dose is increased.

For any antidepressant treatment of generalized anxiety or panic disorder, full therapeutic response may take 6 or more weeks. If antidepressants are discontinued because of ineffectiveness, they should usually be tapered to avoid discontinuation syndromes. This is especially the case for paroxetine and venlafaxine, which may provoke severe anxiety, restlessness, and paresthesias if stopped suddenly.

Benzodiazepines

Benzodiazepines have potent anxiolytic properties and are rapidly effective for severe anxiety. Many patients with panic attacks require initial benzodiazepine treatment while awaiting the development of anxiolytic effects from antidepressants. Lorazepam and oxazepam have no active metabolites and have mean elimination half-lives of 12 and 10 hours, respectively. Lorazepam, 0.5 mg TID (increasing if needed to 1 mg TID) is generally effective for panic symptoms. Oxazepam is usually effective at 10 to 15 mg TID. Individual patients may require higher doses. All patients should be warned about sedation, addiction potential, effects on driving, and the withdrawal that may occur with sudden discontinuation.

Benzodiazepines with very short half-lives (eg, alprazolam) should usually be avoided because of their elevated potential for abuse and their propensity to provoke withdrawal symptoms after sustained use. If any benzodiazepine is used long-term, rebound anxiety may occur when it is discontinued. In general, patients with panic disorder should have benzodiazepine use tapered slowly after 3 to 6 weeks. By that stage of treatment, the anxiolytic effect of antidepressant agents has usually been established. Tapering of benzodiazepines over several weeks is usually well-tolerated.

All benzodiazepines can cause anterograde amnesia, may exacerbate cognitive impairment in the elderly, and can contribute to falls by causing incoordination and muscular weakness. In older patients and in those with impaired hepatic function, benzodiazepines with very long half-lives and active metabolites (eg, diazepam and chlordiazepoxide) should be avoided because of the potential for excessive drug accumulation. On some occasions, however, longer acting benzodiazepines such as clonazepam (half-lives of 18–40 hours) are useful when tapering patients from benzodiazepines with short half-lives, in order to minimize fluctuations in drug levels that may exacerbate withdrawal symptoms.

When starting a benzodiazepine, patients should be counseled about the risks associated with their use, and this should be documented in the chart. Where possible, nonbenzodiazepine agents should be used to manage anxiety. Benzodiazepines are also best avoided in persons with a history of benzodiazepine, alcohol, or other substance abuse, unless there is a specific indication for management of withdrawal symptoms.

Buspirone

The azapirone buspirone, a partial 5-HT$_{1A}$ agonist, is at times effective in the treatment of mild to moderate generalized anxiety. Patients with more severe symptoms, panic disorder, or comorbid depression are best treated with antidepressants. For patients who might benefit from buspirone, the major advantages include minimal sedative effects and no potential for abuse or dependence.

Buspirone is begun at 5 mg TID and slowly increased up to 20 mg TID if necessary. This agent does not produce euphoria, and its anxiolytic effects may not be achieved for 6 weeks. Buspirone is not cross-reactive with benzodiazepines and thus cannot prevent withdrawal from those agents. Moreover, it has no anticonvulsant properties. Potential side effects of buspirone include lightheadedness, nausea, headache, restlessness, insomnia, and fatigue. However, the drug is generally well tolerated with slow dose escalation.

Use of Anxiolytics for Acute Sedation

In emergency situations where severe anxiety leads to agitation or endangerment to self or others, benzodiazepines are often rapidly effective. Lorazepam is well absorbed with intramuscular use, and 1–2 mg intramuscularly calms most patients effectively.

Elderly or medically frail patients should be given 1 mg initially and occasionally may respond to 0.5 mg intramuscularly.

Some anxious patients scheduled for noninvasive procedures (eg, magnetic resonance imaging) also cooperate better if their anxiety is alleviated. In these instances, 0.5 to 2.0 mg of lorazepam is effective and can usually be given orally, 45 minutes before the procedure.

Anxiolytics in Long-Term Care Facilities

As noted in Chapter 17, the use of all psychotropic drugs in long-term care facilities is governed by the "unnecessary drug" regulation of the Omnibus Budget Reconciliation Act of 1987 (OBRA). This regulation requires that any psychotropic drug prescribed in such settings be medically necessary, that the necessity be documented, that treatment response be monitored and documented, and that treatment not extend indefinitely without appropriate attempts to reduce the drug. Use of anxiolytics to manage relatively minor problem behaviors (eg, wandering) that could successfully be addressed by nonpharmacologic means clearly would not meet regulatory requirements.

Reference

Schoevers, R.A., Beekman, A.T.F., Deeg, D.J.H., Jonker, C., van Tilburg, W. (2003). Comorbidity and risk-patterns of depression, generalized anxiety disorder, and mixed anxiety-depression in late life: results from the AMSTEL study. *International Journal of Geriatric Psychiatry* 18: 944–1001.

20

Cholinesterase Inhibitors and Memantine

CONSTANTINE G. LYKETSOS

Several lines of evidence suggest that acetylcholine (ACh) neurotransmission is important to the normal functioning of memory, and loss of ACh-producing cells in the basal forebrain (nucleus basalis) is a consistent finding in patients with Alzheimer's disease and other dementias. The most successful approach to increasing ACh in vivo has been to develop drugs that reduce its degradation by the synaptic enzyme acetylcholinesterase (AChE). Four cholinesterase inhibitors are available to treat memory and other cognitive symptoms in dementia patients. They may also stabilize or prevent the onset of milder non-cognitive neuropsychiatric or behavioral symptoms, although their use as exclusive agents for the more severe forms of the latter is not recommended. A recent Consensus Panel has articulated sound clinical principles regarding the use of these drugs in the context of the broader treatment of Alzheimer's dementia (Lyketsos et al., 2006).

Tacrine, donepezil, rivastigmine, and galantamine have been approved by the U.S. Food and Drug Administration (FDA) for the treatment of Alzheimer's disease. Tacrine should not ordinarily be used in light of the associated high risk of hepatotoxicity, its complex titration, and the availability of better-tolerated alternatives. The other three cholinesterase inhibitors seem similar in efficacy. All appear to modestly improve cognitive symptoms in 15% to 20% of patients, sometimes quite notably. In addition, they may either improve patient function and delay the emergence of behavioral symptoms or reduce the severity of the latter. The evidence does not support their use as single agents to treat more severe neuropsychiatric symptoms such as depression or delusions, although patients with apathy and visual hallucinations may respond.

Any benefit of cholinesterase inhibitors to the long-term progression of dementia has not been shown conclusively. Some studies suggest that they may attenuate the long-term slope of cognitive or functional decline, but those studies have been flawed due to high levels of dropout and the use of historical untreated comparison groups. One brain imaging study, part of a clinical trial, has suggested that they may affect the size of the hippocampus or the integrity of hippocampal neurons. In the absence of replication or a better understanding of the imaging measures involved, these data are not conclusive. At present, the efficacy of cholinesterase inhibitors is limited and may not extend much past 1 or 2 years after starting treatment in most patients. Occasional patients, however, experience more sustained benefits that warrant continued treatment into more advanced dementia stages.

The mechanism of action of some cholinesterase medications has been shown in some cases to be broader than once believed. Rivastigmine is also an inhibitor of butyrylcholinesterase, which may be more important than AChE in the degradation of ACh in later dementia. Galantamine is also an allosteric modulator of the nicotinic ACh receptor. Although these additional mechanisms of action may play a role in the pharmacology of these agents, their clinical relevance not been demonstrated.

In addition to mild to moderate Alzheimer's disease cases, patients with Lewy body dementia likely benefit from cholinesterase inhibitors, as do patients with vascular dementia (many of whom also have Alzheimer's pathology). One of these medications, rivastigmine, is also approved by the FDA for the treatment of the dementia associated with Parkinson's disease ("DPD"). The use of these agents in more advanced dementia is less well supported by clinical trial data, but benefits of their use probably outweigh risks in patients with scores on the Mini-Mental State Examination (MMSE) in the 5 to 10 range who are not very frail and have never taken them before.

The practicalities of the use of cholinesterase inhibitors in dementia are largely a matter of opinion because research to answer day-to-day clinical questions about their use has not been carried out. The preferred approach involves sequential use of these agents with careful monitoring for benefit. Physicians should make an effort not to raise expectations when prescribing these agents; they should explain that it might become necessary to consider discontinuing the medication if there is no convincing evidence of a clinical response. In light of their comparability in efficacy for cognitive and functional symptoms, choices of agent is driven primarily by ease of use, dosing frequency, and side-effect profile.

Donepezil is the recommended first-line agent because is it used once a day, can be titrated to maximal dose after 30 days of treatment, and is generally well tolerated. Donepezil is begun at 5 mg QHS, increasing to 10 mg QHS a month later. Nausea, anorexia, diarrhea, muscle cramps, and insomnia may occur but are usually mild and transient. Donepezil seems to have the best side-effect profile from the point of view of gastrointestinal (GI) symptoms.

Galantamine, the recommended second-line agent, is also used once a day in the extended-release form but requires a 3- to 4-month titration to maximal effective dose. It is best started in the extended-release version at 8 mg daily (with food), and this dose is increased to 16 mg daily after one month, and then 24 mg daily after 2 months. Patients who tolerate it well can be increased to 32 mg daily if they fail to show clear benefit on lower doses. Nausea and vomiting are more common than with donepezil.

Rivastigmine is started at 1.5 mg BID and then increased by 1.5 mg per BID dose every 4 weeks until the effective dose of 6 mg BID is reached. In our experience, it is least well tolerated of the three agents, causing the most nausea, vomiting, and diarrhea. FDA approval came in 2007 for a "patch" delivery formulation of rivastigmine that appears to have fewer side effects.

The side effects of cholinesterase inhibitors reflect increased central and peripheral cholinergic activity. All cause increased gastric acid secretion. Nausea, vomiting, and diarrhea may occur, especially with rapid dose escalation. In more advanced dementia, the GI adverse effects often manifest as refusal to eat or weight loss to which clinicians must be alert. Less commonly cholinesterase inhibitors cause muscle cramps, bradycardia, or exacerbations of asthma. Two clinical trials, one with galantamine in patients with mild cognitive impairment, and the other with donepezil in vascular dementia, have suggested that small increases in mortality occur with cholinesterase inhibitor use. Other trials do not show such a concern, but active investigation is ongoing in this area.

Memantine

The putative action of memantine, approved for marketing in the United States for the treatment of moderate to severe Alzheimer's disease involves the glutamatergic system. Memantine exerts its effects at the glutamate N-methyl-D-aspartate (NMDA) receptor through uncompetitive blockade: the binding site is accessible only if the receptor is activated. Memantine blocks glutamate-activated ion currents—including calcium—through the NMDA receptor, an ion channel. Several clinical trials have reported that memantine slightly delays the progression of Alzheimer's dementia, with beneficial effects on cognition and activities of daily living. There is also evidence that memantine reduces caregiving time in more advanced dementia. Safety data are good, with the most common side effects being dizziness, headaches, and agitation in about 5% of patients. There is also clinical trials evidence to suggest that it can be administered safely with cholinesterase inhibitors, such as donepezil.

The starting dose of memantine is 5 mg in the morning; this is increased by 5 mg per week to a full dose of 10 mg BID after about a month if well tolerated. The titration is facilitated by a titration pack made available by the manufacturer through local pharmacists. Once memantine is started, and assuming it is well tolerated, clinicians often face the quandary of deciding whether or not it is helpful to a given patient. The clinical trials data suggest that about 15% of patients show improvement on memantine, with most of this improvement being above and beyond a placebo response. Eighty-five percent of patients do not improve but may show an attenuation of cognitive or functional decline. Physicians and other clinicians must be prepared for this quandary and must also prepare patients and families for it. The decision to continue or to stop memantine should be individualized and tailored to each patient's situation. A discontinuation trial is often a good idea to help decide if there is continued benefit from this treatment.

Reference

Lyketsos, C.G., Colenda, C., Beck, C., Blank, K., Doriaswamy, M., Kalunian, D., Yaffe, K. (2006). Position statement of the American Association for Geriatric Psychiatry regarding principles of care for patients with dementia due to Alzheimer's disease. *American Journal of Geriatric Psychiatry* 14: 561–72.

21

Electroconvulsive Therapy

JOHN R. LIPSEY

Electroconvulsive therapy (ECT) is a highly effective intervention for severe major depression (American Psychiatric Association Committee on Electroconvulsive Therapy, 2001). ECT is most often used because pharmacotherapy has failed. In certain clinical situations, however, ECT is the initial treatment of choice.

Ten to fifteen percent of patients with major depression fail to respond to antidepressants. Such outcomes may persist despite adequate treatment with multiple classes of antidepressant drugs (Rush et al., 2006) and other pharmacologic augmentation strategies (eg, the addition of lithium to an antidepressant). Eventually, social relationships and work performance decline as patients lose hope and other depressive symptoms worsen in intensity. ECT should be strongly considered for such patients because many may fully recover with it. Those with an episodic, rather than chronic, course of depressive disorder are most likely to respond.

Patients with persistent suicidal intention or actions are often given ECT as primary treatment because it would be dangerous to undergo a potentially prolonged series of medication trials while the patient remained at risk of self-injury. Similarly, those with severe inanition, psychomotor retardation, and depression-related immobility are usually treated with ECT first, to avoid medical complications such as aspiration, atelectasis, pneumonia, other infections, decubitus ulcers, and venous thrombosis. In both of these classes of patients, ECT is much more likely than antidepressants to rapidly improve depressive symptoms.

Although delusionally depressed patients may respond to a combination of an antidepressant and neuroleptic, they are more likely to respond to ECT and to do so rapidly. The mental suffering associated with depressive delusions (eg, of hopelessness, criminality, bodily decay, or self-loathing) is often unbearable, and the patient's response to such beliefs may make behavior impulsive and unpredictable. ECT is the treatment of choice to accelerate recovery and enhance patient safety. Catatonic patients almost always respond quickly to ECT and should be treated with it early. Although a minority of catatonics have a sustained positive response to benzodiazepines, this improvement is usually transient, and ECT is then required. Other medications are rarely effective. Retarded and agitated forms of catatonia are dangerous for the patient, and effective treatment with ECT should not be delayed.

Pharmacologic treatment of mania is usually successful, but cases that fail adequate drug trials usually respond to ECT. Severely agitated manic patients occasionally require ECT within the first few days of treatment because response to pharmacotherapy may not occur promptly enough to ensure patient safety. Similarly, some manic patients are endangered because comorbid medical conditions (eg, congestive heart failure or chronic obstructive pulmonary disease) are exacerbated by agitation and poor treatment compliance. In such situations, ECT is indicated early to reduce the risk of medical deterioration; the medical risks of ECT itself are more predictable, limited to the time of treatment, and generally acceptable with careful anesthetic evaluation and monitoring.

Schizophrenia is infrequently treated with ECT because drug treatment is generally more effective. Severe depressive symptoms in the course of schizophrenia may respond to ECT if other interventions fail, and delusions or hallucinations may rarely respond preferentially to ECT.

Technique of Electroconvulsive Therapy

ECT produces a brief generalized tonic-clonic seizure by means of a controlled electrical stimulus in the setting of general anesthesia. The mechanism by which this seizure activity generates a therapeutic effect remains unknown.

Patients are ventilated with 100% oxygen during the procedure. Routine monitoring includes serial vital signs and pulse oximetry, as well as an electrocardiogram (EKG) and electroencephalogram (EEG) recording. Brief general anesthesia is induced by methohexital or propofol, followed by muscle relaxation with succinylcholine. This muscle relaxation is never complete—rather, the sequelae of the convulsion are prevented without producing a prolonged period of paralysis or preventing observation of the motor seizure. A flexible bite block is placed between the teeth before induction of the seizure.

A constant current brief-pulse square wave electrical stimulus is used to provoke the seizure. This is delivered by means of right unilateral or bitemporal electrodes applied to clean skin surfaces with conducting paste. The seizure that ensues usually lasts 20 to 60 seconds. Seizures reaching 180 seconds (by motor observation or EEG) are terminated with intravenous benzodiazepine or additional anesthetic agent. Recovery following the seizure is rapid, with most patients awakening within 5 to 15 minutes.

Electroconvulsive Therapy Treatment Course and Response

ECT treatments are usually given three times per week, but they may be given two times per week for elderly patients who are more vulnerable to delirium and memory dysfunction. A typical course of ECT is six to twelve treatments, but the number of treatments required varies greatly.

Most patients show some partial improvement by the third or fourth treatment. Early signs of recovery often include an increased activity level, more participation in social interaction, or improvement in sleep or appetite. In delusional patients, initial improvement may be a decrease in preoccupation with delusional beliefs, even though these beliefs may still be held. For many patients, the subjective experience of a better mood may not come until relatively late in the treatment course; thus, they look better before they feel better.

Lack of any improvement by the eighth treatment is a poor prognostic sign. Because most patients are initially treated with unilateral ECT in order to diminish cognitive side effects, consideration should be given to switching to bilateral ECT at this point. Some patients may respond well only to bilateral ECT treatment.

In any case, there is no predetermined number of ECT treatments a patient should receive. Treatment should continue if the patient is showing steady improvement. It should end when the patient has fully recovered.

Electroconvulsive Therapy
for Medically ill Patients

Every patient receiving ECT undergoes a full medical assessment, including a physical examination, comprehensive metabolic panel, complete blood count, chest X-ray, EKG, and pretreatment evaluation by an anesthesiologist. Other laboratory or brain imaging studies are ordered as specifically indicated by the patient's condition.

Conditions associated with substantial increased risk from ECT include coronary artery disease, recent myocardial infarction, severe congestive heart failure, severe cardiac arrhythmias, arterial aneurysm, recent stroke, intracranial tumor, and deep venous thrombosis. In many cases, the risks from these conditions can be adequately reduced by careful anesthesia management if the necessity for ECT is clear. For instance, anesthesia management control of the hypertension and tachycardia associated with ECT reduces the risk of myocardial ischemia in patients with coronary artery disease.

ECT in patients with seizure disorders or Parkinson's disease is of particular interest to neurologists. In patients with epilepsy, the dose of anticonvulsant must be optimized to allow an ECT-induced seizure to occur, yet maintain adequate anticonvulsant effect outside of the treatments. Initially, usual doses of anticonvulsants are continued. If ECT seizures cannot be elicited, the dose of anticonvulsant is reduced. Although there is a risk of prolonged ECT seizures as the dose is reduced, this can be managed with intravenous anticonvulsants. Moreover, ECT itself produces an anticonvulsant effect that increases over the course of treatment.

Patients with Parkinson's disease may show diminished rigidity and reduced "on-off" fluctuations during ECT, and this improvement may last for several weeks after treatment. However, the dose of antiparkinson agents must at times be reduced during ECT to decrease the risk of delirium and treatment-emergent dyskinesias.

Adverse Effects of Electroconvulsive Therapy

Nausea, headache, and muscular aches are common minor side effects of ECT that are managed symptomatically and rarely limit treatment.

A wide variety of cardiac arrhythmias are seen during the treatment and immediately following it. These are related to the parasympathetic-sympathetic outflow caused by the electrically induced seizure, are almost always benign, and generally resolve without any treatment. Rarely, more severe or sustained arrhythmias develop that require specific intervention.

Myocardial infarction, stroke, and cardiac arrest are very rare complications of ECT, and the mortality of ECT is one in ten thousand patients treated. This is the same mortality associated with general anesthesia in minor surgery. Prolonged seizures are occasionally seen in ECT but respond to appropriate treatment with intravenous anticonvulsants. Status epilepticus is rare.

Cognitive side effects are common in ECT and vary greatly among individual patients. Many patients have a brief period of confusion (usually lasting an hour or less) immediately after treatment. This may be related to the ECT stimulus itself, as well as the anesthetic agents used. As the ECT treatment course progresses, anterograde and retrograde amnesia also frequently occurs and is more severe with bilateral electrode placement (Weiner et al., 1986; Sackeim et al., 1993; Lisanby et al., 2000).

Memory dysfunction secondary to ECT is most prominent immediately after a course of treatment is completed. Retrograde amnesia is more pronounced for events closer to the time of treatment than it is for more distant events. Retrograde memory disturbances improve over several weeks to several months, but permanent gaps in memory may occur, especially for events close to the time of treatment. Any difficulties in learning new information resolve within two months of completion of ECT.

A small minority of patients complain of more severe or sustained memory difficulty. The reasons for such complaints are poorly understood, but some may be explained by persisting depression. For most patients, amelioration of depression with ECT results in eventual improvement in attention, concentration, and general cognitive capacity.

Finally, frank delirious states are occasionally caused by ECT, in the absence of other obvious medical precipitants. These are most common in the elderly and in patients on multiple psychotropic medications. Reducing treatment frequency, changing from bilateral to unilateral treatment, and discontinuing unnecessary centrally active medications improve the delirious state.

References

American Psychiatric Association Committee on Electroconvulsive Therapy (2001). *The Practice of Electroconvulsive Therapy: Recommendations for Treatment, Training and Privileging* (2nd ed.). Washington, DC: American Psychiatric Association.

Lisanby, S.H., Maddox, J.H., Prudic, J., Devanand, D.P., Sackeim, H.A. (2000). The effects of electroconvulsive therapy on memory of autobiographical and public events. *Archives of General Psychiatry* 57: 591–2.

Rush, A.J., Trivedi, M.H., Wisniewski, S.R., Stewart, J.W., Nierenberg, A.A., Thase, M.E., Ritz, L., Biggs, M.M., Warden, D., Luther, J.F., Shores-Wilson, K., Niederehe, G., Fava, M., STAR*D Study Team. (2006). Bupropion-SR, sertraline, or venlafaxine-XR after failure of SSRIs for depression. *New England Journal of Medicine* 354: 1231–42.

Sackeim, H.A., Prudic, J., Devanand, D.P., Kiersky, J.E., Fitzsimons, L., Moody, B.J., McElhiney, M.C., Coleman, E.A., Settembrino, J.M. (1993). Effects of stimulus intensity and electrode placement on the efficacy and cognitive effects of electroconvulsive therapy. *New England Journal of Medicine* 328: 839–46.

Weiner, R.D., Rogers, H.J., Davidson, J.R., Squire, L.R. (1986). Effects of stimulus parameters on cognitive side effects. *Annals of the New York Academy of Sciences* 462: 315–25.

22

Psychotherapy

SUSAN W. LEHMANN

To nonpsychiatric physicians the term *psychotherapy* often sounds vague and mysterious. Yet, the art of providing healing through the clinician–patient relationship is as old as medicine itself. Psychotherapy is a form of treatment that uses psychologic techniques within the context of this confiding clinician–patient relationship to treat mental symptoms and relieve emotional distress. Psychotherapy may be the main approach to treatment of identified symptoms, or it may be used as an adjunct to pharmacotherapy.

The clinician–patient relationship at the core of psychotherapy can be distinguished from other confiding relationships a person may have with family members, friends, mentors, and advisors. In psychotherapy, there is a clearly identified provider of care and a recipient of that care. The provider is specially trained to deliver the care in a professional and coherent way, using specific psychologic techniques. Both the provider and the patient focus their attention on the patient's specific problems and work together in partnership to address the elements of psychologic distress and improve the patient's symptoms.

Goals of Psychotherapy

The goal of psychotherapy may differ depending on the patient and his or her situation. Sometimes, the goal of psychotherapy is symptom reduction (eg, to decrease anxiety, improve mood, or reduce friction in an interpersonal relationship). It may be used to help an individual replace unhealthy, counterproductive ways of thinking or reacting with more adaptive ones. In other instances, the goal of psychotherapy may be educational or instructive and involve teaching techniques to expand an individual's coping abilities or communication skills. All forms of psychotherapy develop an individual's self-awareness and help bolster appropriate self-esteem. The therapeutic setting between patient and clinician establishes validation that the patient's concerns are worth addressing and provides a sense of hopefulness that things can improve. As new options are explored and new techniques for dealing with distressing situations are discussed, patients develop an increased sense of mastery and feel less overwhelmed by life circumstances.

Forms of Psychotherapy

Psychotherapy may take three main forms of: (1) individual, (2) couples or family, or (3) group. In individual psychotherapy, a single patient and therapist work together, focusing on the patient's unique attitudes, perceived experiences, and behaviors that are associated with his or her current distress. In couples or family psychotherapy, family members who share a problem are treated together to enhance communication and problem-solving abilities in a socially realistic setting. In group psychotherapy, unrelated patients are treated together so that individuals may benefit from the camaraderie of supporting and learning from others who share similar situations.

All three forms of psychotherapy may be further defined by specific techniques of treatment—supportive, insight-oriented, and cognitive-behavioral. Any or all of these techniques may be used in each form of therapy. In supportive psychotherapy, the emphasis tends to be practical, focuses on the "here and now," and aims to recruit the patient's preexisting psychological strengths to promote recovery. In insight-oriented psychotherapy, the goal of treatment is to help the individual develop greater self-awareness and thereby expand his or her options for responding to challenging situations. In cognitive-behavioral therapy, the goal is to develop specific skills to counteract or replace maladaptive behaviors or ways of reacting.

Indications for Psychotherapy

Psychotherapy is beneficial in a variety of conditions and for a wide range of psychologic complaints. It is a vital cornerstone in the treatment of patients with significant mood disorders, especially depression. A number of well-constructed studies have demonstrated that psychotherapy coupled with antidepressant therapy produces superior results compared to medication alone in patients with serious depressive disorders (Thase et al., 1997; Reynolds et al.; 1999; Pampallona et al., 2004). Psychotherapy is especially essential in the early weeks of pharmacologic treatment of major depression. Although there are many effective antidepressant medications, they all take at least 4 to 6 weeks to achieve full therapeutic activity. During this early period, patients experience high levels of psychologic distress, yet have not experienced the therapeutic benefits from antidepressant therapy. Psychotherapy addresses this suffering and can provide a needed sense of hope and emotional support. Moreover, psychotherapy provides a vehicle for close monitoring of the patient regarding possible progression of depressive symptoms, including the development of suicidal ideation, which may necessitate referral for inpatient treatment.

Psychotherapy is a valuable and effective treatment for patients suffering from milder depressive disorders as well. As described in Chapter 2, demoralization may be a feature of the mental state of many patients with neurologic disorders. Patients with demoralization feel overwhelmed and discouraged by their condition and life circumstances. These feelings may be accompanied by mood changes such as irritability, impatience, despondency, and despair. The emotional distress frequently has an impact on functioning, making it difficult to make decisions and get along with others (family, friends, coworkers). Patients who are demoralized may be less likely to be adherent with physician recommendations regarding their primary neurologic condition. For these patients, psychotherapy may provide a supportive framework in which these feelings are countered and more adaptive stances developed.

Besides depression, anxiety is frequently associated with many neurologic conditions. Anxiety may manifest as self-consciousness related to physical changes engendered by the neurologic disorder such as tremor, dyskinesia, paresis, incoordination, gait unsteadiness, or changes in speech quality. There may be anticipatory anxiety related to fears of incontinence or of falls, or the individual may experience discrete panic attacks. These concerns and other anxious ruminations may inhibit socialization and contribute to social isolation. In addition, the patient may have fears and anxiety about the prognosis, the possibility of dependency, and financial worries. In all of these instances, psychotherapy should be considered to help the patient reduce anxiety and prevent it from causing further disability.

Psychotherapy is also advisable for patients who may be having difficulty dealing with adjustment and relationship issues related to their neurologic disorder. These may include coping with new or altered dependency needs and loss of independence. Such issues may be especially important if there has been a need to curtail working or driving, or if there have been significant role changes within the household due to the patient's neurologic condition.

Finally, neurologists should not overlook the psychologic needs of caregivers involved in the care of their patients with neurologic disorders. There is a high prevalence of depression, anxiety, and emotional distress among caregivers (Pinquart and Sorensen, 2003). Caregivers who feel overwhelmed and depressed by the demands of caring for a family member will have difficulty meeting the needs of the ill individual. Furthermore, they are at increased risk for medical morbidity themselves (Schultz and Beach, 1999). Support groups or individual psychotherapy help caregivers cope more effectively and reduce symptoms of psychologic distress.

Referral for Psychotherapy

Although all physicians provide a supportive relationship with their patients, few offer formal psychotherapy. Moreover, effective and successful psychotherapy is time-intensive. It usually involves at least weekly sessions of 30 to 60 minutes. Most physicians do not have the time to provide this kind of treatment during regular office hours. The referring neurologist should endeavor to refer the individual needing psychotherapy to a licensed professional. This may be a psychiatrist, clinical social worker, or psychologist. Although some people may improve after only a few sessions, others need longer treatment over months. Often the frequency of psychotherapy changes over time, being more frequent in the beginning and less frequent as symptoms improve.

Table 22–1 lists common reasons to refer a patient or family member for psychotherapy.

Table 22.1. When to Refer for Psychotherapy

Consider referral for psychotherapy for a patient or family member who reports:
- Feeling overwhelmed, overstressed, having difficulty coping
- Depression, hopelessness, mood swings, irritability
- High levels of anxiety, panic attacks
- Difficulty following treatment recommendations, missing appointments
- Social isolation, social withdrawal
- More somatic symptoms than expected or less functional than expected

References

Pampallona, S., Bollini, P., Tibaldi, G., Kupelnick, B., Munizza, C. (2004). Combined pharmacotherapy and psychological treatment for depression: a systematic review *Archives of General Psychiatry* 61: 714–9.

Pinquart, M., Sorensen, S. (2003). Differences between caregivers and non-caregivers in psychological health and physical health: a meta-analysis. *Psychology and Aging* 18:250–67.

Reynolds, C.F. III, Frank, E., Perel, J.M., Imber, S.D., Cornes, C., Miller, M.D., Mazumdar, S., Houck, P.R., Dew, M.A., Stack, J.A., Pollock, B.G., Kupfer, D.J. (1999). Nortriptyline and interpersonal psychotherapy as maintenance therapies for recurrent major depression: a randomized controlled trial in patients older than 59 years. *Journal of the American Medical Association.* 281: 39–45.

Schultz, R., Beach, S.R. (1999). Caregiving as a risk factor for mortality: the caregiver health effects study. *Journal of the American Medical Association* 282: 2215–19.

Thase, M.E., Greenhouse, J.B., Frank, E., Reynolds, C.F. III, Pilkonis, P.A., Hurley, K., Grochocinski,V., Kupfer, D.J. (1997). Treatment of major depression with psychotherapy or psychotherapy-pharmacotherapy combinations. *Archives of General Psychiatry* 54: 1009–15.

23

Nonpharmacologic Interventions Other Than Psychotherapy

CONSTANTINE G. LYKETSOS

Several nonpharmacologic interventions are available to the physician for the management of psychiatric disturbances in patients with neurologic disease. These include education, providing day-to-day structure, and caregiver interventions. They are discussed individually in this chapter.

Education

Patient education is a critical aspect of management that can reassure patients, help them better understand what is happening to them, reduce distress, promote a stronger clinician–patient relationship, and enhance adherence to treatment. When treating psychiatric symptoms in a patient with neurologic disease, it is important to set aside time to provide such education.

Several approaches to patient education might be incorporated. For the patient who has limited insight into his or her psychiatric symptoms, it is important to approach education delicately and nonjudgmentally, emphasizing treatment options without directly confronting the patient about the lack of insight. For example, a man might be told that his symptoms of anxiety, irritability, and trouble sleeping represent a "mood disorder" for which effective treatment is available to reduce his suffering. By focusing on doing something to help, the physician avoids conflict and preserves the clinician–patient relationship while asking the patient to keep an open mind about diagnosis and therapy.

For the patient who has better insight, education involves more detailed explanation of the psychiatric diagnosis and the physician's best judgment about its cause. For example, "you are seeing things that are very real to you but that others do not see. I have no doubt that these are real to you, and that they are troubling. Many patients with Parkinson's disease develop such symptoms that we call hallucinations. They may be caused by some of the medication you take for your condition or by the brain damage caused by the Parkinson's disease. I think we might be able to make them better."

Sometimes, and commonly in the context of dementia care, a patient's condition precludes constructive discussion of diagnosis. The patient may be incapable of understanding or may not even recognize that anything is wrong with him. In some cases, the patient may become upset and agitated if a diagnosis is discussed. The physician must then involve an alternative decision maker in the care of the patient and deliver the education to this surrogate.

Other aspects of patient education revolve around the prognosis for psychiatric symptoms and choices among treatment options. Information from several chapters in this book can be used to educate a patient about his or her prognosis or treatments. In all cases, education should be delivered with plenty of time for questions and with careful attention to patient understanding of what is being explained. It is often useful to provide the patient, or surrogate, with written educational materials to take home. If that is done, the physician should ask the patient if he or she has any questions about such materials in a follow-up visit.

A useful resource to locate prepared patient education materials for patients with psychiatric disorders is provided by the National Library of Medicine at www.nlm.nih.gov/medlineplus. This Web site provides patient education information for a range of medical problems. A user-friendly search engine facilitates location of specific topics relevant to psychiatric aspects of neurologic disease (eg, "depression in Parkinson's disease," "apathy"). Materials can be downloaded in easy-to-print format, free of charge.

Providing Day-to-Day Structure

For many patients with psychiatric conditions in the context of neurologic disease, the provision of structure and activities in day-to-day life is an important therapeutic intervention that helps keep symptoms under control and improves quality of life. Patients with cognitive disorders and dementia have trouble organizing their day and may spend their time doing very little. This passive inactivity leads to deconditioning, lack of stimulation, and poor socialization. Patients with apathy, depression, and other motivational problems similarly need external motivators or cues to prevent them from becoming isolated. The additional disability associated with neurologic disease only makes things worse, thus leaving patients more vulnerable to living unstructured, isolated lives. Homebound inactivity may also lead to family conflict, further worsening the patient's condition. Moreover, patients with comorbid psychiatric and neurologic conditions have much trouble completing basic daily living activities (eg, taking medications, preparing meals, keeping house, grooming) often requiring that these be built into a more structured approach to their lives.

The first step in addressing this problem is for the physician to make a detailed review, with the patient and critical informants, of how the patient is spending his or her time. The patient's premorbid activity level and interests, as well as personal wishes regarding his or her current daily schedule and activities, should also be discussed. After this review, the physician has a good sense of how the patient spends his or her time and whether a more specific intervention is needed to provide structure and increase activity level.

The physician might consider "prescribing" the development of a structured daily life schedule. The patient might also develop and implement this himself or herself, with encouragement from the physician and help from a family member.

Motivated family members might sit with the patient weekly to develop (1) a schedule that incorporates basic activities in the home (eg, sleep, medication, and meals schedules) and (2) regular out-of-home activities and social interactions (eg, trips to the mall, visiting family and friends). Occupational therapy consultation, sometimes in the patient's home, should be considered to help develop such a schedule and ways of implementing it. This is especially helpful for patients who have little family support.

If structure out of the home cannot be provided by the family or the patient, or if respite for caregivers requires external support, several options are available. These include psychosocial programs, adult day care, or senior centers. Psychosocial programs, operating in daytime business hours, typically were developed to provide structure and activities for the chronically mentally ill. These programs provide a place to go during the week for long periods, activities, medication oversight, group therapy, and they often have licensed staff on site such as nurses or occasionally physicians. Facilities are increasingly catering to patients with comorbid psychiatric and neurologic disease, especially in those who are younger. Also, a new generation of psychosocial programs targeted at people with brain injuries and behavior problems offers similar services. These programs are well qualified to provide care to the patients in question and can accommodate patients with physical disabilities, or milder behavioral problems. In addition to providing psychosocial care, these treatment settings also facilitate access to resources (eg, social workers) and can ensure medication administration during the day. To locate such programs, the physician might call the local mental health center or county social services, or ask a collaborating psychiatrist.

Senior centers and adult day-care programs typically cater to older people, although many make exceptions depending on resource availability. Senior centers are able to accommodate patients functioning at a higher level by providing them a place to visit and socialize as well as to access higher-level activities (eg, woodworking, art classes, museum excursions). For the most part, senior centers do not offer access to resources such as social workers, and they rely on the participants to show up and participate in activities. In contrast, adult day-care programs provide lower level activities, access to resources, and much more structure. Senior centers typically do not charge for most of their services, whereas adult day-care programs are fee for service, with the occasional availability of free care through Medicaid. The best way to locate individual programs, to find available programs in a given area, or to make a referral is to contact the local County Area Agency on Aging or access its Web site.

Caregiver Interventions

The great majority of patients with comorbid psychiatric and neurologic conditions have one or more caregivers involved in their lives to a lesser or greater degree. These are typically family members, most often spouses, parents, or children. The role of these caregivers in the day-to-day life of these patients is essential. Therefore, it is critical to find out if a patient has a caregiver and to involve that individual in ongoing treatment. If the patient does not have a caregiver and needs one, it may be necessary to help the patient find one.

Involving caregivers greatly facilitates and improves the care of the patient, especially in the long term as the effects of progressive neurologic disease accumulate. Moreover, the relationship with the physician makes a very positive difference to the lives of the caregivers who themselves are at increased risk of becoming frail due to the stressful effects of caregiving. For a more detailed discussion of the effects of caregiving on both the patient and the caregiver, it may be necessary to refer to *Practical Dementia Care* (Rabins, Lyketsos, and Steele, 2006). Occasionally, patients do not agree to have their caregivers involved in their treatment. In such cases, patients should be educated carefully about the importance of caregiver involvement and advised to permit their inclusion. If patients are not capable of making their own health care decisions, then it may be necessary to involve the caregivers against the wishes of the patient as surrogate decision makers.

Two groups of caregiver-targeted interventions may be distinguished: (1) those that are targeted at helping the caregiver

Table 23.1. Listing of Caregiver Interventions

TARGETED AT HELPING THE CAREGIVER PROVIDE BETTER CARE

1. Education about the patient's condition, its causes, prognosis, treatment
2. Education about the caregiving role and how it is different from other roles
3. Teaching specific caregiving skills that may be needed
4. Teaching how to solve problems that arise in day to day care
5. Encouragement and facilitation of long-range planning about the patient's care
6. Clarification of decision-making roles and implementation of advance directives

TARGETED AT HELPING THE CAREGIVER HELP HERSELF

1. Help with finding other caregivers, family or paid, to assist in patient care
2. Referrals to access resources that might help provide care
3. Help with resolving family conflict that arises around the patient's care
4. Encouragement of arrangements for regular respite from the caregiving role
5. Encouragement of attention to personal needs, health, and mental health
6. Provision of emotional support when overwhelmed by caregiving
7. Assurance of easy access of the caregiver to the physician
8. Referral to support and advocacy groups

---

give better care to the patient, and (2) those that are intended to help the caregiver herself (the vast majority of caregivers are women). Table 23–1 provides a list of relevant caregiver interventions. In general, these interventions are self-explanatory. The key to their success is to make sure that the physician considers caregiver involvement as part of the care of the patient and makes sure it occurs during patient office visits. Third-party payers, including Medicare, recognize the importance of caregiver involvement and reimburse these aspects of care, as long as they are medically necessary and targeted at helping the patient. One way to do this is to schedule private time with the caregiver during early visits and at regular intervals, as well as to make sure that the caregiver has the opportunity to speak openly about the patient's condition.

Reference

Rabins, P.V., Lyketsos, C.G., Steele, C.D. (2006). In *Practical Dementia Care*, (2nd ed.). New York. NY: Oxford University Press.

Glossary

Important Mental Phenomena and Symptoms

adjustment disorder: a disturbance brought on by a reaction to an episode of psychological, social, or physical stress (eg, divorce, natural disaster).

affect: the outward expression of a person's emotional state as manifested in their facial expression, posture, and behavior. Important elements of affect include its range and how rapidly it changes.

affective disorder: a disturbance of affect, characterized by extreme emotional responses and persistent mood disturbances. Major depressive disorder and bipolar disorder are types of affective disorders.

agnosia: a disturbance of perception in which individuals are not able to recognize that a set of perceptions represent a previously learned pattern. For example, individuals may be able to see a face and name the parts of the face but not recognize that this face belongs to a specific familiar person (*prosopagnosia*). Similarly, individuals may realize that they cannot remember certain things and that they are having trouble communicating, but they may not realize that these inabilities suggest a medical impairment (*nosagnosia*).

amnesia: a disturbance in memory that may manifest itself as a loss of recall for previously learned events (*retrograde amnesia*) or an inability to form new memories (*anterograde amnesia*).

anhedonia: an inability to find pleasure from experiences or activities that are normally pleasurable.

anxiety: an emotional state characterized by apprehension, tension, uneasiness, and/or worry. It may be associated with tachycardia, sweating, and other physical symptoms.

anxiety disorder: a chronic disturbance marked by an excessive and persistent sense of apprehension, often accompanied by physical symptoms such as sweating and palpitations. Generalized anxiety disorder, obsessive-compulsive

405

disorder, panic disorder, and social phobia are some types of anxiety disorders classified by the DSM-IV.

apathy: a state of reduced interest and initiative.

aphasia: a language disturbance in the patient's ability to comprehend or express speech due to brain lesion.

apraxia: the inability to carry out a learned, complex, motor task, in the absence of paralysis, sensory loss or movement dyscontrol (e.g., tremor, chorea).

attention-deficit hyperactivity disorder: a disorder characterized by a short attention span, excessive activity, or impulsive behavior. The symptoms of the disorder begin early in life.

bipolar mood disorder (formerly called manic depression): an affective disorder characterized by episodes of both mania and depression. Bipolar I disorder is characterized by the occurrence of at least one *manic* or *mixed* mood episode, often preceded by an episode of severe depression. Bipolar II disorder is characterized by an alternating pattern of *hypomania* and major depression.

catastrophic reaction: a sudden emotional and behavioral response to a seemingly minor stimulus that is often seen in brain-damaged individuals when their capacity to respond to a situation is exceeded. For example, a patient with expressive aphasia might cry and become agitated when unable to recall a specific word.

catatonia: a state usually characterized by immobility and mutism, with preservation of consciousness. Catatonia may also be marked by phenomena such as abnormal postures, negativism (ie, refusing to do what is asked, doing the opposite of what is asked), echolalia, echopraxia, and motor ambivalence (repeatedly initiating, but not completing, an act).

compulsion: an intrusive repetitive action that is difficult to resist without anxiety. Compulsions may be repetition of certain simple acts (eg, checking, counting, tapping) or more complex ones (eg, washing hands, cleaning house) or consist of complex rituals (brushing teeth in a certain way). Typically, compulsions are associated with obsessions and distract the person from other mental activities.

conversion disorder: a somatoform disorder that describes neurologic or other general medical symptoms affecting sensation (eg, blindness, deafness) or voluntary motor skills (paralysis, seizures, urine retention) in the absence of a physical explanation or cause.

delirium: a widespread cognitive disturbance consisting of deficits of attention, arousal, consciousness, memory, orientation, perception, and speech or language.

delusion: a fixed, false, idiosyncratic belief. Common types of delusions include persecutory (paranoid), grandiose, nihilistic, guilt, and bodily ideas.

dementia: a cognitive disorder marked by acquired global cognitive decline in the absence of delirium. The most common cause is Alzheimer's disease.

demoralization: a normal state of sadness and discouragement in response to adversity. When the patient's situation improves, the demoralization abates.

depression: a state of sadness or low mood which may also be accompanied by tearfulness, a constricted affect, paucity of speech, pessimistic thinking, and a slumped posture.

disinhibition: the loss of previously developed behavioral restraint resulting in actions that are unexpected, out of context, or socially inappropriate.

dysmnesia: a disturbance in memory in which the capacity for memory is present but the processing of memory is impaired. For example, patients might be able to learn lists of words but have difficulty retrieving them so that they perform better on recognition tasks than on recall tasks.

dysphoria: an unpleasant mood state (eg, sadness, anxiety, foreboding, excitement).

dysthymia: a depressive disorder consisting of a chronic, sustained pattern of "down" or "low" days outnumbering symptom-free days.

emotional incontinence: a sudden, exaggerated expression of emotion that may or may not occur in response to a stimulus. Examples include pathologic laughing and crying when an individual unexpectedly laughs or cries but reports the absence of sad or happy mood. It often occurs when there is damage to subcortical brain structures such as in pseudobulbar palsy and Parkinson's disease. A more recent term developed by a panel of experts is "intermittent emotional expressive disorder."

euphoria: a state of elevated mood, which may be accompanied by a sense of heightened well-being or confidence in one's abilities.

euthymia: a neutral mood state, neither sad nor happy nor anxious.

flight of ideas: the very rapid succession of loosely related ideas, often with a "push" to get the ideas out, so that interrupting the patient is difficult; it is typically associated with mania.

hallucination: a perception without a stimulus, in any sensory modality.

ictal emotion: any suddenly occurring and quickly disappearing emotional reaction, but especially depression and anxiety.

illusion: a misinterpretation of a stimulus, in any sensory modality.

impulse control disorder: a disturbance characterized by the inability to resist an urge or temptation to do something that will harm oneself or others; a sense of increasing tension or arousal preceding the act; and a feeling of relief, pleasure, or gratification during or on completion of the act.

lability: the degree and speed of changeability in a person's mood. Mood-labile persons rapidly change moods (eg, from happy to neutral to sad) in response to minimal stimuli.

language disorder: a disturbance in the comprehension or use of language reflected in the patient's speech or writing. Examples include *aphasia* and *paraphrasia*.

level of consciousness: the degree of clarity of awareness of the environment. This dimension ranges from alert and attentive to comatose. It may manifest with hyper- or hypovigilance.

loosening of associations (also called derailment): where the sequence of the talk is not logical or linear and the patient's talk does not follow a coherent path.

major depression (also called unipolar depression): a mood disorder in which the patient is depressed or irritable nearly all the time or loses interest in almost everything. These feelings last for more than 2 weeks, are associated with several other symptoms, and cause significant distress or impaired functioning.

mania: a pathologic mood state characterized by an elated, euphoric, or irritable mood that is often unstable. The mood elevation is associated with increased psychomotor activity, restlessness, agitation, sleep disturbance, and poor judgment. Patients are also overconfident, grandiose, and may be delusional, and they exhibit hallucinations or thought disorder.

mood: an individual's current, predominant emotional state. Examples include sadness (depression), anxiety, irritability, happiness, excitement, frustration, and boredom.

obsession: an intrusive, repetitive urge or thought that is difficult to resist without anxiety. Obsessions may or may not be associated with compulsions. Examples include the intrusive idea that something bad is about to happen, that one's hands are dirty, or that a certain sequence or actions must be followed to prevent harm from coming to a loved one.

obsessive-compulsive disorder: an anxiety disorder characterized by recurrent, uncontrollable obsessions and/or compulsions.

panic disorder (also called episodic paroxysmal anxiety): an anxiety disorder consisting of recurrent, uncued panic attacks. Many of the symptoms characteristic of panic disorder are reported in patients with complex partial seizures.

paranoia: a commonly used term referring to suspiciousness or persecutory delusions. In the original Greek, it refers to a tendency to misinterpret events and people as being hostile and directed against the person.

pathologic laughing and crying: see emotional incontinence.

personality disorder: a disorder characterized by long-lasting, maladaptive patterns of behavior and thought that severely limit the patient's ability to function on a day-to-day basis.

phobia: a disproportionate fear of specific objects (such as, snakes, the sight of blood) (*specific phobia*), or situations, such as being seen in public (*social phobia*), or being in situations from where it is difficult to escape (*agoraphobia*).

post-traumatic stress disorder: an anxiety disorder that develops after the patient witnesses or is confronted with one or more events involving actual or threatened death or injury, or involving a threat to the physical integrity of oneself or others.

pseudobulbar affect: see emotional incontinence.

psychogenic non-epileptic seizure: a manifestation or a form of *conversion disorder* that may take many forms. In particular, it can mimic any sort of epileptic seizure.

psychosis: a mental state characterized by delusions, hallucinations, or formal thought disorder.

schizophrenia: a severe, chronic disorder marked by delusions, hallucinations, thought disorder, and disintegration of personality and social functioning.

self-attitude: an individual's sense of his or her self worth or confidence. Impairments in self-attitude might be positive or negative. A diminished self-attitude could be manifest as reduced confidence, guilt, feeling a burden, and worthlessness. Elevations in self-attitude could be manifest as overconfidence and grandiosity.

sleep disturbance: a disorder in sleep that interferes with mental and emotional functioning. Insomnia, sleep apnea, and narcolepsy are common sleep disturbances.

somatization disorder: a somatoform disorder in which patients have multiple (typically more than 10) physical symptoms (eg, back pain, neck pain, joint pain) for which they persistently seek medical attention.

somatoform disorder: any disorder characterized by physical complaints for which no adequate physical explanation can be found. Examples include *conversion disorder* and *somatization disorder.*

suicidal ideation: thoughts of committing suicide. These can range from planning to actual attempts at suicide.

tangentiality: a pattern of response to questions in which the patient repeatedly gives answers that are not directly responsive to the questions asked.

thought disorder: a disturbance in the flow or sequencing of thought as reflected in the patient's speech or writing. Examples include *loosening of associations* and *tangentiality.*

vital sense: an individual's subjective sense of their state of energy and well-being. Reductions in vital sense might manifest in a feeling of exhaustion or illness. Elevations in vital sense might manifest in a feeling or vigor and fitness.

Index

AACE (American Association of Clinical Endocrinologists), 354t, 355

Abuse, drug. *See* Substance abuse

Acetylcholine, 376

Acetylcholinesterase (AChE), 376

Acetylcholinesterase inhibitors, 152

Acquired immunodeficiency syndrome (AIDS), 314

Acquired Involuntary Movement Scale (AIMS), 353

Acute brain syndrome. *See* Delirium

Acute confusional state. *See* Delirium

AD. *See* Alzheimer's disease

ADA (American Diabetes Association), 354t, 355

Adderall (amphetamine/ dextroamphetamine), 340t

Addiction, 113t

ADHD. *See* Attention deficit hyperactivity disorder

Adult day-care programs, 401–402

AEDs. *See* Anti-epileptic drugs

Affect. *See* Mood

Aggression
acute, antipsychotics for, 355–356
differential diagnosis, 175
in epilepsy, 174–175
in frontotemporal dementia, 238t, 239

Agitation
acute, antipsychotics for, 355–356
in dementia, 58
in frontotemporal dementia, 239
in hyperactive-hyperalert delirium, 57
pharmacotherapy, 94, 244t

Agranulocytosis, 212, 351

AIDS (acquired immunodeficiency syndrome), 314

AIMS (Acquired Involuntary Movement Scale), 353

Alcohol withdrawal, 57

Alertness, in dementia, 57

Allodynia, 102t

Alprazolam, 372

ALS (amyotrophic lateral sclerosis), 135, 236, 237

Alzheimer's disease (AD), 218–232
agitation/aggression, 223, 232
apathy, 222–223, 231–232
catastrophic reactions, 224, 232
delirium, 55
delusions, 220–221, 227, 230
dementia, 58, 68–69
depression, 218–220, 225–227
executive dysfunction syndrome, 222, 230–231
hallucinations, 220–221, 227, 230